Clinical Problems in Oncology

Clinical Problems in Oncology

A Practical Guide to Management

EDITED BY

Sing Yu Moorcraft, MB BCh, MRCP

Clinical Research Fellow in Medical Oncology
The Royal Marsden NHS Foundation Trust
London, UK

Daniel L.Y. Lee, MB BCh, MRCP

Specialist Registrar in Medical Oncology
St James' Institute of Oncology
Leeds, UK

David Cunningham, MD, FRCP, FMedSci

Consultant Medical Oncologist
The Royal Marsden NHS Foundation Trust
London, UK

WILEY Blackwell

This edition first published 2014 © 2014 by John Wiley & Sons, Ltd

Registered Office
John Wiley & Sons, Ltd, The Atrium, Southern Gate, Chichester, West Sussex PO19 8SQ, UK

Editorial Offices
9600 Garsington Road, Oxford OX4 2DQ, UK
The Atrium, Southern Gate, Chichester, West Sussex PO19 8SQ, UK
111 River Street, Hoboken, NJ 07030-5774, USA

For details of our global editorial offices, for customer services and for information about how
to apply for permission to reuse the copyright material in this book please see our website at
www.wiley.com/wiley-blackwell

The right of the author to be identified as the author of this work has been asserted in accordance with
the UK Copyright, Designs and Patents Act 1988.

Library of Congress Cataloging-in-Publication Data
Clinical problems in oncology : a practical guide to management / edited by Sing Yu Moorcraft,
Daniel L.Y. Lee, David Cunningham.
    p. ; cm.
  Includes bibliographical references and index.
  ISBN 978-1-118-67382-9
  I. Moorcraft, Sing Yu, editor of compilation.   II. Lee, Daniel L. Y., editor of compilation.
III. Cunningham, David, 1954 December 4– editor of compilation.
  [DNLM: 1. Neoplasms–Handbooks.   2. Clinical Medicine–methods–Handbooks. QZ 39]
  RC261
  616.99′4–dc23
                              2014001178
A catalogue record for this book is available from the British Library.

Wiley also publishes its books in a variety of electronic formats. Some content that appears in print may
not be available in electronic books.

Set in 9/11.5pt Meridien by SPi Publisher Services, Pondicherry, India
Printed and bound in Malaysia by Vivar Printing Sdn Bhd

1   2014

Contents

List of contributors

Emma Dugdale, MB ChB, MRCP, FRCR
Specialist Registrar in Clinical Oncology, St James's Institute of Oncology, Leeds, UK

Alexandra Gilbert, BSc, MBBS, MRCP
National Institute for Health Research Doctoral Research Fellow in Clinical Oncology,
St James' Institute of Oncology, Leeds, UK

Daniel L.Y. Lee, MB BCh, MRCP
Specialist Registrar in Medical Oncology, St James' Institute of Oncology, Leeds, UK

Juanita Lopez, MB BChir, MRCP, PhD
Specialist Registrar in Medical Oncology, The Royal Marsden NHS Foundation Trust,
London, UK

Sing Yu Moorcraft, MB BCh, MRCP
Clinical Research Fellow in Medical Oncology, The Royal Marsden NHS Foundation Trust,
London, UK

Karen Neoh, MBChB, MRCP
Academic Clinical Fellow in Palliative Medicine, St Gemma's Academic Unit of Palliative
Care, Leeds, UK

Alexandra Pender, MB BCh, MRCP
Academic Clinical Fellow in Medical Oncology, The Royal Marsden NHS Foundation Trust,
London, UK

Robin Prestwich, FRCR, PhD
Consultant Clinical Oncologist, St James' Institute of Oncology, Leeds, UK

Samantha Turnbull, MB ChB, MRCP
Specialist Registrar in Medical Oncology, St James' Institute of Oncology, Leeds, UK

Preface

Clinical Problems in Oncology: A Practical Guide to Management was written by a group of trainees who found that there was no good source of information to guide them through the day-to-day management of patients with cancer.

The book, which is also available electronically, aims to provide a clear and yet concise description of how to deal with the day-to-day challenges of working within an oncology team. This includes essential background, such as the design and conduct of clinical trials, assessment of tumour response, evaluation of the performance status of patients and an overview of the concept of personalised medicine. There are also chapters outlining how to treat tumour-related symptoms and manage the side effects of conventional chemotherapy and the new class of targeted agents. The chapters on radiotherapy provide a grounding in this important aspect of cancer care, including practical solutions to assist clinicians looking after patients receiving this treatment, and there is also a detailed description of the management of oncological emergencies.

The objective of the authors was to provide a comprehensive source of information that would guide the trainee through their time on the ward, clinic and acute medical assessment unit. We have therefore included information that trainees will need to successfully function in these environments, ranging from the dose of drugs that would be typically used, through to guidance on the practical procedures that are frequently used to treat patients with cancer. We hope a copy of the book will find its way onto wards and clinics throughout the country and will become established as a reliable and comprehensive clinical guide to assist busy trainees.

Professor David Cunningham

Acknowledgements

We would like to thank Dr Kimberley Goldstein-Jackson and Niamh Cunningham for taking the time to read the manuscript and for their constructive comments. We would also like to thank Jane Ashton and Emily Wighton for reviewing the manuscript from a pharmacist's perspective and Dr Liz O'Mahony for her comments on the Psychiatric disorders section. Finally, but by no means least, we are indebted to our families and friends, particularly John Moorcraft and Shaune Teasdale, for their support and patience during the preparation of this manuscript.

List of abbreviations

5-FU	5-fluorouracil
A&E	accident and emergency
ABG	arterial blood gas
ACE	angiotensin converting enzyme
ADL	activities of daily living
ADT	androgen deprivation therapy
AE	adverse event
AF	atrial fibrillation
AFP	alpha-fetoprotein
ALK	anaplastic lymphoma kinase
ALP	alkaline phosphatase
ALT	alanine aminotransferase
AR	adverse reaction
AST	aspartate aminotransferase
ATE	arterial thromboembolism
BCG	Bacillus Calmette-Guérin
BD	bis di (twice daily)
BMI	body mass index
BNF	British National Formulary
BP	blood pressure
BRCA1	breast cancer gene 1
BRCA2	breast cancer gene 2
BTA	bladder tumour antigen
CA	carbohydrate antigen
CBD	common bile duct
CCF	congestive cardiac failure
CDF	Cancer Drugs Fund
CEA	carcinoembryonic antigen
CID	chemotherapy-induced diarrhoea
COPD	chronic obstructive pulmonary disease
CML	chronic myeloid leukaemia
CNS	central nervous system
CPAP	continuous positive airway pressure
CR	complete response
CRP	C-reactive protein
CRPC	castration-resistant prostate cancer
CSF	cerebrospinal fluid
CT	computerised tomography
CTCAE	Common Terminology Criteria for Adverse Events
CTPA	computed tomography pulmonary angiogram
CVC	central venous catheter

CXR	chest X-ray
dB	decibel
DIC	disseminated intravascular coagulation
DPD	dihydropyrimidine dehydrogenase
DNA	deoxyribonucleic acid
DVT	deep vein thrombosis
ECG	electrocardiogram
ECOG	Eastern Cooperative Oncology Group
EDTA	(51)Cr-ethylenediaminetetra acetic acid plasma clearance
EEG	electroencephalogram
EGFR	epidermal growth factor receptor
ENT	ear, nose and throat
ER	oestrogen receptor
ERCP	endoscopic retrograde cholangio-pancreatography
ESR	erythrocyte sedimentation rate
FBC	full blood count
FDA	Food and Drug Administration
FEV$_1$	forced expiratory volume in first second
FFP	fresh frozen plasma
FGFR	fibroblast growth factor receptor
FISH	fluorescence in situ hybridisation
FSH	follicle-stimulating hormone
FVC	forced vital capacity
g	gram
GBM	glioblastoma multiforme
GCP	Good Clinical Practice
GCS	Glasgow Coma Scale
GCSF	granulocyte colony-stimulating factor
GFR	glomerular filtration rate
GGT	gamma-glutamyltransferase
GI	gastrointestinal
GIST	gastrointestinal stromal tumour
GLP1	glucagon-like peptide-1
GnRH	gonadotrophin releasing hormone
GOJ	gastro-oesophageal junction
GP	general practitioner
Hb	haemoglobin
HCC	hepatocellular carcinoma
hCG	human chorionic gonadotrophin
HDU	High Dependency Unit
HER2	human epidermal growth factor receptor 2/aka *neu*
HIV	human immunodeficiency virus
HRCT	high resolution computerised tomography
HRT	hormone replacement therapy
ICP	intracranial pressure
IFR	individual funding request
IG	immunoglobulin
IGF-1	insulin-like growth factor-1
IHC	immunohistochemistry

IM	intramuscular
IMRT	intensity-modulated radiation therapy
INR	international normalized ratio (prothrombin ratio)
IPPV	intermittent positive pressure ventilation
ITU	Intensive Therapy Unit
IU	international unit
IV	intravenous
IVC	inferior vena cava
K	potassium
kg	kilogram
KRAS	v-Ki-ras2 Kirsten rat sarcoma viral oncogene homolog
KUB	kidneys, ureter, bladder
L	litre
LCP	Liverpool Care Pathway
LDH	lactate dehydrogenase
LFT	liver function test
LH	luteinising hormone
LHRH	luteinising hormone releasing hormone
LLN	lower limit of normal
LMWH	low molecular weight heparin
LP	lumbar puncture
LVEF	left ventricular ejection fraction
mane	in the morning
mcg	micrograms
MDT	multidisciplinary team meeting
MESNA	sodium-2-mercaptoethane
MHRA	Medicines and Healthcare products Regulatory Agency
µg	microgram
mg	milligram
MI	myocardial infarction
min(s)	minute(s)
ml	millilitre
mmHg	millimetres of mercury
MMR	mismatch repair (of DNA)
MMR	measles, mumps, rubella
MR	modified release
MR	magnetic resonance
MRA	magnetic resonance angiography
MRCP	magnetic resonance cholangio-pancreatography
MRI	magnetic resonance imaging
MSI	microsatellite instability
MSU	midstream urine
mTOR	mammalian target of rapamycin
MUGA	multi-gated acquisition scan
Na	sodium
NBM	nil by mouth
ng	nanogram
NG	nasogastric tube
NHL	non-Hodgkin's lymphoma

NHS	National Health Service
NICE	National Institute for Health and Care Excellence
nocte	at night
NSAID	non-steroidal anti-inflammatory drug
NSCLC	non-small-cell lung cancer
NSE	neuron-specific enolase
OD	omni di (once daily)
OGD	oesophageogastroduodenoscopy
OS	overall survival
OT	occupational therapist
PARP	poly (ADP-ribose) polymerase
PD	progressive disease
PDGFR	platelet derived growth factor receptor
PE	pulmonary embolism
PEFR	peak expiratory flow rate
PEG	percutaneous endoscopic gastrostomy
PET	positron-emission tomography
PFS	progression-free survival
PI3K	phosphatidylinositol 3-kinase
PICC	peripherally inserted central catheter
PO	per os (by mouth)
PPI	proton pump inhibitor
PR	partial response
PR	per rectum (by the rectum)
PR	progesterone receptor
PRLS	posterior reversible leukoencephalopathy syndrome
PRN	pro re nata
PS	performance status
PSA	prostate-specific antigen
PT	prothrombin time
PTC	percutaneous transhepatic cholangiography
PTEN	phosphatase and tensin homolog deleted on chromosome 10
PTH	parathyroid hormone
QDS	quater in die (four times a day)
RANK	receptor activator of NF-kB
RCC	renal cell carcinoma
RCT	randomised controlled trial
RECIST	Response Evaluation Criteria In Solid Tumours
RFA	radiofrequency ablation
RIG	radiologically inserted gastrostomy
RUQ	right upper quadrant
SAE	serious adverse event
SALT	speech and language therapy
SAR	serious adverse reaction
SC	subcutaneous
SCF	supraclavicular fossa
SCLC	small-cell lung cancer
SD	stable disease
SIGN	Scottish Intercollegiate Guidelines Network

SL	sublingual
SOB	short of breath
SOBOE	short of breath on exertion
SR	slow release
SSRI	selective serotonin reuptake inhibitors
SUSAR	suspected unexpected adverse reaction
SVC	superior vena cava
TACE	transarterial chemoembolisation
TDS	ter die sumendus (three times a day)
TFTs	thyroid function tests
TKI	tyrosine kinase inhibitor
TNM	tumour, lymph nodes, metastasis
TPN	total parenteral nutrition
TSH	thyroid-stimulating hormone
U	unit
U&E	urea and electrolytes
UK	United Kingdom
ULN	upper limit of normal
USA	United States of America
USS	ultrasound scan
UTI	urinary tract infection
VATS	video-assisted thoracic surgery
VEGF	vascular endothelial growth factor
VTE	venous thromboembolism
VZIG	varicella zoster immunoglobulin
WBC	white blood cell
WHO	World Health Organisation

CHAPTER 1

Introduction to clinical problems in oncology

Sing Yu Moorcraft

The Royal Marsden NHS Foundation Trust, UK

CHAPTER MENU
General approach to the management of oncology patients, 2
Performance status, 6
Tumour markers, 6

Cancer is currently a major healthcare problem. For example, in the UK, approximately 33% of the population will develop some form of cancer during their lifetime. A person's risk of developing cancer is dependent on age and therefore the importance of oncology is likely to grow even further in the coming decades as the average age of the population increases. Oncology is one of the fastest developing specialities in medicine, with increasingly complex treatments entering daily practice and a significant number of patients in clinical trials. In the UK, the specialty is comprised of clinical oncology and medical oncology. The main difference is that clinical oncologists deliver radiotherapy, while medical oncologists do not and have historically been more heavily involved in drug research and clinical trials.

Patients may present to their oncology team, local hospital, A&E or GP with symptoms due to their cancer (e.g. pain), secondary complications (e.g. bowel obstruction) or side effects from their treatment. This book aims to provide practical guidance on how to manage the most commonly occurring problems experienced by oncology patients. However, this book is not designed to replace local or national guidelines and patients who require admission to hospital should be discussed with their oncology team or the acute oncology team in accordance with local procedures.

Clinical Problems in Oncology: A Practical Guide to Management, First Edition.
Edited by Sing Yu Moorcraft, Daniel L.Y. Lee and David Cunningham.
© 2014 John Wiley & Sons, Ltd. Published 2014 by John Wiley & Sons, Ltd.

General approach to the management of oncology patients

Types of treatment

Oncology treatments can be local or systemic. Local treatments include surgery and radiotherapy. Systemic treatments include chemotherapy, endocrine treatments, immunotherapy and targeted therapies (e.g. monoclonal antibodies or small molecules which target specific receptors or cell signalling pathways).

This book provides guidance on the management of toxicities associated with oncology treatment. It is important to consider the aims of treatment when deciding on the most appropriate management strategy. The aims of treatment can be:

- *Curative*: treatment given as the definitive treatment for cure.
- *Radical*: usually refers to chemotherapy or chemoradiotherapy given with curative intent.
- *Neoadjuvant*: treatment given before a definitive treatment with the aim to facilitate the procedure and/or improve the chances of curing the patient.
- *Adjuvant*: treatment given after a definitive treatment, with the aim to reduce the risk of recurrence (and therefore increase the chances of curing the patient) by destroying micrometastatic disease.
- *Palliative*: the aims of treatment are to improve patients' symptoms and quality of life. The treatment may (but not necessarily) prolong the patient's life and will not cure the patient.

The management of toxicities should be discussed with the patient's oncology team, but in general, if a patient is receiving treatment with curative intent, it is important to try to minimise dose delays and reductions, whenever possible, to maintain treatment efficacy. However, in patients receiving palliative treatment, quality of life is the most important consideration.

Tumour types and extent of disease

In oncology, treatment decisions are often heavily influenced by both the type and extent of a patient's tumour. This involves grading and staging their disease.

- *Grading*: the grade of a tumour gives an indication of how well differentiated a tumour is. This often reflects the aggressiveness of the tumour, with grade I being the most differentiated and grade IV being the least differentiated.
- *Staging*: staging is used to assess the extent of disease. Some cancers have their own specialised staging systems, but many are staged by the TNM staging system. In TNM staging, the T usually represents tumour size or depth, the N reflects nodal involvement (which may be number of nodes, size of nodes or pattern of nodal involvement) and the M indicates the presence or absence of metastatic disease.

Some cancers have a predictable pattern of nodal spread and therefore some patients undergo a sentinel lymph node biopsy to determine the presence of nodal involvement. The sentinel node is the first lymph node that a cancer drains to and if it is clear of tumour then it is unlikely that lymph nodes further down the chain are involved.

Other important tumour characteristics
- *Hormone/endocrine sensitivity*: some cancers, such as breast cancer, can be hormone sensitive.
- *Increased receptor expression*: some cell surface receptors are overexpressed in certain cancer cells, for example HER2 positive breast or gastric cancers.
- *Presence or absence of specific mutations*: specific mutations have been linked to the development/progression of cancer. These mutations can be targeted by drugs, for example vemurafenib for BRAF mutation positive metastatic melanoma.

Decision making in cancer patients
Decision making in cancer patients can be complex. The following questions provide a framework to aid in making these decisions.
1 What is the histology/type of cancer? i.e. 'what is it?'
   This impacts on prognosis and treatment, for example some types of cancer are sensitive to radiotherapy (e.g. squamous cell carcinomas), whereas others are relatively radiation resistant.
2 What is the stage of their cancer? i.e. 'where is it?'
   (a) This also impacts on prognosis and treatment.
   (b) In general, localised disease is treated with local therapies, whereas systemic disease is treated with systemic agents.
3 Is it potentially curable (based on tumour histology and staging)?
4 If we could potentially cure their cancer, what would the treatment involve? (e.g. surgery +/− chemotherapy +/− radiotherapy).
   (a) Would neoadjuvant therapy be beneficial?
   Neoadjuvant therapy may increase the chance of cure if the patient responds to treatment (e.g. by shrinking a tumour so that it can be surgically removed with clear margins). However, there is a risk of the patient's cancer progressing if they do not respond to neoadjuvant therapy.
   (b) Would adjuvant therapy be beneficial?
   This is often a complicated decision as the patient has already had a radical treatment aiming for cure. This treatment alone may have cured the patient. However, some patients will be cured by the addition of adjuvant treatment.
      The individual patient will not know if they personally benefited from the adjuvant treatment as the benefit is determined from population statistics. There is no biochemical or radiological evidence to show an immediate benefit of treatment.

This can be difficult to explain to patients and the choice of statistics used to explain benefits and risks can influence their decisions regarding treatment.

Decision-making aids (such as www.adjuvantonline.com) can assist with decision making and explanations.

Factors to consider when making decisions regarding adjuvant therapy include:

The presence of risk factors for local recurrence, for example large tumours, close surgical margins, nodal involvement. Adjuvant radiotherapy may be indicated for these patients.

The presence of risk factors for haematogenous spread, for example high grade tumours, lymphovascular invasion, nodal involvement. Adjuvant chemotherapy may be appropriate to reduce the risk of developing metastatic disease.

The pattern of lymphatic spread:

   (i) If this is predictable then radiotherapy may be appropriate to eradicate subclinical disease in the next echelon of nodes.

   (ii) If this is not predictable then systemic therapy is more appropriate.

(c) What are the potential side effects and complications of treatment?

(d) Is the patient fit enough for treatment? Consider age and comorbidities.

(e) What are the patient's priorities?

   (i) Different patients have different views on treatment. Some patients would prefer to have a treatment with a small chance of cure but significant side effects, whereas for others their quality of life is more important.

   (ii) It is important to balance the potential benefits of treatment with both the short and long-term side effects and risks. This is particularly important when considering adjuvant therapies.

5 If the cancer is not curable (either due to the disease itself or due to the patient's suitability for curative treatment), what are the aims of possible treatment options? For example, symptom control, slowing of disease progression, prevention of complications.

(a) What would the treatment involve?

(b) What is the likely response rate/improvement in survival?

(c) What are the potential side effects and complications of treatment?

(d) Is the patient fit enough for treatment? Consider age and comorbidities.

(e) What are the patient's priorities?

   (i) It is important that the patient understands the potential benefits and risks of treatment. Their initial expectations may not be realistic and may alter following an informed discussion.

   (ii) Different patients have different views on treatment. Some patients would prefer to have a treatment with a small chance of response and a small improvement in overall survival but significant side effects, whereas for other patients their quality of life is more important.

Assessing response to treatment

There are a number of different ways of assessing whether a patient is responding to a treatment. If the patient has clinically measurable disease (e.g. a breast lump) then this can be regularly measured and compared to previous measurements. Some cancers have tumour markers that correlate with response to treatment, for example PSA in patients with prostate cancer. In other patients, response assessment involves imaging (e.g. with CT scans, bone scans, PET scans). There are defined criteria for the radiological assessment of response, such as the RECIST 1.1 criteria (Response Evaluation Criteria In Solid Tumours). This assesses both target lesions and non-target lesions:

- *Target lesion* = a lesion that can be accurately measured in at least one dimension with a longest diameter that is ≥ 10 mm with CT or ≥ 20 mm by chest X-ray.
- *Non-target lesion* = all other lesions, including small lesions, for example leptomeningeal disease, ascites, pleural and pericardial effusions.

RECIST 1.1 criteria for evaluation of target lesions
- *Complete response (CR)* = disappearance of all target lesions. Any pathological lymph nodes must have a reduction in short axis to < 10 mm.
- *Partial response (PR)* = at least a 30% decrease in the sum of diameters of target lesions, taking as reference the baseline sum diameters.
- *Stable disease (SD)* = neither sufficient shrinkage to qualify for PR nor sufficient increase to qualify for PD, taking as reference the smallest sum diameters.
- *Progressive disease (PD)* = at least a 20% increase in the sum of diameters of target lesions, taking as reference the smallest sum diameter recorded since the treatment started (the sum must also demonstrate an absolute increase of at least 5 mm) or the appearance of one or more new lesions.

RECIST 1.1 criteria for evaluation of non-target lesions
- *Complete response (CR)* = disappearance of all non-target lesions and normalisation of tumour marker level. All lymph nodes must be non-pathological in size (< 10 mm short axis).
- *Incomplete response/stable disease (SD)* = persistence of one or more non-target lesion(s) or/and maintenance of tumour marker level above the normal limits.
- *Progressive disease (PD)* = appearance of one or more new lesions and/or unequivocal progression of existing non-target lesions.

References

Cancer Research UK. All cancers combined Key Facts. Available from: http://info.cancer researchuk.org/cancerstats/keyfacts/Allcancerscombined/ (accessed 1 January 2014).

Eisenhauer EA, Therasse P, Bogaerts J, Schwartz LH, Sargent D, Ford R, *et al*. New response evaluation criteria in solid tumours: revised RECIST guideline (version 1.1). *European Journal of Cancer*. 2009. 45(2): 228–47. Epub 23 December 2008.

Table 1.1 Performance status.

Score (%)	Karnofsky performance status	Score	WHO/ECOG performance status
100	Normal, no signs of disease.	0	Asymptomatic, fully active and able to carry out all pre-disease activities without restriction.
90	Capable of normal activity, a few symptoms or signs of disease.	1	Symptomatic, restricted in physically strenuous activity but ambulatory and able to carry out light or sedentary work.
80	Normal activity with some difficulty. Some symptoms or signs.		
70	Self-caring, not capable of normal activity or work.	2	Capable of all self-care but unable to carry out any work activities; < 50% in bed during the day.
60	Needs some help with care; can take care of most personal requirements.		
50	Help required often, frequent medical care needed.	3	Capable of only limited self-care; > 50% in bed during the day.
40	Disabled, requires special care and help.		
30	Severely disabled, hospital admission needed but no risk of death.	4	Completely disabled and cannot do any self-care. Totally confined to bed or chair.
20	Very ill, needs urgent admission and requires supportive care.		
10	Moribund, rapidly progressive fatal disease.		
0	Death.	5	Death.

Adapted from Ma C, *et al. European Journal of Cancer.* (2010). 46: 3175–83. Reproduced with permission of Elsevier.

Performance status

Performance status (PS) is used to try to quantify patients' physical well-being and help guide treatment decisions. PS should be routinely documented for all oncology patients. There are a number of scoring systems in use (see Table 1.1).

Tumour markers

Overview
- Tumour markers are substances, usually proteins, which are produced by cancer cells or normal tissues in response to cancer growth.
- Some are relevant to one type of cancer, others to a number of different cancers.
- Tumour markers can also be elevated by non-cancerous conditions and are therefore not used on their own to diagnose cancer.

- Not all patients with cancer have elevated tumour markers and so a negative result does not necessarily exclude the presence of cancer.

Current uses of tumour markers

- *Screening*: their role in screening programmes is not fully established due to low specificity and/or low levels seen at early stages of disease.
- *Monitoring of high risk patients*: they may be useful in the monitoring of patients who are at particularly high risk of specific cancers due to a strong family history/gene mutations.
- *Diagnosis*: they can *assist* with diagnosis and guide further investigations (e.g. an elevated Ca125 might be suggestive of ovarian cancer rather than other pathology).
- *Staging*: they can have a role in staging tumours to assess the extent of disease (e.g. elevated LDH is part of the staging system for melanoma).
- *Determining prognosis*: they can be an indicator of a patient's prognosis.
- *Assessing response to treatment/monitoring for disease recurrence*: if a patient has elevated markers, then the markers can be used to assess response to treatment and to monitor for signs of treatment resistance and disease progression (i.e. if the level drops then this is suggestive of a response to treatment, if the level then starts rising again then the treatment may be losing efficacy). If a patient did not have elevated markers prior to treatment then they cannot be used to assess response.

Common tumour markers

New potential tumour markers are constantly being evaluated and incorporated into clinical practice. Table 1.2 provides a guide to the most commonly used tumour markers. A full discussion of the use of specific markers in each cancer type is beyond the scope of this book.

Tumour markers most commonly measured for specific cancers

- *Breast*: Ca15-3, CEA, Ca125
- *Colon*: CEA, Ca19-9
- *Germ cell*: AFP, LDH, hCG
- *Hepatocellular*: AFP
- *Ovarian*: Ca125, CEA
- *Prostate*: PSA
- *Upper GI/pancreatic*: Ca19-9, CEA

Circulating tumour cells/DNA

- Circulating tumour cells are tumour cells that are found in the peripheral circulation in low concentrations. These cells have potential as markers of response to treatment, assessment of prognosis and monitoring for recurrence.
- Circulating tumour DNA is cell-free DNA carrying tumour specific alterations. This DNA is found in the peripheral circulation and has potential as a marker of response to treatment and prognosis.

Table 1.2 Common tumour markers.

Tumour marker	Usual reference range	Associated cancers (italics indicate the most relevant)	Associated other conditions	Aid diagnosis	Response assessment	Staging	Prognosis	Monitor for recurrence
AFP (α-fetoprotein)	0–10 ng/mL or 0–12 µg/L	*HCC, germ cell tumours,* hepatoblastoma, hepatobiliary, gastric, lung, colorectal	Pregnancy, hepatitis, cirrhosis, biliary tract obstruction, alcoholic liver disease, ataxia telangiectasia, hereditary tyrosinaemia	X	X			X
β2-microglobulin	< 2.5 mg/L.	*Multiple myeloma, lymphoma*	Many other conditions, including Crohn's disease, hepatitis and renal disease				X	
BTA (bladder tumour antigen)	Urine is either positive or negative	*Bladder*	Renal stones, UTI	X				X
Ca15-3	0–5 to 0–40 U/ml	*Breast,* ovarian, lung	Benign breast conditions, hepatitis, chronic liver disease, colitis, dermatological conditions		X			X
Ca19-9	very variable, from 0–37 U/ml to 0–100 U/ml	*Pancreatic, colorectal, gastric,* hepatocellular, oesophageal, ovarian	Pancreatitis, inflammatory bowel disease, cholangitis, cholestasis, chronic liver disease, diabetes, irritable bowel syndrome, jaundice, cystic fibrosis		X			X

Tumour marker	Usual reference range	Associated cancers (italics indicate the most relevant)	Associated other conditions	Aid diagnosis	Response assessment	Staging	Prognosis	Monitor for recurrence
Ca125	0–35 U/ml	*Ovarian*, breast, cervical, endometrial, hepatocellular, lung, non-Hodgkin's lymphoma, pancreas, peritoneal, uterine, any advanced adenocarcinoma	Endometriosis, menstruation, inflammatory pelvic disease, post-laparoscopy, peritoneal inflammation, non-malignant ascites, hepatitis, chronic liver disease, pancreatitis, respiratory disease (e.g. pneumonia, pleural inflammation), colitis, diverticulitis, irritable bowel syndrome, heart failure, pericarditis, diabetes, ovarian hyperstimulation, pregnancy, recurrent ischaemic strokes, arthritis, sarcoidosis, systemic lupus erythematosus, acute urinary retention, cystic fibrosis		X	X		X
Calcitonin	< 5–12 pg/ml	*Medullary thyroid carcinoma*, lung cancer, leukaemia	Thyroiditis, pernicious anaemia	X	X			X

Continued

Table 1.2 Continued

Tumour marker	Usual reference range	Associated cancers (italics indicate the most relevant)	Associated other conditions	Aid diagnosis	Response assessment	Staging	Prognosis	Monitor for recurrence
CEA (carcinoembryonic antigen)	0–2.5 ng/ml (non-smoker) to 0–5.0 ng/mL (smoker)	Bowel, lung, breast, thyroid, pancreatic, liver, cervix, bladder, mesothelioma, oesophageal	Hepatitis, respiratory diseases (e.g. COPD, pneumonia, pleural inflammation), colitis, pancreatitis, higher in cigarette smokers, chronic liver disease (e.g. cirrhosis, chronic active hepatitis), diverticulitis, irritable bowel syndrome, jaundice, renal disease		X			X
Chromogranin A	< 50 ng/mL, results vary by laboratory	Neuroendocrine tumours		X	X			
hCG (human chorionic gonadotrophin)	0–5 IU/L	Testicular, trophoblastic, lung	Pregnancy, testicular failure, cannabis use, menopause, pituitary adenoma, after termination of pregnancy	X	X			X
LDH (lactate dehydrogenase)	very variable	Melanoma, lymphoma, testicular cancer, germ cell tumours	Damage to an organ (e.g. MI)		X	X	X	X

Tumour marker	Usual reference range	Associated cancers (italics indicate the most relevant)	Associated other conditions	Aid diagnosis	Response assessment	Staging	Prognosis	Monitor for recurrence
NSE (neuron-specific enolase)	> 9 ug/mL	*Neuroendocrine tumours*			X			
PSA (prostate specific antigen)	0–4 ng/mL but some advocate age-related reference ranges	*Prostate*	Benign prostatic hypertrophy, ejaculation, prostatitis, increasing age, 5-α reductase inhibitors (e.g. finasteride), catheterisation, digital rectal examination, cystoscopy, prostatic massage/biopsy/USS, acute urinary retention, UTI	X	X			X
Thyroglobulin	Variable depending on assay used	*Thyroid*	Other thyroid diseases					X (and to detect residual disease)

Other relevant sections of this book
Chapter 10, section on personalised medicine

References

American Association for Clinical Chemistry. Tumour markers. Available from: http://www. labtestsonline.org.uk/understanding/analytes/tumor-markers/ (accessed 1 January 2014).

American Cancer Society. Tumour markers 2011. Available from: http://www.cancer.org/ Treatment/UnderstandingYourDiagnosis/ExamsandTestDescriptions/TumorMarkers/index (accessed 1 January 2014).

Dawson SJ, Tsui DW, Murtaza M, Biggs H, Rueda OM, Chin SF, *et al.* Analysis of circulating tumor DNA to monitor metastatic breast cancer. *The New England Journal of Medicine.* 2013. 368(13): 1199–209. Epub 13 March 2013.

Duffy M, McGing P. *Guidelines for the Use of Tumour Markers.* Scientific Committee of the Association of Clinical Biochemists in Ireland (ACBI). 2005.

Sleijfer S, Gratama JW, Sieuwerts AM, Kraan J, Martens JW, Foekens JA. Circulating tumour cell detection on its way to routine diagnostic implementation? *European Journal of Cancer.* 2007. 43(18): 2645–50.

Sturgeon CM, Lai LC, Duffy MJ. Serum tumour markers: how to order and interpret them. *British Medical Journal.* 2009. 339:b3527.

CHAPTER 2

Oncological emergencies

Daniel L.Y. Lee
St James' Institute of Oncology, UK

Anaphylaxis and hypersensitivity reactions

Definition
- Hypersensitivity and anaphylaxis are immunologically triggered responses. Anaphylaxis can broadly be defined as a severe, life-threatening, generalised or systemic hypersensitivity reaction.
- There are two types of reaction, one is IgE mediated and the other is not. There has recently been a move away from these distinct diagnoses, that of anaphylaxis and anaphylactoid reactions respectively, to sub-categorisation within an overarching diagnosis of anaphylaxis.

Causes
- All intravenous infusions are at some risk of a hypersensitivity reaction or anaphylaxis. The overall incidence is around 5%; however, some are much more high risk.

Clinical Problems in Oncology: A Practical Guide to Management, First Edition.
Edited by Sing Yu Moorcraft, Daniel L.Y. Lee and David Cunningham.
© 2014 John Wiley & Sons, Ltd. Published 2014 by John Wiley & Sons, Ltd.

- *High risk infusions include*: platinum and taxane chemotherapies (e.g. cisplatin, carboplatin, paclitaxel, docetaxel), some monoclonal antibody therapies (e.g. rituximab).
- *Other causes include*: antibiotics, NSAIDs, vaccines, contrast media, foods, insect stings, skin preparations and latex.

Symptoms and signs
- Patient education is paramount, and early symptoms may be as vague as feeling 'unwell' or 'not normal'.
- Early diagnosis improves outcomes and shortens the possible effects, so vigilance of the treating team is important.
- Acute reactions can occur within seconds of exposure and can progress rapidly, slowly or in a biphasic manner. Rarely, reactions can occur after a few hours or persist for more than 24 hours.
- Beta-blockers may increase the severity of the reaction and antagonise the effect of adrenaline. Adrenaline can cause severe hypertension and bradycardia in patients taking non-cardioselective beta-blockers.

Symptoms can range in severity and are most commonly divided into two groups:
1 Mild symptoms only, without any respiratory symptoms.
2 Clinical signs of shock with possible respiratory distress, stridor, wheeze or laryngeal oedema.

Management
Specific treatment will depend on the severity of the reaction and the drug which is being infused. Each department should have guidance on the local protocol, but general guidance is given below.

Localised hypersensitivity reaction
- Assess symptoms and observations.
- Consider antihistamine and/or corticosteroid use (see anaphylaxis treatment section below for doses).
- Repeat observations every 15 minutes for one hour.

Anaphylaxis
- Stop the IV infusion and keep the IV access.
- Call for help and prepare resuscitation trolley for use.
- Assess airway, breathing and circulation, along with consciousness (GCS).
- Lay the patient flat or in the Trendelenberg position (i.e. feet elevated).
- Oxygen – 15 litres/minute via a non-rebreath mask.
- *Adrenaline*:
  ○ Intramuscular injection (1 mg/ml, 1:1000 dilution) into antero-lateral thigh, 0.5 mg every five minutes (treatment of choice).

- Intravenous 50 mcg (0.5 ml, 1:10,000 dilution) boluses according to response – if repeated boluses required, start an adrenaline infusion. This is usually only given in specialist units (e.g. HDU, ITU or theatres) for patients with profound shock that is immediately life threatening.
- *Fluids*: start with a fluid challenge of 500–1000 ml of crystalloid. Over two litres of fluid may extravasate within the first five minutes, so large volumes may be needed.
- *Corticosteroids*: 200 mg hydrocortisone stat IM or slow IV.
- *Anti-histamines*: 10 mg chlorpheniramine stat IM or slow IV.
- Monitor pulse oximetry, blood pressure and perform an ECG.
- Consider admission to a high-level bed if vasopressor or ventilatory support is needed.
- *Other drugs*:
  - Glucagon may be useful in the treatment of anaphylaxis in patients on beta-blockers.
  - Atropine may be useful for bradycardia.
  - Bronchodilators (e.g. salbutamol, ipratropium) may be useful if a patient has asthmatic symptoms.
- *Investigations*: mast cell tryptase – at least one sample after the onset of symptoms (do not delay resuscitation to take the sample). Ideally, also take another sample 1–2 hours after the start of symptoms and a third sample at convalescence or at 24 hours. This can help to confirm the diagnosis of anaphylaxis.

Observation and biphasic reactions

- A period of observation is recommended after an anaphylactic reaction. This may be from four to six hours, to an admission, depending on the severity of the reaction.
- There is the possibility of the recurrence of symptoms after the effects of the adrenaline have worn off, although these are usually milder than the initial attack. A biphasic reaction is the recurrence of symptoms after the complete resolution of symptoms. This can occur in 3–20% of patients after an anaphylactic reaction.
- At discharge, consider prescribing anti-histamines and oral steroids for up to three days to help treat urticaria (may also decrease the risk of a further reaction).

Ongoing management and retreatment

After the acute episode has abated further treatment with the offending drug may be considered. This is dependent on the grade of the reaction and the 'value' of pursuing further treatment with the same drug, or the benefits of any possible alternatives. There may be the possibility of increasing premedication regimens for the reaction or reducing the infusion rate. All such decisions should be undertaken by a senior member of the treating team. Refer to local guidelines regarding drug re-challenges and for desensitisation protocols.

References

Gleich GJ, Leiferman KM. Anaphylaxis: implications of monoclonal antibody use in oncology. *Oncology* (Williston Park). 2009. 23(2 Suppl. 1): 7–13.

Resuscitation Council (UK) Emergency treatment of anaphylactic reactions guidelines for healthcare providers (annotated July 2012). Available from: http://www.resus.org.uk/pages/reaction.htm (accessed 1 January 2014).

Viale PH. Management of hypersensitivity reactions: a nursing perspective. *Oncology* (Williston Park). 2009. 23(2 Suppl. 1): 26–30.

Bleeding

Overview

Bleeding can occur in up to 10% of patients with advanced cancer. This may increase to up to 30% in those with a haematological malignancy.

There are multiple causes for bleeding in cancer patients:

- Related to the cancer:
  - Varies dependent on the size, type and location of the primary tumour and the presence of lymphadenopathy or metastases.
  - Higher risk tumours include head and neck cancers, pelvic malignancies and fungating tumours, particularly if there is direct vascular invasion or damage from the cancer.
- Related to cancer treatment:
  - Chemotherapy – thrombocytopenia.
  - Radiotherapy – bleeding secondary to inflammation or tumour shrinkage.
  - Surgery.
- Related to comorbidities or other treatments:
  - Anticoagulants.
  - Liver impairment with subsequent coagulation deficiency.
  - Concurrent infection can raise the risk of bleeding due to inflammation. Antibiotic treatment may lower the risk.

Clinical presentation

The presentation can vary markedly:

- Sub-acute or occult bleed:
  - Presenting as iron-deficiency anaemia
  - Anaemia beyond that expected from systemic therapies
  - Relating to the site of bleed, for example subarachnoid haemorrhage, intra-femoral bleed post fracture
  - Bleeding metastases (most commonly from malignant melanoma or RCC)
- Visible bleed:
  - Bruising
  - Minor bleeding
  - Major/catastrophic bleeding

Clinical assessment

Appropriate management will depend on assessing:
- Cancer history and treatment intent:
  - Prior surgery
  - Systemic treatment – discuss with senior if unsure of related bleeding risk
- Time and severity of bleed:
  - Patient consciousness
  - Observations: pulse, BP, oxygen saturations, visible evidence of bleed
- Identify the site of bleeding from history and examination.
  Note: a minor bleed may herald further more severe bleeding.
- Bloods including: FBC, U&E, LFT, coagulation, group and save.

Management
General measures

Patients receiving adjuvant or curative treatment should be treated as per any other patient, with prompt assessment and intervention as needed. Major catastrophic haemorrhage is rare in cancer patients, but should be assessed in an acute environment and with the use of appropriate local protocols. Most emergency departments will have a specific catastrophic haemorrhage algorithm. Blood tests and IV access should be sought early and IV fluids administered as appropriate. IV fluids may further dilute the blood, so consider the use of blood products (see section on systemic interventions).

Particular consideration should be given to the patients' prior treatment and the bleeding risk associated with this, for example after surgery. There are situations where patients at the end of life may have an unexpected or predicted catastrophic bleeding event. These should be managed with a very different approach, as detailed in the next section.

Local interventions
- Packing:
  - Consider in nasal, vaginal or rectal bleed.
  - Haemostatic agents (e.g. topical sulcralfate, topical tranexamic acid) may be useful.
  - Dressings provide direct compression and can be soaked in tranexamic acid to try and stem the bleeding further.
- Endoscopy:
  - Particularly useful as it is able to visualise and treat multiple sources of bleeding.
  - Consider in upper GI, lung and bladder bleeds.
- Interventional radiology:
  Transcutaneous arterial embolisation with beads/particles, glue or coils:
  - Restricted by patient factors and site of bleed.
  - Requires good patient selection to improve outcomes.
  - Benefit reported in patients with head and neck, pelvis, lung, liver and GI tract cancers.

- Radiotherapy:
  - Most commonly used for bleeding in cancers of the lung, vagina, skin, rectum and bladder.
  - May be considered in head and neck cancers and in upper GI cancers.
  - There is a delay between treatment and effect, so not considered in the acute setting.
- Surgery:
  - May be appropriate with good performance status and prognosis.
  - Particularly important in adjuvant patients with possible bleed secondary to resection.
  - Reserved for those who have failed conservative measures in advanced cancer.

Systemic interventions

Vitamin K:
  - IV is quicker but associated with more 'over-correction', usually at doses between 2.5 and 10 mg.
  - SC and oral administration are also effective if time is not of the essence.
- Vasopressin/desmopressin:
  - Continuous infusions are reported to control half of patients with upper-GI malignancy-related bleeding.
  - Associated with myocardial, mesenteric and cerebral circulation ischaemia.
- Somatostatin analogues (e.g. octreotide): used in upper GI bleeds, but no reports for efficacy in cancer patients.
- Anti-fibrinolytic agents (e.g. tranexamic acid):
  - Act through reduced fibrin clot breakdown.
  - Cautious use in those with previous thrombotic event, renal failure (accumulation) and those with a cardiac stent.
  - Can be associated with GI side-effects (e.g. nausea, vomiting).
- Blood products (e.g. platelets, fresh frozen plasma, coagulation factors, packed red blood cells):
  - Platelets – increased risk of bleeding if < 20, severe risk if < 10. May need four to six bags of platelets to reduce active bleeding – discuss with local bleed service or haematologist.
  - Fresh frozen plasma – selected for:
    - Coagulation deficiencies
    - Urgent reversal of INR in patients on warfarin
    - Urgent intervention needed (e.g. thoracic surgery)
    - Treatment of disseminated intravascular coagulation (DIC) when appropriate

Disseminated intravascular coagulopathy (DIC)

Associated with malignancy, sepsis and trauma. There is increased thrombin formation (with associated decreased fibrinogen, PT and APTT) and increased fibrinolysis (with associated increased d-dimer). There is an associated poor prognosis. The basis of treatment is:

- Treatment of underlying condition (e.g. sepsis, malignancy)
- Haemodynamic support
- Platelet and FFP only if actively bleeding
- Discussion with haematologist regarding further evaluation and management (e.g. use of heparin, blood films)

End of life considerations/catastrophic bleed

Advanced planning is crucial in palliation of expected catastrophic bleed. Patients undergoing palliation should have their chances of an acute catastrophic bleed identified early. An early, sensitive discussion with the family and patient about their wishes is paramount and can provide forewarning and reassurance. 'Do not attempt resuscitation' orders should be discussed and completed prior to any event.

Patients who are particularly at risk are those with:
- Terminal head and neck cancer
- Pelvic malignancy
- Patients who presented with bleeding (e.g. haemoptysis)

The central focus of intervention is:
- A calm approach to patient and family to reduce distress
- Dark towels to soak up bleeding and provide direct pressure
- Use of sedation (e.g. SC midazolam, lorazepam) for distress in the terminal event
- Review of medications such as anticoagulation and NSAIDs
- Care in a side room and timely 'do not resuscitate' decision

Other relevant sections of this book

Chapter 3, sections on anaemia, thrombocytopenia

References

Hulme B, Wilcox S. Yorkshire Palliative Medicine Clinical Guidelines Group: Guidelines on the management of bleeding for palliative care patients with cancer (2008). Available at: http://www.palliativedrugs.com (registration required) (accessed 1 January 2014).

Nauck F, Alt-Epping B. Crises in palliative care – a comprehensive approach. *Lancet Oncology*. 2008. 9(11): 1086–91.

Pereira J, Phan T. Management of bleeding in patients with advanced cancer. *The Oncologist*. 2004. 9(5): 561–70.

Central airway obstruction and stridor

Definition

- *Central airway obstruction* (CAO): the central airways are defined as the trachea, main and lobular bronchi. These may become obstructed via an intraluminal, luminal or extraluminal pathology. The grading of tracheal obstruction is shown in Table 2.1.

Table 2.1 CTCAE (V4.03) grading of tracheal obstruction.

Grade	Criteria
1	Partial symptomatic obstruction on examination (e.g. visual, radiologic or endoscopic).
2	Symptomatic (e.g. noisy airway breathing), no respiratory distress, medical intervention indicated (e.g. steroids), limiting ADL.
3	Stridor, radiologic or endoscopic intervention indicated (e.g. stent, laser); limiting self-care ADL.
4	Life-threatening airway compromise; urgent intervention indicated (e.g. tracheotomy or intubation).
5	Death.

From the website of the National Cancer Institute (http://www.cancer.gov).

Table 2.2 CTCAE (V4.03) grading of stridor.

Grade	Criteria
1	—
2	—
3	Respiratory distress limiting self-care ADL; medical intervention indicated.
4	Life-threatening airway compromise; urgent intervention indicated (e.g. tracheotomy or intubation).
5	Death.

From the website of the National Cancer Institute (http://www.cancer.gov).

- *Stridor*: this is a harsh noise associated with respiration due to reduction in lumen of upper airway tracts. The grading of stridor is shown in Table 2.2.
  - If there is stridor and dyspnoea at rest, the central airways are usually narrowed to <25% of their cross-sectional area.
  - The causes and treatment for stridor in children are very different from that seen in adults. This chapter will focus on adult cases only.

Causes

CAO can be the result of malignant or non-malignant causes. Malignancy is the most common pathology, and the most common malignant pathology leading to CAO is lung cancer. Lung cancer can obstruct the airway intraluminally or through extraluminal compression.

Malignant causes include:
- Lung cancer
- Metastatic cancer – colon, breast, oesophagus, kidney and melanoma
- Metastatic lymphadenopathy

Non-malignant processes include:
- Laryngeal pathology – anaphylaxis, acute epiglottitis
- Inhaled foreign bodies, food or blood clots
- Chronic medical conditions affecting the lung – TB stricture, Wegener's granulo-matosis, sarcoidosis
- Secondary to previous trauma to the airways – post-endotracheal tube insertion, post tracheostomy, chemical burns, post-bronchial sleeve resection
- Idiopathic

Symptoms

Symptoms are dependent upon the degree of airway stenosis. In some cases, symptoms can develop rapidly and become life threatening. Symptoms include:
- Wheeze
- Stridor
  - Can be exertional or at rest
  - May be on inspiration, expiration or biphasic, depending on the site of cause
- Haemoptysis
- Chest pain
- Post-stenotic pneumonia may be evident on CXR or suggested by recurrent episodes of pneumonia

Investigation

- Radiology – most patients will have undergone a CXR as part of their initial assessment. A CT thorax will best determine the site and degree of stenosis. In patients who are not previously known to have cancer, it may also provide diagnostic use. 3D reconstruction sequences of the central airways have been cited as the gold standard, but are not readily available in all centres.
- Bronchoscopy – allows direct visualisation of the airways to identify the site of stenosis and dimensions. It may allow intervention in some cases, such as clearing of mucous plugs. In undiagnosed cases, it may also provide histological confir-mation of cancer.
- Concomitant exacerbating factors, such as anaemia, COPD or asthma should also be sought and managed appropriately.

Management

There are multiple interventional procedures now available in the management of CAO. The optimum choice is dependent upon a number of patient factors (such as performance status and wishes), cancer and prognostic factors and local avail-ability. Optimum intervention selection should involve an MDT, if time allows.

General management

- Avoid respiratory depressants (e.g. sedatives) and muscle relaxants.
- Oxygen supplementation may reduce respiratory effort.
- High-dose steroids are commonly used (e.g. 8 mg OD dexamethasone IV/PO with PPI cover) but with little evidence.

- Heliox (8:2 or 7:3) has been used in an attempt to reduce airway turbulence associated with CAO and stridor. Its use is supported by results from small case series, but further evidence is required. Any likely benefit should be seen at an early stage.
- In severe cases (e.g. reduced pO2 or respiratory fatigue), discuss with ITU regarding extra respiratory support.
- Early ENT input may be required for lesions around the epiglottis or vocal cords as patients may require a tracheostomy.
- Do not attempt to instrument the airway without expert help.

Specific anti-cancer treatments
- For those cases with a mild degree of CAO, usually without the presence of stridor, chemotherapy or radiotherapy may be the first choice of treatment.
- Chemotherapy is particularly useful in SCLC or lymphoma, but also commonly used in non-severe cases with alternate cancer types that may respond to systemic treatment (e.g. NSCLC).
- Radiosensitive tumours (e.g. NSCLC, thyroid and tracheal tumours) may be treated with radiotherapy, either prior to systemic therapy or concomitantly/ sequentially with chemotherapy or endoscopic procedures.

Endoscopic procedures
- Airway stent – available more readily in most areas than the alternatives discussed here.
  - The ability to place the stent will depend on the exact location of obstruction and whether a stent can be viably placed. Common contraindications include lesions proximal to bifurcation of the airways. However, Y-shaped stents have been developed for placement at the carina.
  - Stent related issues include: mucostasis, stent migration, colonisation with bacteria or fungi and possible subsequent pneumonia/lung abscesses.
    Re-stenosis due to tumour overgrowth or excessive granulation tissue formation may be overcome with a further stent, cryotherapy or argon plasma coagulation (APC).
- Laser resection – particularly useful for central lesions with endobronchial tumour growth. This may be combined with stenting, brachytherapy or external beam radiotherapy to reduce tumour re-growth into the airway.
- Electrocautery – APC, which is a form of electrocautery, may control local tumour growth and relieve obstruction as well as provide local haemostatic control.
- Cryotherapy – a super-cooled tip (−89 °C) is placed in direct contact with the tumour and may debulk the mass so as to relieve the obstruction. It is less effective than either laser or electrocautery at controlling bleeding in the immediate to short term.
- Intraluminal brachytherapy – effects are delayed, so not suitable in life-threatening circumstances. Usually used as part of a multi-modality treatment. Palliative brachytherapy may be considered in patients who have non-life threatening airway

compromise, and are not able to undergo radiotherapy or surgery (either due to fitness or because they have already received maximal treatment with this modality).

- Airway dilatation – short-lived in malignant processes, but may be useful in benign processes (such as post-surgical stenosis of the airways).

References

Gompelmann D, Eberhardt R, Herth FJF. Advanced malignant lung disease: what the specialist can offer. *Respiration*. 2011. 82(2): 111–23.

Feller-Kopman DJ, O'Donnell C. Physiology and clinical use of heliox. In: Hollingsworth H (ed.) *UpToDate*. UpToDate, Waltham, MA. 2013.

Williamson JP, Phillips MJ, Hillman DR and Eastwood PR. Managing obstruction of the central airways. *Internal Medicine Journal*. 2010. 40(6): 399–410.

Extravasation

Definition

Extravasation is the leakage of a pharmacological or biological agent from the infusion site into the surrounding tissue. The grading of extravasation is shown in Table 2.3.

The incidence of extravasation is unclear and there is variability in the guidelines of its management. Chemotherapeutic agents can be classified into categories based on their potential to cause damage and this is central to the management of extravasation. These categories are:

- *Vesicant*: causes tissue necrosis leading to severe and lasting injury. It may affect the full thickness of the skin and underlying structures.
- *Irritant*: causes a localised inflammatory response leading to discomfort, burning, tingling or phlebitis at the cannulation site or tracking along the vein. This is a short-term complication without the tissue necrosis seen with vesicant drugs.
- *Non-vesicant/irritant*: no local inflammation.

However, these categories are not absolute and may depend on the volume of drug extravasated and the concentration of the infusion (e.g. a classically irritant drug can cause a vesicant reaction). Chemotherapeutic agents and their extravasation potential are listed in Table 2.4.

Risk factors and prevention of extravasation

- Risk factors include:
  - Difficult IV access (e.g. small, mobile or fragile veins, obesity)
  - Long infusion times
  - Site of cannulation

Table 2.3 CTCAE (V4.03) grading of extravasation.

Grade	Criteria
1	—
2	Erythema with associated symptoms (e.g. oedema, pain, induration, phlebitis).
3	Ulceration or necrosis; severe tissue damage; operative intervention indicated.
4	Life-threatening consequences; urgent intervention indicated.
5	Death.

From the website of the National Cancer Institute (http://www.cancer.gov).

Table 2.4 Chemotherapeutic categories Adapted from Perez Fidalgo JA et al. Ann Oncol 2012; 23:vii167–73. Reproduced with permission of Oxford University Press.

DNA-binding Vesicants	Non-DNA-binding Vesicants	Irritants	Non-Vesicants
Alkylating Agents	**Vinca Alkaloids**	**Alkylating Agents**	Asparaginase
Mecholretamine	Vinblastine	Ifosfamide	Bleomycin[3]
Bendamustine[1]	Vincristine	Streptozocin	Bortezomib
Carmustine[2]	Vindesine	Dacarbazine[2]	Cladiribine
	Vinorelbine	Melphalan	Cytarabine
Anthracyclines			Cyclophosphamide
Doxorubicin	**Taxanes**	**Anthracyclines (other)**	Fludarabine
Daunorubicin	Docetaxel (rare)	Liposomal doxorubicin	Gemcitabine
Epirubicin	Paclitaxel (rare)	Liposomal daunorubicin	Interferons
Idarubicin		Mitoxantrone	Interleukin-2
	Others		Methotrexate
Others (Antibiotics)	Trabectedin	**Topoisomerase II inhibitors**	Monoclonal antibodies
Amsacrine		Etoposide	Pemetrexed
Dactinomycin		Teniposide	Raltitrexed
Mitomycin C			Temsirolimus
Mitoxantrone[2]		**Antimetabolites**	Thiothepa[3]
		5-FU	
		Platinum Salts	
		Carboplatin	
		Cisplatin[2]	
		Oxaliplatin[2]	
		Topoisomerase I inhibitors	
		Irinotecan	
		Topotecan	
		Others	
		Ixabepilone	
		Arsenic trioxide	
		Melphalan	
		Trastuzumab	

[1]Bendamustine is classified as a vesicant but reports have since described soft tissue damage on extravasation.
[2]May have vesicant or irritant properties, dependent upon the volume of the drug extravasated. Greater volume or concentration of the drug is associated with higher vesicant potential.
[3]May have irritant properties, dependent upon the volume of the drug extravasated.

- Prevention of extravasation: choice of cannulation site, if these cannot be avoided then consider a central line:
  - Choose a new site rather than a previous site
  - Choose a large vein in the forearm
  - Use local warming to dilate the vein
  - Never place the cannula in the inner wrist
  - Never place over a joint or in an area affected by lymphoedema
  - Avoid sites of previous radiation therapy or surgery

Diagnosis
Early signs that a drug may be extravasating include:
  - Tingling, burning, erythema/blanching and discomfort or swelling at the cannulation site.
  - Medical staff may notice a reduction in the flow rate or increased resistance on manual administration of medications via the cannula. Many infusion devices are set up to alarm in this scenario.
  - Patients should be informed to alert staff quickly if these symptoms occur. This is particularly important for vesicant drugs.
- Late signs include blistering, necrosis and ulceration around the site of cannulation. This can occur up to two to three days after the infusion, or later in some instances.
- Care should be taken with the following patients during the infusion or bolus:
  - Patients with peripheral neuropathy (and thus reduced sensation).
  - Patients with thrombosed veins from previous treatments.
  - When cannulation is ipsilateral to a mastectomy, axillary lymph node clearance or in an arm affected by lymphoedema.

Differential diagnoses
- Extravasation is the most important diagnosis if local site irritation or reaction occurs.
- Some drugs may cause a local reaction or a chemical phlebitis which is not related to extravasation. These are listed in Table 2.5.

Management
Each chemotherapy unit should have a nurse experienced in managing extravasation and an extravasation kit for reference and these should be consulted at diagnosis. It is important to identify the vesicant or irritant potential of the extravasated drug, as this can greatly alter the management, for example cold compress application to vinka alkaloid extravasation is associated with poorer outcomes.

General measures
- Stop and disconnect infusion.
- Leave the cannula in place.
- Do not flush the cannula.

Table 2.5 Chemotherapeutic agents that may cause a local reaction.

Local skin reactions	Chemical phlebitis
Aspariginase	Amsacrin
Cisplatin	Carmustine
Daunorubicin	Dacarbazine
Epirubicin	Epirubicin
Fludarabine	5-FU (as continual infusion in combination with cisplatin)
Mechlorethamine	Gemcitabine
Melphalan	Mechlorethamine
	Vinorelbine

- Identify the extravasated agent and check for differential diagnoses such as local itching, erythema or urticaria (see Table 2.5).
- Gentle aspiration of the agent – attempt to aspirate as much as possible.
- Mark the outline of the affected area for further monitoring.
- Avoid manual pressure over the area and then remove the cannula.
- Elevate the limb and provide analgesia.

Non-vesicant drugs
Apply a dry compress to cannula site.

Vesicant or irritant drugs
- *Localise and neutralise*: for anthracyclines, antibiotics (mitomycin, dactinomycin) and alkylating agents (see Table 2.4):
  - Localise: apply a dry cold compress for 20 minutes QDS for 1–2 days.
  - Neutralise: DMSO (see below).
- *Disperse and dilute*: for vinka alkaloids, taxanes and platinum salts:
  - Disperse: apply a dry warm compress for 20 minutes QDS for 1–2 days.
  - Dilute: agents to increase resorption: vinka alkaloids and taxanes – hyaluronidase (see below).
- *Hyaluronidase*
This is an enzyme that degrades hyaluronic acid and thus improves the absorption of the agent. It is often included in protocols as part of the 'disperse and dilute' arm. Particularly useful in vinca alkaloid extravasation but also in paclitaxel and ifosfamide extravasation. Dosing differs between protocols.
- *Corticosteroids*:
  - The subcutaneous injection of steroids at the extravasation site has been shown to increase necrosis rate and is not recommended.
  - Topical 1% hydrocortisone remains on many protocols to reduce non-specific inflammation.
  - It is important not to use corticosteroids in vinka alkaloid extravasation as this is associated with worsening of necrosis.

- *Dimethyl sulfoxide (DMSO)*:
  - This is a topical agent that increases the local removal of the extravasated drug.
  - Used in anthracycline, mitomycin and platinum salt extravasation.
  - A 50% preparation more commonly used, as 99% preparation is associated with local erythema, which can make further assessment of the extravasation site difficult.
  - Use every four hours for the first 24 hours then four times per day for seven days, alternating with topical hydrocortisone 1%.
- *Dexrazoxane*:
  - An iron binding agent used to reduce the formation of anthracycline-iron complexes. This is an intravenous infusion which should be started within six hours of the extravasation event.
  - Included in some anthracycline extravasation guidelines. The availability of dexrazoxane varies across the UK, as not all trusts have incorporated it into their extravasation guidelines. For example, the Scottish Medicines Consortium did not pass this agent in 2008 due to economic constraints, so check local trust/network guidelines.

Central venous device extravasation

Extravasations are much more commonly associated with peripheral access, but can rarely be associated with central venous devices. As this is such a rare event, little literature has been produced for its management.

- The extravasated solution may accumulate in the mediastinum, pleura or sub-cutaneous area of the chest or neck.
- The most common presenting symptom is acute thoracic pain.
- The diagnosis is clinical, but can be confirmed on thoracic CT scan.
- Management includes:
  - Stopping the infusion.
  - Aspirating as much solution as possible through the device.
  - Consideration of surgical drainage of remaining solution is recommended.
  - Usually a conservative approach is undertaken, including the use of antibiotics, intravenous corticosteroids and analgesia.

Recall injury

Paclitaxel has been shown to demonstrate a recall reaction at the site of previous extravasation when next infused. This is similar to the 'recall reaction' seen in areas of radiotherapy skin toxicity on anthracycline use. This has also been reported with doxorubicin and epirubicin.

Surgical referral

- One third of extravasations may progress to unresolved tissue necrosis or pain lasting more than ten days. Both of these outcomes warrant surgical management.

• Surgical management may involve excision of all involved tissue and a skin graft to recover the affected area. The re-graft is usually delayed by 2–3 days.
• Referral should be made to the local plastic surgical unit if a severe extravasation is expected, or if the affected site fails to settle on follow up.

References

Bertelli, G. Prevention and management of extravasation of cytotoxic drugs. *Drug Safety*. 1995. 12(4): 245–255.

Payne AS, Savarese DMF. Extravasation injury from chemotherapy and other non-neoplastic vesicants. In: Ross ME (ed.) *UpToDate*. UpToDate, Waltham, MA, 2013.

Perez Fidalgo JA, Fabregat LG, Cervantes A, Margulies A, Vidall C, Roila F, and on behalf of the ESMO Guidelines Working Group. Management of chemotherapy extravasation: ESMO-EONS Clinical Practice Guidelines. *Annals of Oncology*. 2012. 23(Suppl. 7): vii, 167–173.

Schulmeister L. Extravasation management: clinical update. *Seminars Oncology Nursing*. 2011. 2(1): 82–90.

Thomson D. Adult chemotherapy extravasation policy. Yorkshire Cancer Network (2012). Available from: http://www.yorkshire-cancer-net.org.uk (accessed 1 January 2014).

Febrile neutropenia

Definition

• NICE defines febrile neutropenia as a temperature of 38°C or higher on one occasion at home or in hospital, where the absolute neutrophil count is $0.5 \times 10^9/l$ or below.
• Caution should be exercised in those who may be about to become neutropenic, and those with a temperature below 36°C. Many hospitals would initially treat these patients with the febrile neutropenia protocol.

Background

• Particularly important on days 7–14 post chemotherapy, but very regimen dependent.
• The possibility of neutropenic sepsis is also affected by the use of other related treatments (e.g. radiotherapy, biological therapies and surgery).
• Patients may present with few localising signs, so watch out for the 'generally unwell' patient on chemotherapy.
• Young patients with good reserve may have very limited signs of sepsis on presentation.
• Pyrexia may be masked by high dose steroids and analgesics. Patients may present with hypothermia (temperature < 36°C).
• Patients may appear clinically well but can deteriorate very rapidly.
• If patients present generally unwell, or with signs of sepsis, shortly before the expected period of neutropenia they may be treated in accordance with the neutropenic guidelines despite the presenting neutrophil count.

Table 2.6 CTCAE (V4.03) grading of neutropenic sepsis.

Grade	Criteria
1	—
2	—
3	ANC < 1.00×10^9/l with a single temperature of > 38.5°C or a sustained temperature of ≥ 38°C for more than one hour.
4	Life-threatening consequences (e.g. haemodynamic collapse).
5	Death.

From the website of the National Cancer Institute (http://www.cancer.gov).

Assessment
- Signs of sepsis, history and examination to identify possible source: particular attention to lines, oral cavity, CNS, chest, abdomen, skin, wounds and urine.
- Consider comorbidities.
- Do NOT undertake a PR examination.
- Assess severity. The CTCAE grading of neutropenic sepsis is shown in Table 2.6. Note the differences from the definition of febrile neutropenia used in NICE 2012 guidelines, which are used as per the definition above.

Management
- *Culture*: any suspected site of infection from history or examination: blood cultures – peripheral and line cultures, urine sample and any other possible source.
- *Antibiotics*: broad-spectrum antibiotics *within one hour of presentation* – do not wait for blood tests as each hour's delay is associated with higher mortality.
  - Follow local protocol on antibiotic use:
    - Common regimens include: IV Tazocin® 4.5 g TDS.
    - If there are signs of systemic sepsis and haemodynamic instability then consider adding gentamicin (5 mg/kg) (caution in renal impairment).
    - Consider adding:
      - Vancomycin IV 1 g BD to cover for line infections.
      - Aciclovir if there any concerns regarding herpes zoster/varicella infection. The dose depends on infection and route.
      - Fluconazole 100 mg OD PO – if suspecting fungal infection or oral candida.
    - When switching to oral antibiotics, a commonly used regime is co-amoxiclav 625 mg TDS PO with ciprofloxacin 500 mg BD PO for seven days. This changes according to local antibiotic resistance rates.
  - Calculate patient's Multinational Association of Supportive Care in Cancer (MASCC) score. This is a scoring system that identifies patients at low risk of complications. The higher the score, the lower the risk of complications.
    - Score >21: low risk and oral antibiotics at home or within a short-stay facility may be appropriate.
    - Score <21: need for admission and IV antibiotics.

○ Points are allocated according to the following factors: age (2 points if < 60 years), underlying diagnosis (5 points if the patient has a solid tumour or has a haematological malignancy but has not had a previous fungal infection), absence of COPD (4 points), burden of illness (5 points for no or mild symptoms, 3 points for moderate symptoms), absence of hypotension (5 points), absence of dehydration (3 points), and whether they are an outpatient (2 points).

- *Supportive medications*: IV fluids to ensure normotension and adequate renal perfusion. Consider hourly fluid balance on any septic patient.
- *Level of care*: involve intensive care teams or outreach early if appropriate. If unsure, discuss this immediately with a senior colleague.
- *Granulocyte-Colony Stimulating Factors* (GCSF):
  ○ If they have been given as part of the patient's chemotherapy schedule then they should be continued.
  ○ Consider daily GCSF (e.g. filgrastim 300 mcg SC OD) if the patient has any of the following: shock/severe sepsis, comorbidities, a complicated infection (e.g. colitis), probable lengthy duration of neutropenia or in 'curative' treatments (to ensure future treatments are not overly delayed).

Future cancer management
- Further anti-cancer treatment will depend on the severity of, and the recovery from, the infection.
- The primary treating team (and acute oncology team if available) should be informed of any admission, with neutropenic sepsis as a priority, and also of their discharge.
- Management options include dose delay or reduction, further adjuvants (such as GCSF or antibiotics) or switching systemic treatments.
- In severe cases, particularly in palliative patients with few options, no further systemic treatment may be instigated. Ideally this should be discussed between the primary treating team and the patient after the acute episode.

References

Carmona-Bayonas A, Gómez J, González-Billalabeitia E, Canteras M, Navarrete A, Gonzálvez ML, Vicente V, *et al*. Prognostic evaluation of febrile neutropenia in apparently stable adult cancer patients. *British Journal of Cancer*. 2011. 105(5): 612–17.

Klastersky J, Paesmans M, Rubenstein EB, Boyer M, Elting L, Feld R, *et al*. The Multinational Association for Supportive Care in Cancer risk index: a multinational scoring system for identifying low-risk febrile neutropenic cancer patients. *Journal of Clinical Oncology*. 2000. 18(16): 3038–51.

National Institute for Health and Care Excellence. *Neutropenic Sepsis* (CG151). National Institute for Health and Care Excellence: London. 2012.

Hypercalcaemia

The normal range of total calcium is usually 2.12–2.65 mmol/L. Hypercalcaemia is defined as the elevation of serum calcium, after correction for albumin. The grading of hypercalcaemia is shown in Table 2.7.

Table 2.7 CTCAE (V4.03) grading of hypercalcaemia.

Grade	Criteria
1	Corrected serum calcium of > ULN – 11.5 mg/dL; > ULN – 2.9 mmol/L; ionised calcium > ULN – 1.5 mmol/L.
2	Corrected serum calcium of > 11.5–12.5 mg/dL; > 2.9–3.1 mmol/L; ionised calcium > 1.5–1.6 mmol/L; symptomatic.
3	Corrected serum calcium of > 12.5–13.5 mg/dL; > 3.1–3.4 mmol/L; ionised calcium > 1.6–1.8 mmol/L; hospitalisation indicated.
4	Corrected serum calcium of > 13.5 mg/dL; > 3.4 mmol/L; ionised calcium > 1.8 mmol/L; life-threatening consequence.
5	Death.

From the website of the National Cancer Institute (http://www.cancer.gov).

Symptoms/signs

- Hypercalcaemia may be asymptomatic or may be associated with symptoms, depending on the level of calcium and the rate of change in the calcium concentration.
- The symptoms of hypercalcaemia do not correlate well with the level of calcium found on biochemistry.
- The most common symptoms are malaise and fatigue. Other symptoms include nausea, vomiting, polydipsia, polyuria and constipation. Hyporeflexia and weight loss can also occur.
- Increasingly high calcium levels are associated with renal failure, confusion, seizures, coma and death.
- Early detection can be difficult due to the constellation of symptoms and conditions in patients with metastatic disease. However, the early detection and treatment of hypercalcaemia can lead to significant improvements in the patient's quality of life.

Causes

- The rate of hypercalcaemia in adult cancer patients can be as high as 20%. It is most common in patients with multiple myeloma, lung or breast cancer.
- Normal calcium homeostasis is controlled by parathyroid hormone (PTH), calcitriol and normal functioning kidneys. Cancer-associated hypercalcaemia has two possible mechanisms:
  - The most common is the direct osteolytic activity of a primary or secondary cancer in the bones, increasing bone resorption.
  - The excretion of parathyroid-like hormone from cancer cells, increasing bone resorption and leading to a rise in calcium levels. In this humoral mechanism, the calcium level can rise independently of the presence of any bone metastases.
- The majority of cases are therefore caused by bone metastases, but a dual mechanism may account for 11% of cancer-associated cases.
- Consider non-cancer related causes (e.g. hyperparathyroidism), especially in patients in complete remission.

Management
General management
Most patients with hypercalcaemia will be treated as below, allowing good resolution of symptoms and improvements in their quality of life. However, some patients with incurable and untreatable disease (e.g. where no further lines of treatment are appropriate) may opt not to treat their hypercalcaemia. This decision should be taken by a senior colleague at an early point, when the patient's consciousness and reasoning are not compromised by their symptoms.

Intravenous fluids
- Initial treatment is IV fluid replenishment as the osmotic effect seen with hypercalcaemia leads to hypovolaemia.
- Up to 3–4 litres of fluid (usually 0.9% sodium chloride) may be needed within the first 24 hours.
- Diuretics are solely used for the management of fluid overload from treatment and not to increase urine output or to force a diuresis.
- Correct hypokalaemia and hypomagnesaemia.

Bisphosphonates
- Bisphosphonates may be used after initial IV hydration has been completed.
- Bisphosphonate choice may be influenced by the primary cancer, severity of symptoms and local provision. Zoledronic acid is a more potent agent and ibandronic acid is available orally, which is more tolerable to patients in the long term.
- The dose and rate of bisphosphonate infusion may need to be reduced in patients with renal impairment.
- Common choices are:
  - Pamidronate: the dose and rate is dependent on the serum calcium concentration, for example:
    - Calcium 3.0–3.4 mmol/l: 30 mg IV in 250 ml of 0.9% normal saline over two hours
    - Calcium 3.41–4.0 mmol/l: 60 mg IV in 500 ml of 0.9% normal saline over four hours
    - Calcium >4.0 mmol/l: 90 mg IV in 500 ml of 0.9% normal saline over six hours
  - Zoledronic acid: 4 mg in 100 ml of 0.9% sodium chloride over 15 minutes
  - Ibandronate
- Side effects include: malaise, flu-like symptoms, anaemia, headache and osteonecrosis of the jaw.
- Plasma calcium levels start to fall after 48 hours and continue to fall for the next six days.
- Hypercalcaemia that is unresponsive to bisphosphonates is a poor prognostic sign and should be discussed with a senior.

Other treatments
- Glucocorticoids – only useful in hypercalcaemia due to particular types of lymphomas and granulomatous disease. May provide very short-term control in those who are symptomatic.
- Renal dialysis – only used in patients with severe hypercalcaemia who are fit enough for dialysis.
- Calcitonin – may be tried if bisphosphonates are ineffective, but reductions in calcium levels are likely to be small and transient. The usual dose is 100 units SC or IM every 6–8 hours, titrated according to response (maximum 400 units every 6–8 hours).
- A clinical trial is currently assessing the efficacy of denosumab for bisphosphonate-resistant hypercalcaemia.

Systemic anti-cancer treatment
- Chemotherapy or hormone therapy may be used to control the cancer and thus reduce osteolytic activity. This would usually occur after rehydration and the use of a bisphosphonate as appropriate.
- The continuing use of bisphosphonates has been shown to reduce further hypercalcaemia or skeletal-related events in some cancers, and may therefore be used alongside chemotherapy.

Contributory factors and comorbidities
Further factors that may affect hypercalcaemia include:
- Calcium resorption from the bone increases with increasing immobility.
- Dehydration may reduce the kidneys' ability to excrete calcium. This will be exacerbated by anorexia, nausea, vomiting and diarrhoea.
- Some hormonal therapies are known to increase calcium levels (such as anti-oestrogens and androgen therapies).
- Thiazide diuretics increase kidney calcium resorption and may exacerbate or precipitate hypercalcaemia.

References

Macmillan: Zolendronic acid. 2013. Available from: http://www.macmillan.org.uk/Cancer information/Cancertreatment/Treatmenttypes/Supportivetherapies/Bisphosphonates/Zoledronicacid.aspx (accessed 1 January 2014).

Soyfoo MS, Brenner K, Paesmans M, Body JJ. Non-Malignant causes of hypercalcaemia in cancer patients: a frequent and neglected occurrence. *Support Care Cancer*. 2013. 21(5): 1415–9.

Stewart AF. Hypercalcemia associated with cancer. *New England Journal of Medicine*. 2005. 352(4): 373–9.

Woodward EJ, Coleman RE. Prevention and treatment of bone metastases. *Current Pharmaceutical Design*. 2010. 16(27): 2998–3006.

Non-neutropenic sepsis

Definitions
- *Sepsis*: microbial invasion of a normally sterile environment. If this leads to hypoperfusion or dysfunction of at least one organ then this is termed *severe sepsis*.
- *Septic shock* is where severe sepsis is combined with hypotension or the requirement for vasopressors despite adequate fluid resuscitation.

The CTCAE grading system has specific grades for each site of infection. A general overview is provided in Table 2.8.

Presentation and management
Assessment
- Assess risk factors for sepsis: for example central venous access devices, comorbidities such as COPD and diabetes.
- The initial assessment for any patient currently/recently receiving active treatment should be as that for neutropenic sepsis. If the patient is subsequently found not to be neutropenic, and not in danger of shortly becoming neutropenic, then they should be treated as per any other medical patient with an infection.
- If a patient is receiving treatment that does not cause neutropenia then they may be assessed as any other patient, but be mindful of the possible impact of the cancer, or its treatment, on the presentation and natural history of any infection.

Diagnosis
- Presentation is highly variable dependent on a multitude of factors, including comorbidities and the infective organism. The diagnosis of sepsis can be complex, but the international Surviving Sepsis Campaign aims to standardise this and is summarised in Table 2.9.

Table 2.8 General overview of CTCAE (V4.03) grading of infection.

Grade	Criteria
1	—
2	Requires local or oral intervention (e.g. anti-fungals or antibiotics).
3	Requires intravenous intervention (e.g. anti-fungals or antibiotics), radiological or operative intervention.
4	Life-threatening consequences.
5	Death.

From the website of the National Cancer Institute (http://www.cancer.gov).

Table 2.9 Diagnostic criteria for sepsis.

Documented or suspected infection and some of the following:	
General variables	Fever (> 38.3°C) or hypothermia (< 36°C). Tachycardia (> 90 beats/minute). Tachypnoea. Altered mental status. Significantly positive fluid balance (> 20 ml/kg over 24 hours). Hyperglycaemia (> 7.7mmol/L) in absence of diabetes.
Inflammatory variables	White cell count: > 12×10⁹/L or < 4×10⁹/L. Raised CRP. Raised plasma procalcitonin.
Haemodynamic variables	Arterial hypotension (< 90 mm/Hg).
Organ dysfunction variables	Arterial hypoxaemia. Acute oliguria (urine output < 0.5/kg/hr for at least 2 hours) despite adequate hydration. Creatinine increase/acute kidney injury. Deranged coagulation (INR > 1.5). Ileus (absent bowel sounds). Thrombocytopenia (platelet count < 100×10⁹/L). Raised bilirubin (> 70 µmol/L).
Tissue perfusion variables	Hyperlactataemia (> 4 mmol/L). Decreased capillary refill or mottling.

Adapted from Dellinger RP, *et al. Critical Care Medicine.* 2013. 41: 580–637. Reproduced with permission of Lippincott Williams and Wilkins.

- Appropriate and timely diagnosis is dependent upon the initial suspicion of infection. Sites to consider include:
  - Head and neck – including meninges, sinuses, orbits, oral and ear cavities
  - GI tract – from the mouth to the rectum
  - Respiratory system
  - Genito-urinary system
  - Central nervous system
  - Skin
  - Indwelling devices:
    - Vascular access sites
    - Stents – including ureteric, colonic and biliary
    - Catheters
  - Site of cancer – consider fistulae, collections and abscesses
  - Has the patient had prior surgical intervention?

Investigations
- Investigations should be targeted at confirming the diagnosis of sepsis and at identifying the source of infection.

- Blood cultures should be taken (both peripherally and from any central lines *in situ*) before administration of antibiotics.
- Radiological investigations should target the most likely site of infection.

Treatment
- Early antibiotics are associated with increased survival; the aim should be to provide antibiotics within an hour. These should be based empirically on the most likely source of infection in accordance with local antibiotic policy.
- Involve intensive care teams or outreach early if appropriate. If unsure, discuss this immediately with a senior colleague.
- It is important to determine if the episode of sepsis is going to impact on planned or ongoing treatment. This should be discussed with the treating team during admission so a plan is in place prior to discharge.

Other relevant sections of this book
Chapter 2 section on neutropenic sepsis

References

Dellinger RP, Levy MM, Rhodes A, Annane D, Gerlach H, Opal S, *et al*. Surviving Sepsis Campaign: International guidelines for management of severe sepsis and septic shock: 2012. *Critical Care Medicine*. 2013. 41(2): 580–637.

Lever A, Mackenzie I. Sepsis: definition, epidemiology, and diagnosis. *British Medical Journal*. 2007. 335(7625): 879–883.

Raised intracranial pressure and seizures

Raised intracranial pressure (ICP)
Raised ICP may arise as a result of the cancer itself or from treatment complications. Clinical difficulties occur when the cerebrospinal fluid flow is interrupted, usually at the third or fourth ventricle level. This may lead to compression of the brainstem or cerebellum and can lead to coning.

Causes
- *Primary:*
  - Brain tumour – primary or metastases
  - Leukaemia
  - Intracranial haemorrhage – note that intracranial metastases may bleed, particularly in malignant melanoma or RCC
  - Hydrocephalus
  - Ischaemic stroke
  - Idiopathic or benign intracranial hypertension
  - Venous sinus thrombus
  - Intracranial infection

- *Secondary:*
  - Cerebral oedema – post-operative, post-radiotherapy or as a result of rapid changes in biochemistry
  - Hypertension or hypotension
  - Airway blockage
  - Prolonged seizure
  - Shunt blockage
  - Drugs – including chemotherapy (see below)

Symptoms and signs

Raised ICP has a range of symptoms, which can change depending on the level and rate of change in pressure.

Classical symptoms include:
- Headache – such as a morning headache or a headache exacerbated with a change in posture or with coughing
- Vomiting
- Change in vision
- Change in personality or mood (most usually noticed by relatives)
- Fluctuating level of consciousness
- Ataxia or motor disturbance
- Abnormal pupils
- Seizures

Severely raised ICP is associated with:
- Cushing's response (bradycardia and hypertension) – this is a pre-terminal event.
- Papilloedema with any degree of decrease in consciousness level – this constitutes a true oncological emergency.
- Sunsetting – eyes deviated medially and inferiorly – critically raised intracranial pressure.

Management

- Definitive management will depend on the aetiology. It is important to assess any risk factors (e.g. known intracranial metastases or ongoing cranial irradiation).
- Assess airway, breathing, circulation and GCS.
- Tilt patient to 20–30 degree angle.
- Check bloods, including FBC, clotting, U&E and blood sugars.
- Consider mannitol (0.5–1.0 g/kg) – maximal effect within 20 to 60 minutes. Used in moderate to severe cases.
- Consider dexamethasone 8 mg BD or 4 mg QDS to reduce vasogenic oedema. The effects typically start within hours (maximal effect within days). Useful in malignancy related raised ICP, but can result in deterioration in raised ICP secondary to trauma.
- Consider surgical decompression for masses leading to raised ICP – dependent on surgical suitability (e.g. performance status and comorbidities) and overall prognosis from the patient's underlying malignancy.

- If febrile:
  - Antibiotics, antifungals, antivirals – often empirical at time of assessment.
  - Antipyretics – paracetamol in preference to NSAIDs, especially if intracranial haemorrhage is a possibility.
- CT head – should be undertaken urgently when the patient has been stabilised.
- Further management may include radiotherapy (including gamma-knife or stereotactic radiotherapy), surgery, systemic therapy or best supportive care.

Seizures

Seizures occur in around 13% of people with cancer, although this significantly changes depending on whether the patient is an adult or child, and the type of cancer being treated.

Mass-associated seizures

- The most common malignant cause of seizure is a primary brain tumour, followed by metastases.
- In metastases, the most common primary cancer is lung cancer (both NSCLC and SCLC), followed by breast, skin and colon cancers.
- The metastasis is most commonly parenchymal but can be leptomeningeal.
- Alternate causes include brain abscesses, granulomatous and demyelinating diseases.

Drug-induced seizures

- Rare, mainly seen in phase I and II trials or as part of myeloablative treatments.
- Associated with high doses of chemotherapy and/or renal or hepatic dysfunction.
- Drugs include:
  - Cisplatin – rare, occurs 5–15 days after infusion. May be associated with reversible posterior leucoencephalopathy syndrome. Often associated with electrolyte disturbance, particularly magnesium deficiency.
  - Busulphan – readily crosses the blood–brain barrier and associated with seizures in some susceptible individuals.
  - Chlorambucil – seizures associated with overdosing of the drug.
  - 5-FU – very rare, possible associated with dihydropyrimidine dehydrogenase deficiency.
  - Interferon-α – seizures occur in 1–4% people. Associated with disrupted blood–brain barrier and vasogenic brain oedema leading to a lower seizure threshold.
  - Others – many other anti-cancer drugs have case reports linked to seizures. Other commonly used drugs in cancer patients include octreotide and ondansetron.

Seizures due to metabolic disturbance

- Metabolic disturbances are an important cause of seizures as the treatment is aimed at correcting the metabolic disturbance rather than commencing anti-epileptic medication. However, it can be difficult to determine the exact cause in the acute episode.

- The metabolic cause may be drug-induced, for example bisphosphonate use leading to a hypocalcaemic seizure.
- Very rarely, seizure may be the presentation of an insulinoma or phaeochromocytoma.

Neurological paraneoplastic syndromes
- Rare, non-metastatic complication of cancer.
- Limbic encephalitis – involves complex partial seizures or status epilepticus associated with prominent memory and behavioural disorders. Seizures may be refractory to medical treatment. Associated with small cell lung cancer and testicular cancer.

Cerebrovascular events
- Stroke is the second most common brain disorder identified on autopsy of patients with cancer. One series demonstrated 8% of cancer patients with a stroke had a seizure.
- Brain haemorrhage may cause seizures – these can be associated with metastatic melanoma, renal cancer and choriocarcinoma, which are at risk of haemorrhagic metastases.
- Venous sinus thrombosis may present with a seizure and can be associated with direct invasion of the venous sinuses.

Cranial irradiation
- Seizures are associated with both acute radiation encephalopathy and delayed radiation necrosis.
- Often refractory to medical treatment.

Investigation and treatment of seizures in cancer patients
Investigations
- History and temporal relationship between seizure and diagnosis or treatment are important, but may not give an absolute diagnosis.
- Useful investigations include:
  - U&Es.
  - MRI head with contrast is the gold standard imaging technique.
  - Consider a lumbar puncture, if there are no contraindications and on discussion with senior physician.

Acute treatment of a seizure
- Check airway, breathing and circulation.
- Ensure supply of oxygen and IV access.
- If seizure occurs during chemotherapy infusion – stop infusion.
- Time seizure and ensure the patient cannot harm themselves on surrounding objects.

- NICE guidelines recommend ONE of:
  - Diazepam 10–20 mg rectally, repeated after 15 minutes if necessary.
  - Midazolam 10 mg buccally.
  - Lorazepam 0.1 mg/kg (usually a bolus of 4 mg IV), repeated after 10–20 minutes.
- Continue to monitor in lateral position (recovery position).
- Regular anti-epileptics should be given if these are already in use by the patient. Emergency use of anti-epileptics for sustained control or for status epilepticus are as follows: phenytoin infusion at a dose of 15–18 mg/kg at a rate of 50 mg/minute and/or phenobarbitone bolus of 10–15 mg/kg at a rate of 100 mg/minute.
- Seek senior support – further investigation can be complex and neurologist support regarding long-term management is important. Note, some anti-epileptics will affect the metabolism of chemotherapy and this should be considered with the primary treating team and the neurologist.
- Note: in those with a space occupying lesion, long-term anti-epileptic therapy is recommended after the *first* seizure.

Cautions
- Phenytoin used together with cranial irradiation can lead to phenytoin hypersensitivity reactions such as rash leading to erythema multiforme. Abates on discontinuation of anti-epileptic.
- Valproate and certain chemotherapies (e.g. cisplatin) – can lead to enhanced myelosuppression.

Long-term anti-epilepsy treatment
- Only indicated for patients with a structural parenchymal lesion.
- May only need prophylaxis if seizures are related to the treatment.
- Radiotherapy, surgery or steroids may help with the management of seizures due to brain metastases.
- There is no benefit to using prophylactic anti-epileptics in those with brain metastases.

References

National Institute for Health and Care Excellence. *The Epilepsies: the Diagnosis and Management of the Epilepsies in Adults and Children in Primary and Secondary Care* (CG137). NICE: London. January 2012.

Rangel-Catillo L, Gopinath S, Robertson CS. Management of intracranial hypertension. *Neurological Clinics*. 2008. 26(2): 521–41.

Singh G, Rees JH, Sander JW. Seizures and epilepsy in oncological practice: causes, course, mechanisms and treatment. *Journal of Neurology, Neurosurgery & Psychiatry*. 2007. 78(4): 342–349.

Yeomanson D, Phillips R. Guidelines for the management of raised intracranial pressure in children and young people with malignancy. Yorkshire and Humber Children's and Young People's Cancer Network. May 2009. Available from: http://www.yorkshire-cancer-net.org.uk/html/publications/guidelines_cyp_clinical.php (accessed 1 January 2014).

Spinal cord compression

Definition

Vertebral collapse or instability due to metastatic disease or direct extension of the tumour leading to pressure on the spinal cord or cauda equina. This can either lead to neurological deficit, or may threaten to cause this in the near future.

Metastatic spinal cord compression (MSCC) is an acute oncological emergency, where early intervention can help preserve and maintain neurological function and thus enable greater patient independence.

Presentation

Evidence suggests that there are often significant delays in the diagnosis of MSCC, with almost half of patients unable to walk by the time of diagnosis. A prospective observational study of three Scottish cancer centres found a median delay of two months from a patient presenting to a health professional with a relevant symptom to development of a compression syndrome.

Common symptoms at presentation are summarised in Table 2.10. Careful history taking and examination is required, including examination for a sensory level (see Figure 2.1).

- Back pain is the most prevalent symptom and may precede other symptoms by up to two months.
- A small proportion of MSCC present without back pain. Suggestive neurological deficits in a patient with known bone metastases should lead to suspicion of MSCC.
- The cauda equina lies below the spinal cord and contains the lumbar and sacral nerve roots. Compression here can lead to cauda equina syndrome. This may be associated with back pain, urinary incontinence/retention, loss of anal tone and faecal incontinence, sexual disturbance, saddle anaesthesia and sciatic nerve root pain.

Table 2.10 Clinical features at presentation.

Symptom	Proportion of patients affected at diagnosis
Back pain	95%
Limb weakness	85%
Sensory deficit	40–90%
Dermatomal level	50%
Bladder or bowel dysfunction	40–50%

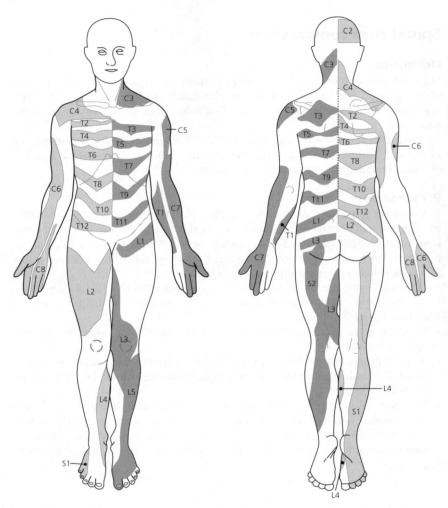

Figure 2.1 Dermatomal distributions. There is individual variation in the distribution of dermatomes. This figure illustrates the likely distribution of dermatomes, but there is overlap between dermatomes areas of increased individual variability. Blank areas illustrate areas of greatest variability and overlap. Source: Lee MWL. *et al Clinical Anatomy*. 2008. 21(5): 363–73. Reproduced with permission of John Wiley and Sons. To see a colour version of this figure, see Plate 2.1.

Risk factors

High risk patients include:
- Patients with a prior history of MSCC
- Patients with known bone metastases
- Patients with the following conditions:
  ◦ Castration-resistant prostate cancer

- ○ Metastatic renal cancer
- ○ Metastatic lung cancer (of any cell type)
- ○ Metastatic breast cancer
- ○ Myeloma

All patients with known risk factors should be informed about the risk of developing MSCC and provided with information about what to do should they develop any symptoms of concern.

Early detection of spinal metastases

NICE recommends contacting the MSCC coordinator (often a specialist nurse or Clinical Oncology SpR) to discuss possible spinal metastases. MRI whole spine is indicated within a week for the following symptoms:

- Pain in the thoracic or cervical spine
- Progressive lumbar spinal pain
- Severe unremitting lower spinal pain
- Spinal pain aggravated by straining (e.g. coughing or sneezing)
- Localised spinal tenderness
- Nocturnal spinal pain preventing sleep

MSCC as an oncological emergency

An urgent *MRI whole spine* (within 24 hours) is indicated if any of the following symptoms are present:

- Neurological symptoms, including radicular pain, limb weakness, difficulty walking, sensory loss or bowel or bladder dysfunction.
- Neurological signs of spinal cord or cauda equina compression: such as sensory level.

MRI whole spine is required as the level of compression can be four levels below or two levels higher than the clinical deficit and up to 85% of cases have multi-level compression. If MRI is contraindicated, then CT myelogram should be discussed with the MSCC co-ordinator and the radiology department.

If MSCC is suspected then each of the following steps should be carried out:

- Analgesia:
  - ○ As per the WHO analgesia ladder. Care should be taken to ensure the patient has access to services to adjust doses as needed, for example with a flare of pain secondary to radiotherapy or after surgery.
  - ○ Consider referral to the palliative care team/pain team if pain is unresponsive to basic analgesia.
- Corticosteroids:
  - ○ 16 mg dexamethasone (orally or IV) should be given on first suspicion of MSCC and before any further investigations, unless contraindicated (e.g. significant suspicion of lymphoma in cases where MSCC is the primary presentation).
  - ○ Continue with 16 mg dexamethasone daily until definitive treatment is undertaken (or decision not to offer definitive treatment) and then reduce the dose gradually over 5–7 days.

- PPI cover should be used to reduce the occurrence of gastritis and upper GI bleed whilst on high dose steroids.
- The dose may have to be re-escalated if neurological deficit reappears. This should be to the last dose where symptoms were controlled.
- Spinal stability – if patients have severe mechanical pain suggestive of spinal instability or evidence of spinal instability on imaging, neutral spine alignment (which entails bed rest and manoeuvres such as 'logrolling') is recommended until definitive treatment has been undertaken. Cautious remobilisation can then start after treatment.
- Additional treatments – in patients who are likely to experience a period of reduced mobility consider prophylactic treatment with LMWH or compression stockings.

Treatment
Once MSCC has been confirmed, definitive treatment should begin with 24 hours and should be available seven days of the week. This requires discussion with the MSCC co-ordinator who should discuss the following definitive treatment options. Definitive treatments include:

- *Radiotherapy* – the mainstay of treatment for the majority of patients. Radiotherapy should commence within 24 hours of diagnosis.
  - Indications: multiple sites of spinal metastases or levels of compression, radio-sensitive tumours, poor performance status or prognosis.
  - Radiotherapy dosing is variable between networks and trusts and may involve 8 Gy in a single fraction or 20 Gy in 5 fractions; the SCORAD trial is currently investigating the optimum dosing schedule. Patients with a good prognosis and no prior radiotherapy to that site may have doses ranging from 20 Gy in 5 fractions to 30 Gy in 10 fractions.
  - Retreatment with radiotherapy is considered if the last treatment was over three months previously and the maximum tolerated dose has not been reached.
- *Spinal surgery* – consider in patients with spinal instability, radioresistant tumours or in those who have reached the maximum dose of radiotherapy.
  - Surgical decompression is not appropriate in many patients, often due to multiple levels of cord compression, poor performance status or poor overall prognosis. The Tokuhashi scoring system is a prognostic tool, which helps to determine those who are fit enough for surgery and with an expected prognosis of at least three months.
  - Surgery may determine the histology in new presentations of cancer.
  - If the patient is para- or tetraplegic then surgery should only be offered for mechanical pain which is not responding to analgesia.
  - If the spine is unstable but the patient is unsuitable for surgery, consider external spinal support (such as a halo vest).
  - Post-operative radiotherapy will be offered to all patients routinely once the wound has healed if they have a satisfactory response to surgery.
- *Vertebroplasty or kyphoplasty* – should be considered in those with vertebral body collapse or mechanical pain resistant to conventional analgesia and no neurological compromise. This requires careful discussion with the patient and the treating oncologist.

- No definitive treatment may be considered in those with a very poor prognosis, or who have complete tetra- or paraplegia and good pain control.

Important treatments alongside the above definitive treatments include:

- Bisphosphonates – should be offered to all MSCC patients with a breast cancer or myeloma diagnosis, and to prostate cancer patients who have not responded to conventional analgesia. Not routinely used in patients with alternate cancer diagnoses as prophylaxis, but may be used for bone pain.
- Bowel and bladder dysfunction – urinary catheterisation should be considered in those with urinary incontinence. Bowel management includes diet change, stool softeners and laxatives or constipating agents as required.

Management after definitive treatment

Strong multidisciplinary input is often necessary after treatment for MSCC. Issues to be considered include:

- Discharge plans should start early and enable the patient to return home if possible; this may require intensive occupational therapy and physiotherapy input.
- Future treatment – discussions should be undertaken with the primary treating team about the possibility of any other or systemic treatment that may be deemed appropriate.
- Palliative care input for those with complex symptoms either directly from their MSCC or their overall cancer burden.

References

Lee MWL, McPhee RW, Stringer MD. An evidence-based approach to human dermatomes. *Clinical Anatomy*. 2008. 21(5): 363–73.

McCurdy MT, Shanholtz CB. Oncologic emergencies. *Critical Care Medicine*. 2012. 40(7): 2212–22.

National Institute for Health and Care Excellence. *Metastatic Spinal Cord Compression* (CG75). National Institute for Health and Care Excellence: London. 2008.

Turner R. Clinical Guidelines: Metastatic Spinal Cord Compression. Yorkshire Cancer Network. September 2012. Available from: http://www.yorkshire-cancer-net.org.uk/html/publications/guidelines_mscc.php (accessed 1 January 2014).

Superior vena cava obstruction

Superior vena cava obstruction (SVCO) is a clinical syndrome which results from the obstruction of the superior vena cava. This is most usually a result of external compression (> 80% cases), direct invasion of the SVC or by thrombus within the SVC.

Causes

- A malignant cause is the most common aetiology; most of these are secondary to lung cancer (squamous cell and small cell), accounting for up to 80% of malignancy-associated cases. SCLC is more common than NSCLC in causing SVCO.
- The remaining malignancy-associated diagnoses include lymphoma, metastatic breast cancer, germ-cell tumours, thymoma and mesothelioma.

Presentation

- SVCO usually develops insidiously. Symptoms are varied and depend on the development of collateral veins and the rate of compression of the SVC.
- *Symptoms*:
  - Dyspnoea (the most common symptom).
  - Swelling of the head, neck and arms.
  - Hoarseness and/or cough.
  - Headache and particularly facial oedema can be signs of raised ICP; this can lead to syncope, confusion and coma.
  - Symptoms may be exacerbated by lying flat or stooping forwards.
- *Signs include*:
  - Venous distension in the neck and chest wall.
  - Facial oedema.
  - Plethoric facies.
  - Cyanosis.

Investigations

SVCO is the first presentation of cancer in up to 60% of all cases of SVCO. Unless there are life-threatening complications, these new presentations should be investigated for the type and extent of cancer before definitive treatment is started for the SVCO itself.

Radiological investigations can help determine the extent and site of SVCO, help identify the primary cancer and the extent of disease as well as identify a possible suitable site for a biopsy.

- CXR: the most readily accessible imaging and will often identify a lung cancer source.
- CT thorax (with or without neck): most readily identifies the site of obstruction and helps stage the cancer.
- Venogram: if CT is unable to identify a point of external compression. It may also be used as part of any stent assessment.

Particular investigations may be considered in new cancer diagnoses; this is most usually after radiological determination of the likely primary and extent of disease and is best managed with a multidisciplinary team approach:

- Cytology: may be available from pleural fluid or fine-needle aspiration of a lymph node.
- CT biopsy: this may be necessary to safely confirm the diagnosis, for example for peripheral lung lesions.
- Bronchoscopy: this may provide histological/cytological information.
- Mediastinoscopy: this may yield results if no other disease is more easily or safely accessible.

Treatment

If a patient is acutely symptomatic then urgent treatment is indicated. Particularly concerning symptoms include stridor (especially if there is concomitant central airways obstruction), confusion or reduced GCS.

For urgent cases:
- Sitting the patient upright helps reduce the intracranial pressure.
- Oxygen therapy as appropriate.
- Dexamethasone with appropriate PPI-cover: usual doses are dexamethasone 16 mg OD or 8 mg BD with lansoprazole 30 mg OD.
- CXR and CT thorax should be undertaken urgently.
- Urgent stent insertion – this provides the most rapid relief of symptoms (see below).
- Thrombolysis – treatment of choice with or without stenting if thrombus is the cause of the SVCO.
- Radiotherapy – used less commonly in the acute situation, but can be appropriate if prognosis and performance status allow. Particularly useful in recurrent SVCO due to SCLC relapse.

The definitive treatment for most patients is taken depending on the extent and type of their malignancy. Options include:
- Endovascular stenting – this is most commonly a percutaneous procedure undertaken by interventional radiology. It can provide symptom relief within 48–76 hours. Stenting is the most commonly used intervention in acutely symptomatic patients.
  - It is especially useful if the patient has respiratory distress or signs of severe raised intracranial hypertension such as reduced GCS or coma.
  - It may be used alongside or in place of systemic thrombolysis in thrombus obstruction.
  - It may be the mainstay of treatment in chemo- or radio-insensitive disease.
  - There is a relatively low rate of re-obstruction after stent placement at around 10%. Re-obstruction is usually secondary to tumour overgrowth or thrombus. In these cases thrombolysis or a further stent may be used.
- Chemotherapy – in relatively asymptomatic patients who have a chemo-sensitive cancer, this may be the first treatment choice. If the patient has a reasonable performance status it can be the mainstay of treatment for many SCLC and lymphoma patients.
- Radiotherapy – considered in patients who are not experiencing severe symptoms as the time lag until treatment effect may be a number of weeks. Particularly useful as an adjunct to other therapies in lung cancer or used on relapse of SVCO due to cancer.
- Combination of the above options, tailored to the patient and their cancer.
- Surgery – rarely appropriate due to the extent and location of disease.

References

Gompelmann D, Eberhardt R, Herth FJF. Advanced malignant lung disease: what the specialist can offer. *Respiration: Thematic Review Series*. 2011. 82(2): 111–23.

Hague J, Tippett R. Endovascular techniques in palliative care. *Clinical Oncology*. 2010. 22(9): 771–80.

Samphao S, Eremin JM, Eremin O. Oncological emergencies: clinical importance and principles of management. *European Journal of Cancer Care*. 2010. 19(6): 707–13.

Wilson LD, Detterbeck FC, Yahalom J. Clinical practice. Superior vena cava syndrome with malignant causes. *New England Journal of Medicine*. 2007. 356(18): 1862–9.

Transfusion reactions

Acute transfusion reactions are rare but potentially life threatening. It is important to recognise the symptoms and signs that might signify a transfusion reaction promptly and manage this appropriately.

Symptoms/signs include:
- Fever, chills or rigors
- Tachycardia, hyper- or hypotension
- Collapse
- Flushing or urticaria
- Bone, muscle, chest and/or abdominal pain
- SOB or respiratory distress
- Nausea or feeling generally unwell

If any of these symptoms occur:
- STOP the infusion.
- Take observations: temperature, pulse, BP, respiratory rate, oxygen saturation.
- Check the patient's details against the compatibility tag or label.

Mild fever only
- Temperature rise of up to 1.5°C from baseline.
- Patient otherwise well.
- Administer 500 mg–1 g of paracetamol.
- Restart infusion at slower rate with frequent observations.

Urticaria/mild allergic reaction only
- Administer chlorpheniramine 10 mg, slowly IV.
- Restart infusion at slower rate with frequent observations.

ABO incompatibility
- STOP transfusion altogether.
- Remove unit being transfused and giving set and return these to Blood Bank.
- Start IV saline infusion.
- Monitor urine output and maintain above 100 ml/hour – with furosemide support if necessary.
- Treat DIC as needed.
- Inform transfusion department/on-call haematologist.

Severe allergic reaction
- *Symptoms/signs*: bronchospasm, angioedema, abdominal pain and/or hypotension.
- STOP transfusion.

- Remove unit being transfused and giving set and return to Blood Bank with any unused units.
- Administer chlorpheniramine 10 mg IV, slowly.
- Administer oxygen and salbutamol nebuliser.
- If severe hypotension: adrenaline 0.5 mg IM (0.5 ml of 1 in 1000 dilution).
- Send clotted sample to transfusion laboratory.
- Saline infusion.

Haemolytic reaction or bacterial infection of unit of transfusion

- Consider if: temperature >39°C or rise >2°C and/or systemically unwell.
- STOP transfusion.
- Remove unit being transfused and giving set and return to Blood Bank with any unused units.
- Take blood cultures, repeat blood group/cross-match/FBC, coagulation screen, biochemistry and urinalysis.
- Monitor urine output.
- Start broad spectrum antibiotic if bacterial infection suspected.
- Commence oxygen and fluid support.
- Seek haematological and ITU support/advice.

Acute dyspnoea/hypotension

- Check blood gas, CXR and assess CVP.
- Raised CVP – possible transfusion-associated circulatory overload (TACO):
  - Clinical features: Acute LVF: tachycardia, hypotension, raised JVP
  - Management:
    - Stop transfusion
    - Give oxygen and furosemide 40–80 mg IV
    - Future transfusion: slow with furosemide cover (20–40 mg IV)
- Normal CVP – possible transfusion related acute-lung injury (TRALI):
  - Clinical features:
    - Acute LVF with/without fever and chills
    - Typically within six hours of transfusion
    - CXR: bilateral nodular infiltrates
  - Management:
    - Discontinue transfusion
    - 100% oxygen administration
    - Treat as ARDS – discuss with ITU and consider ventilation if hypoxia sustained
    - Avoid diuretics
    - Inform transfusion unit – donor may need to be contacted and taken off register

Other relevant sections of this book

Chapter 2 section on anaphylaxis and hypersensitivity reactions

References

McClelland BDL. *Handbook of Transfusion Medicine*. The Stationery Office: London. 2007.

Tinegate H, Birchall J, Gray A, Haggas R, Massey E, Norfolk D, *et al*. Guideline on the investigation and management of acute transfusion reactions. BCSH Blood Transfusion Task Force. *British Journal of Haematology*. 2012. 159(2): 143–153.

Tumour lysis syndrome

Definition

Tumour lysis syndrome (TLS) is a constellation of hyperuricaemia, hyperkalaemia, hyperphosphataemia and hypocalcaemia in response to tumour cells releasing their contents into the bloodstream. This can occur spontaneously or in response to treatment. The grading of TLS is shown in Table 2.11.

TLS can lead to AKI as the result of two processes:

- Nucleic acids are metabolised into hypoxanthine, xanthine and then uric acid. These products can precipitate anywhere in the kidney.
- Crystal-induced tissue damage occurs due to precipitation of calcium phosphate, uric acid and xanthine in the renal tubule.

Classification

TLS is currently classified using the Cairo and Bishop system; this separates cases into laboratory and clinical classifications.

1 Laboratory TLS – metabolic changes within three days before or seven days after initiation of therapy. Requires *two or more* of:
   (a) Hyperuricaemia (uric acid >8 mg/dl or 475 μmol/L).
   (b) Hyperphosphataemia (phosphate >4.5 mg/dl or 1.5 mmol/L).
   (c) Hyperkalaemia (potassium >6.0 mmol/L).
   (d) Hypocalcaemia (corrected calcium <7 mg/dL or 1.75 mmol/L; or ionised calcium <1.12).

Table 2.11 CTCAE (V4.03) grading of tumour lysis syndrome.

Grade	Criteria
1	—
2	—
3	Present.
4	Life-threatening consequences; urgent intervention indicated.
5	Death.

From the website of the National Cancer Institute (http://www.cancer.gov).

2 Clinical TLS – requires criteria for laboratory TLS to be met with the addition of one of the following:
  (a) Cardiac dysrhythmia or sudden death probably or definitely caused by hyperkalaemia.
  (b) Cardiac dysrhythmia, sudden death, seizure, neuromuscular instability (such as tetany, paraesthesias, muscle twitching, Trousseau's sign, Chvostek's sign, laryngospasm or bronchospasm), hypotension or heart failure probably or definitely due to hypocalcaemia.
  (c) Increase in serum creatinine by 0.3 mg/dl (or a single value over 1.5 times upper limit of normal range if no baseline test available); or oliguria (urine output <0.5 ml/kg/hr for six hours).

Causes
- There is great variability in the rates of TLS depending on the tumour, patient and treatment factors.
- Haematological malignancies are most commonly associated with TLS, but solid tumour cases are increasingly associated with reports of TLS secondary to more effective treatments.
- The most commonly associated malignancy associated with TLS is Burkitt's lymphoma, followed by other high-grade non-Hodgkins lymphomas, AML and ALL.

Risk assessment
- Most standard cases undergoing oncological treatment will have prophylaxis built into their treatment protocols, for most solid tumours this is dependent on adequate hydration only.
- Risk factors for TLS are listed in Table 2.12. If a patient is deemed high risk then discuss with a senior colleague:
  o High potential for cell lysis or moderate potential for cell lysis and high tumour burden – consider rasburicase.
  o Tumour burden not high/potential for cell lysis is not very high – consider allopurinol.

Table 2.12 Risk factors for developing tumour lysis syndrome.

Cancer mass	Cell lysis potential	Patient factors	Supportive care
Bulky tumour or extensive metastases	High rate of cell proliferation	Nephropathy before cancer diagnosis	Inadequate hydration
Bone marrow involvement	Cancer-cell sensitivity to treatment	Dehydration	Exogenous potassium
Renal infiltration or outflow tract obstruction	Intensity of initial anticancer treatment	Acidic urine	Exogenous phosphate
		Exposure to nephrotoxins	Delayed uric acid removal (delayed allopurinol/ rasburicase)

Management

Diagnosis requires a low clinical index of suspicion. TLS may occur prior to the commencement of treatment and thus baseline investigations are important.

Blood tests

- Moderate risk patients – daily bloods.
- High risk patients – blood tests may be needed every 8–12 hours.
- Blood tests should continue over the period of highest risk for TLS, in haematological cases this can extend to seven days. The blood tests required are:
  - Biochemistry: urea, creatinine, potassium, albumin and calcium
  - Uric acid level
  - Phosphate level

Established TLS requires early and aggressive treatment, including:

- Discussion with a senior/consultant.
- Aggressive hydration (3 litres/m² per day).
- Correction of hyperkalaemia.
- ECG monitoring.
- Rasburicase 0.2 mg/kg IV once daily (in 50 ml sodium chloride 0.9% over 30 minutes) for 3–5 days.
  - Stop allopurinol if this has been started – it will reduce the effectiveness of rasburicase.
- TLS screen (as above) six hourly.
- Do NOT correct asymptomatic hypocalcaemia in presence of hyperphosphataemia (as this will lead to increased renal calcium phosphate deposition).
- Closely monitor the patient's fluid balance and discuss the patient with the renal and intensive care teams: haemofiltration/dialysis may be indicated, especially if oliguria is unresponsive to aggressive fluid management. Indications for haemodialysis/filtration are the same as for non-TLS patients, but due to the rapid accumulation of electrolytes it may be started at an earlier point.

Other relevant sections of this book

Chapter 7 Electrolyte abnormalities

References

Howard SC, Jones DP, Pui C-H. The tumor lysis syndrome. *New England Journal of Medicine.* 2011. 364(19): 1844–54.

North East Yorkshire and Humber Clinical Alliance (Cancer). Prevention and Management of Tumour Lysis Syndrome in Haematological and some Oncology Malignancies. 2012. Available from: http://www.hyccn.nhs.uk/NetworkGuidelinesAndPublications/Chemotherapy AndPharmacy.htm (accessed 1 Janaury 2014).

CHAPTER 3

Side effects and complications of cancer and its treatment

Alexandra Pender[1], Sing Yu Moorcraft[1] and Daniel L.Y. Lee[2]

[1] *The Royal Marsden NHS Foundation Trust, UK*
[2] *St James' Institute of Oncology, UK*

CHAPTER MENU

Clinical Problems in Oncology: A Practical Guide to Management, First Edition.
Edited by Sing Yu Moorcraft, Daniel L.Y. Lee and David Cunningham.
© 2014 John Wiley & Sons, Ltd. Published 2014 by John Wiley & Sons, Ltd.

Overview of toxicity management

Oncology treatments can cause significant toxicities, which may be life-threatening, significantly impact on patients' quality of life or necessitate changes to their treatment. The severity and type of toxicity varies from patient to patient, even if they are receiving the same dose.

Most hospitals have local guidelines on the management of specific toxicities and clinical trial protocols also provide detailed guidance on toxicity management. This section of the book does NOT aim to replace these but rather to provide further advice on toxicity assessment and management.

Assessment and documentation of toxicities
- It is important to accurately assess toxicities. Patients may be reluctant to report side effects or underplay their severity because they do not want their dose to be reduced or their treatment delayed. Alternatively, other patients may overstate the severity of side effects because they may not realise the potential consequences of dose delays or dose reductions on treatment efficacy.
- Toxicities should be recorded using an internationally accepted scoring system such as the National Cancer Institute Common Terminology Criteria for Adverse Events (CTCAE), which is available from: http://www.eortc.be/services/doc/ctc/.

Advice to patients
- Most patients are advised to contact their oncology centre directly if they experience any side effects. Patients should also be advised to report any side effects to their oncology team when they are reviewed in clinic.
- Patients should be advised to bring information about their treatment (e.g. which drugs they are receiving, when the last dose was administered) if they need to be seen in an emergency setting.
- Oral chemotherapy carries the same risks as IV chemotherapy and oral targeted drugs also have significant toxicities that should not be underestimated.

Principles of toxicity management

1 Supportive care
- **(a)** Supportive care aims to minimise treatment toxicities and should always be considered as it is important to try to maintain dose intensity.
- **(b)** Supportive care may include premedication to prevent chemotherapy-induced nausea and vomiting, prophylactic GCSF to prevent profound or prolonged neutropenia or treatment directed at toxicities when they occur, for example loperamide for diarrhoea.

2 Dose reductions
- **(a)** Drugs may be given at a fixed dose or the dose may be calculated according to a patient's body surface area, weight or renal function.
- **(b)** A dose reduction may be indicated under certain circumstances, for example severe toxicity, cumulative toxicity (e.g. peripheral neuropathy secondary to oxaliplatin), repeated dose delays due to toxicity, or in accordance with haematological or biochemical parameters.
- **(c)** The amount by which a dose should be reduced is usually indicated in local guidelines/trial protocols. This is usually expressed as a percentage (e.g. a 25% dose reduction).
- **(d)** In general, dose reductions due to toxicity should not be re-escalated in subsequent cycles.

3 Dose delays
- **(a)** Doses may be delayed because a patient is too unwell for treatment at the scheduled time (e.g. due to infection). Doses may also be delayed in asymptomatic patients due to abnormal haematological or biochemical parameters (e.g. low platelet or neutrophil counts).
- **(b)** Most chemotherapy protocols require haematological values to be above specified cut-off points for chemotherapy to be administered (e.g. platelets may need to be ≥ 75 or 100 and neutrophil counts may need to be ≥ 1.0 or 1.5 depending on the chemotherapy regime). If the values are below these set parameters then treatment may need to be delayed until their counts improve (typically a delay of one week for practical purposes).
- **(c)** Some schedules involve weekly chemotherapy and therefore a dose may be completely omitted rather than delayed.

4 Discontinuation of one or more drugs
- **(a)** If toxicities cannot be managed successfully following implementation of one or more of the above strategies, then treatment may need to be discontinued.
- **(b)** Some toxicities may be so severe that re-challenging the patient with a particular drug is not appropriate.
- **(c)** If patients are receiving more than one drug then it is important to consider the most likely cause of toxicity. It may not be necessary to reduce the dose or discontinue all of the drugs in a multi-drug regime.

Effects of dose reductions and/or delays on treatment efficacy

Chemotherapy/targeted therapies

- The *dose intensity* is the amount of drug delivered per unit time ($mg/m^2/week$).
- Reduced dose intensity may lead to reduced treatment efficacy. A clear relationship between dose intensity and clinical outcomes has been demonstrated in a number of cancers.

Radiotherapy

- Radiotherapy causes tumour cell death, but the surviving cells grow more rapidly and repopulate the tumour. This repopulation becomes accelerated approximately 28 days after starting radiotherapy.
- Therefore, any delays in treatment that lengthen the overall treatment duration lead to increased tumour repopulation and can cause treatment failure. This is particularly important in certain tumour types (e.g. tumour control in patients with squamous head and neck cancers decreases by 1–2% for each day that treatment is prolonged).
- If treatment is delayed for any reason then the schedule may need to be adjusted to compensate for the missed fractions.

The balance between toxicity management and maintaining dose intensity

- Consider the aims of treatment when assessing and managing treatment-induced toxicity:
  - In patients receiving treatment with curative intent, it is particularly important to try to minimise dose delays and reductions whenever possible.
  - In patients receiving palliative treatment, quality of life is the most important consideration.
- Consider the magnitude of benefit from chemotherapy and balance this with the risks of toxicity (including cumulative toxicities, e.g. permanent peripheral neuropathy).

References

Dale RG, Hendry JH, Jones B, Robertson AG, Deehan C, Sinclair JA. Practical methods for compensating for missed treatment days in radiotherapy, with particular reference to head and neck schedules. *Clinical Oncology* (R Coll Radiol). 2002. 14(5): 382–93.

Foote M. The importance of planned dose of chemotherapy on time: do we need to change our clinical practice? *Oncologist.* 1998. 3(5): 365–8.

Kim JJ, Tannock IF. Repopulation of cancer cells during therapy: an important cause of treatment failure. *Nature Reviews Cancer.* 2005. 5(7): 516–25.

Nguyen LN, Ang KK. Radiotherapy for cancer of the head and neck: altered fractionation regimens. *Lancet Oncology.* 2002. 3(11): 693–701.

Abnormal liver function tests

Abnormal liver function
- Deranged liver function can present on blood biochemistry or clinically.
- The investigations that are most commonly used are ALT, AST, ALP, GGT and bilirubin. The grading of abnormalities in LFTs is shown in Table 3.1.
- Liver synthetic function is best assessed using PT or INR and serum albumin.
- Significantly raised ALT, AST and ALP with a normal or near normal bilirubin, is suggestive of an intrahepatic ('hepatitic') cause of liver dysfunction.
- Significantly raised ALP and bilirubin with a normal or mildly elevated AST or ALT, is suggestive of an obstruction in the biliary tree causing liver dysfunction ('obstructive' liver dysfunction).

Assessment
- History:
  - Remember to take a drug history (including herbal and over-the-counter preparations).
  - Note any recent illnesses or procedures.
- Symptoms/signs:
  - Hepatitic liver dysfunction: malaise, jaundice, icteric sclerae, and pruritus.
  - Obstructive liver dysfunction: as above, plus pale stools and dark urine.
  - Associated symptoms, for example fever.
- The Child-Pugh score and the Model for End-Stage Liver Disease (MELD) scores can be used to evaluate risk of mortality in chronic liver dysfunction. The MELD

Table 3.1 CTCAE (V4.03) grading of abnormal liver function tests.

Grade	ALT increased	ALP increased	Blood bilirubin increased	GGT increased	INR increased
1	> ULN – 3.0 x ULN	> ULN – 2.5 x ULN	> ULN – 1.5 x ULN	> ULN – 2.5 x ULN	> 1–1.5 x ULN; > 1–1.5 times above baseline if anticoagulated
2	> 3.0–5.0 x ULN	> 2.5–5.0 x ULN	> 1.5–3.0 x ULN	> 2.5–5.0 x ULN	> 1.5–2.5 x ULN; > 1.5–2.5 times above baseline if anticoagulated
3	> 5.0–20.0 x ULN	> 5.0–20.0 x ULN	> 3.0–10.0 x ULN	> 5.0–20.0 x ULN	> 2.5 x ULN; > 2.5 times above baseline if anticoagulated
4	> 20.0 x ULN	> 20.0 x ULN	> 10.0 x ULN	> 20.0 x ULN	

ULN=upper limit of normal.
From the website of the National Cancer Institute (http://www.cancer.gov).

score uses serum bilirubin, creatinine and INR. The Child-Pugh Score uses serum bilirubin, INR, albumin and the presence of ascites or hepatic encephalopathy.

Causes of hepatitic liver dysfunction
- Intrahepatic malignancy
- Anti-cancer drug toxicity
  - Tyrosine kinase inhibitors can cause severe hepatotoxicity, particularly sunitinib, pazopanib, lapatinib and regorafenib:
    - Onset of toxicity is usually within the first eight weeks of use, but can be delayed.
    - Usually reversible on withdrawal of drug.
    - Long-term complications such as cirrhosis are uncommon.
  - Abiraterone.
  - Tamoxifen.
- Other drugs
  - Corticosteroids (rare).
  - Antibiotics.
  - Herbal and dietary supplements.
  - Paracetamol.
- Biliary sepsis can cause liver dysfunction, but is more likely to cause an obstructive pattern of biochemical abnormalities.
- Severe sepsis and hepatic ischaemia.
- Portal vein thrombosis.
- Viral hepatitis:
  - Reactivation of hepatitis viruses can occur with chemotherapy regimens containing rituximab and steroids.
  - It is imperative that hepatitis serology is negative prior to commencing these treatments.
  - Reactivation of the hepatitis B virus and subsequent fulminant hepatitis has a higher mortality rate than acute hepatitis B.
- Radiofrequency ablation (RFA) of HCC or liver metastases.
- Transarterial chemo-embolisation (TACE) of HCC or liver metastases.
- SIRspheres® treatment for liver metastases.

Causes of obstructive liver dysfunction
- Extrahepatic obstruction of biliary tree:
  - Pancreatic head mass
  - Porta hepatis lymphadenopathy
  - Ampulla of Vater lesion
  - Blockage of common bile duct (CBD) stent
  - CBD stricture (benign or malignant)
  - Other biliary pathology, for example primary biliary cirrhosis, primary sclerosing cholangitis
  - Gallstones

- Intrahepatic obstruction of biliary tree:
  - Cholangiocarcinoma
  - Intra-hepatic malignant disease – primary or metastatic disease
- Steatohepatitis
- Oxaliplatin-induced sinusoidal obstruction (rare)
- Capecitabine can cause an isolated hyperbilirubinaemia
- Gilbert's syndrome

Investigations
- Suspected biliary obstruction – USS of liver and biliary tree to establish the level and cause of obstruction. If ultrasound is not helpful, consider CT or MRI.
- Suspected venous thrombosis – doppler scans of the hepatic and portal veins.
- If no clear obstructive cause is found, evaluation of conjugated and unconjugated bilirubin may determine whether there is a pre-hepatic cause of hyperbilirubinaemia.

Management
- Consider stopping hepatotoxic medication.
- Administer specific antidote if appropriate (e.g. N-acetylcysteine for paracetamol overdose).
- Abnormal clotting may need to be corrected if there is a significant risk of bleeding or a procedure is planned.
- Treat the underlying cause if possible.
- Seek hepatology advice if significant liver dysfunction or evidence of acute liver failure.
- Biliary obstruction:
  - Extrahepatic: consider ERCP and retrograde biliary stenting.
  - Intrahepatic: consider percutaneous drainage and stent insertion.
  - Patients with biliary obstruction are at risk of biliary sepsis and so there should be a low threshold for initiation of antibiotics until the obstruction is relieved.

Prescribing and liver function
- Caution should be exercised when prescribing chemotherapy for patients with intrahepatic disease and compromised liver function. Drugs may be contraindicated or require dose reductions. Advice from pharmacy may be required.
- Patients with Gilbert's syndrome or an isolated hyperbilirubinaemia require an irinotecan dose modification as this may represent a liver enzyme polymorphism that enhances irinotecan toxicity.
- Consider the risks of thrombocytopenia and bleeding if liver dysfunction is accompanied by deranged clotting.

Other relevant sections of this book
Chapter 9, sections on biliary drains and stents, chemoembolisation, radioembolisation (SIR-Spheres®), radiofrequency ablation (RFA)

References

Asrani SK, Kim WR. Model for end stage liver disease: end of the first decade. *Clinics in Liver Disease*. 2011. 15(4): 685–698.

Cholongitas E, Papetheodoridis GV, Vangeli M, Terreni N, Patch D, Burroughs AK. Systematic review: the model for end-stage liver disease – should it replace Child-Pugh's classification for assessing prognosis in cirrhosis? *Alimentary Pharmacology and Therapeutics*. 2005. 22(11–12): 1079–89.

King PD, Perry MC. Hepatotoxicity of chemotherapy. *Oncologist*. 2001. 6(2): 162–176.

Ohishi W, Chayama K. Prevention of hepatitis B virus reactivation in immunosuppressive therapy or chemotherapy. *Clinical and Experimental Nephrology*. 2011. 15(5): 634–40.

Shah RR, Morganroth J, Shah DR. Hepatotoxicity of tyrosine kinase inhibitors: clinical and regulatory perspectives. *Drug Safety*. 2013. 36(7): 491–503.

Vietor NO, George BJ. Oxaliplatin-induced hepatocellular injury and ototoxicity: a review of the literature and report of unusual side effects of a commonly used chemotherapeutic agent. *Journal of Oncology Pharmacy Practice*. 2012. 18(3): 355–9.

Alopecia

Alopecia is defined as a disorder characterised by a decrease in density of hair compared to normal for a given individual at a given age and body location. The grading of alopecia is shown in Table 3.2. Hair loss may affect patients' eyebrows, eyelashes, nasal hair, moustache, beard, chest, underarm, leg and pubic hair, as well as their scalp.

Symptoms and signs
- *Anagen effluvium*:
  - Involves the loss of growing (anagen) hairs. The majority of hairs are in this phase and therefore this causes profound hair loss.
  - Usually starts within two weeks and is usually nearly complete within 1–2 months after starting treatment.
- *Telogen effluvium*:
  - Usually results in hair thinning of < 50% of the scalp.
  - This is usually worst 3–4 months after starting chemotherapy and although distressing for the patient is less noticeable to others.
- Consider the psychological impact, which can be significant (and cause some patients to decline potentially curative treatment). Hair loss is one of the most distressing side effects of chemotherapy for both women and men, serving as a constant physical reminder of their cancer, identifying them to others as a cancer patient and affecting their body image and self-esteem.

Causes
- *Chemotherapy*:
  - Severity depends on drug combination, dose, duration, route of administration and the patient's individual response.

Table 3.2 CTCAE (V4.03) grading of alopecia.

Grade	Criteria
1	Hair loss of up to 50% of normal for that individual that is not obvious from a distance but only on close inspection; a different hair style may be required to cover the hair loss but it does not require a wig or hair piece to camouflage.
2	Hair loss of >50% normal for that individual that is readily apparent to others; a wig or hair piece is necessary if the patient desires to completely camouflage the hair loss; associated with psychosocial impact.
3	—
4	—
5	—

From the website of the National Cancer Institute (http://www.cancer.gov).

- ○ Drugs that cause alopecia include: doxorubicin, daunorubicin, epirubicin, cyclophosphamide, ifosfamide, etoposide, topotecan, irinotecan, vincristine, vinblastine, bleomycin, paclitaxel, docetaxel and 5-FU (mild).
- *Targeted drugs*:
  - ○ EGFR inhibitors can cause changes in hair texture, slower growth of scalp hair, trichomegaly of eyelashes and both scarring and non-scarring alopecia.
  - ○ Dasatinib and sunitinib can cause reversible hair depigmentation but do not cause alopecia.
- *Radiotherapy*: causes hair loss within the radiation field.

Management
Scalp cooling
- Scalp cooling with cryogel caps or caps connected to cooling devices can limit hair loss in 50–80% of patients. It may be less effective for patients with impaired liver function due to the potential for persistently high circulating drug levels.
- Scalp cooling causes vasoconstriction, which reduces the amount of drug received by hair follicles. The decreased temperature also leads to a reduction in the metabolic rate of hair follicles.
- Scalp cooling can be uncomfortable and also leads to longer hospital stays as cooling needs to start at least 15 minutes prior to chemotherapy and continue for at least 30 minutes after chemotherapy.
- Scalp cooling is not suitable for all patients (e.g. patients receiving very high dose chemotherapy or patients having continuous chemotherapy via a pump). There is a theoretical risk of scalp metastases, but the risk is very small. Scalp cooling is not recommended for patients with haematological malignancies.

General management
- Avoid bleaching, perming or colouring hair as this can weaken it and worsen hair loss.
- Protect the scalp from heat/sun and the cold.

- Camouflage hair loss with a wig, scarf, hat or turban.
- Wigs:
  - May be made of synthetic materials or animal or human hair.
  - Some patients prefer to obtain a wig before hair loss occurs so that it can be matched to their normal hair colour and texture.
  - NHS wigs are free in Wales and Scotland and for certain groups of patients in England.
- Consider using false eyelashes/eyebrows, redrawing eyebrows with an eyebrow pencil or specialist eyebrow tattoos.

Hair re-growth

- Hair usually starts re-growing 1–3 months after completing chemotherapy. Permanent alopecia following chemotherapy is rare but can occur.
- Hair may grow back a different colour, texture or waviness.
- Hair can usually be tinted or permed once it is about three inches long if the patient's scalp is healthy. Advise patients to seek professional advice to check that colours/perms, etc. will not damage the hair or cause an allergic reaction.
- A 2% topical minoxidil solution is not effective in preventing hair loss but has shown promise in accelerating hair regrowth following chemotherapy.
- Hair usually starts to grow back within 3–6 months of finishing radiotherapy but this depends on the radiation dose and duration. However, hair does not always grow back after radiotherapy, may grow back in patches or not as thickly as before.

References

Chon SY, Champion RW, Geddes ER, Rashid RM. Chemotherapy-induced alopecia. *Journal of the American Academy of Dermatology*. 2012. 67(1): e37–47.

Katsimbri P, Bamias A, Pavlidis N. Prevention of chemotherapy-induced alopecia using an effective scalp cooling system. *European Journal of Cancer*. 2000. 36(6): 766–71.

Macmillan Cancer Support. Cancer treatments and hair loss. 2012. Available from: http://www.macmillan.org.uk/Cancerinformation/Livingwithandaftercancer/Symptomssideeffects/Hairloss/Hairloss.aspx

Yeager CE, Olsen EA. Treatment of chemotherapy-induced alopecia. *Dermatologic Therapy*. 2011. 24(4): 432–42.

Anaemia

Anaemia is common amongst cancer patients, affecting over 40% of patients. The severity of anaemia due to treatment varies between individual patients and the grading of anaemia is shown in Table 3.3.

Anaemia can significantly impact on quality of life and influence the biology of the tumour and its response to treatment, particularly in radiotherapy.

Table 3.3 CTCAE (V4.03) grading of anaemia.

Grade	Criteria
1	Haemoglobin < LLN – 100 g/L or < LLN – 10 g/dL
2	Haemoglobin < 100–80 g/L or < 10.0–8.0 g/dL
3	Haemoglobin < 80 g/L or < 8.0 g/dL; transfusion indicated
4	Life-threatening consequences; urgent intervention indicated
5	Death

LLN = lower limit of normal.
From the website of the National Cancer Institute (http://www.cancer.gov).

Cancer-related anaemia also has prognostic value, with reduced haemoglobin levels at the start of treatment associated with worse outcomes.

Causes
Anaemia is usually multi-factorial and can be broadly divided into three categories which are intrinsically intra-linked. Comorbidities are also important, with hereditary anaemia, chronic renal insufficiency and inflammatory conditions contributing to anaemia. The categories are:
- *Blood loss*:
  - Overt or occult blood loss: GI, head and neck, genitourinary, uterine cancers
  - Bleeding into tumours: for example sarcoma, bulky melanomas, hepatomas, ovarian cancer and adrenocortical tumours
  - Coagulopathies: resulting from cancer or treatment
- *Reduced red cell production*:
  - Bone metastases: stem cell destruction secondary to invasion – most commonly seen in breast and prostate cancer patients
  - Secondary to chemotherapy, particularly with platinum agents – most commonly seen in lung and ovarian cancer patients
  - Secondary to radiotherapy – bone marrow stem cells are very sensitive to radiation
  - Haematological malignancies
  - Cytokine or chemical mediated mechanism by tumour
  - Surgical bowel resection: leading to malnutrition or malabsorption of essential vitamins/nutrients (e.g. B12 or folate)
- *Reduced red cell survival*:
  - Antibody production: for example CLL, lymphoma and some solid tumours may lead to immune haemolytic anaemia
  - Hypersplenism
  - Microangiopathic haemolytic anaemia: resulting from procoagulant factors released by some solid tumours (e.g. gastric, breast, pancreatic, colon and prostate cancers)

Symptoms and signs

The symptoms experienced vary depending on the rate of blood loss and the patient's capacity to accommodate this. Older patients and those with coronary artery disease may present with symptoms of hypoxia to the brain and heart.

- *Symptoms*: fatigue, reduced exercise capacity, dyspnoea, decreased appetite, dizziness, syncope, vertigo, tinnitus or headache
- *Signs*: pallor, jaundice (if haemolysis is present), tachycardia, tachypnoea, hypotension, reduced capillary refill

Investigations

- FBC
- Iron, transferrin saturation and ferritin
- B12, folate
- Reticulocyte count
- Bone marrow evaluation – important for persistent anaemia
- Urine dipstick, faecal occult blood

Management
General management

- Treat underlying cause and stem any bleeding
- Address nutrition
- Aim to maintain an Hb of $\geq 120\,g/L$ in patients undergoing radical radiotherapy for head and neck, oesophageal or cervical cancer. An Hb $< 120\,g/L$ may reduce treatment effectiveness.

Red cell infusion

- Urgent transfusion in severe haemorrhage, electively planned for chronic symptomatic anaemia.
- One adult unit should raise the haemoglobin level by $10\,g/L$ (or $1\,g/dL$).
- Risks and side effects – transfusion reactions, congestive cardiac failure, iron overload, viral or bacterial infection.
- Some patients may require irradiated and/or CMV negative blood:
  - Irradiated blood is required for:
    - All patients with Hodgkin's lymphoma
    - After treatment with fludarabine, pentostatin or cladribine
    - Stem cell transplant patients from prior to harvesting and for six months post-transplant until lymphocytes >1.
  - CMV negative blood is required for:
    - All new patients with AML, ALL, non-Hodgkin's lymphoma and CML and other candidates for stem cell transplant
    - CMV negative stem cell transplant recipients
    - CLL patients < 70 years (unless not a candidate for alemtuzumab)
    - Pregnant women

Erythropoietin-stimulating agents (ESA)

- ESA initially demonstrated reduced blood transfusion rates and increased quality of life but Phase III trials have shown mixed results.
- Associated with increased mortality during treatment and thereafter; increased venous thrombo-embolism (VTE) and possible tumour progression (although this has been contested more recently).
- NICE guidelines (2008) – for use in ovarian cancer patients with Hb <80 g/L or in severe persistent anaemia without ability to transfuse blood. This guideline is currently under further review.
- Current advice is to use only in anaemia secondary to cancer treatment and to use with caution in curative patients. Further research is required regarding the safety of ESAs, particularly into the possibility of an association with tumour progression.

Iron replacement

- Iron supplementation may be required for anaemic patients.
- Data suggest IV iron concomitantly with ESA may improve Hb response compared to oral iron or no iron.
- Oral iron is limited by oral tolerance (primarily GI side-effects) and there is debate over its effectiveness.

Refusal of blood products

Some patients will have concerns about the use of blood products. This may stem from a concern regarding the complications of blood transfusion, such as reactions or infections, or a religious belief. The largest community within Britain who do not wish to receive blood products are the Jehovah's Witnesses.

In these circumstances, the wishes of the patient should be sought early. Alternative products may be discussed if appropriate, such as albumin or coagulant factors. Each person may have a different view on each individual product.

The GMC is clear that a patient with capacity should have their wishes respected. There should be a clear discussion about the consequences of refusing treatment and this should be recorded accurately in the patient's notes. A patient with capacity may decline any treatment, independently of the consequences.

Treatment

- In emergency situations check if an advanced directive is in the notes or carried by the patient. This should be respected. Friends or relatives may accompany a patient unable to give or withhold consent; if they raise concern that treatment should not be given then appropriate measures should be undertaken to check if there is an advanced directive in place.
- Elective surgery may be undertaken; this should be in close liaison with the patient, a liaison officer and the blood transfusion service.

Palliative care

In advanced cancer, up to 70% of patients are anaemic. The utility of blood transfusion in these patients should be balanced against symptoms and prognosis. Blood transfusion has inherent risks and the logistics of administering transfusion may not be appropriate in terminal care.

It was noted in a recent Cochrane review that fatigue and dyspnoea may quickly dissipate following blood transfusion but this effect starts to reduce after approximately 14 days. There was a noted increase in 14-day mortality after blood transfusion. This has raised the question about the appropriateness of blood transfusion in advanced cancer, particularly within a hospice setting, and further studies are required to identify the benefit on quality of life.

Other relevant sections of this book

Chapter 2, section on transfusion reactions

References

Dicato M and Plawny L. Erythropoietin in cancer patients: pros and cons. *Current Opinion in Oncology*. 2010. 22(4): 307–311.

Dicato M, Plawny L, Diederick M. Anemia in cancer. *Annals of Oncology*. 2010. 21(7): 167–172.

General Medical Council. *Consent: Patients and Doctors Making Decisions Together*. GMC: London. 2008.

McClelland BDL. *Handbook of Transfusion Medicine*. United Kingdom Blood Service, fourth edition. TSO Publishers: London. 2007.

Mercadante S, Gebbia V, Marrazzo A, Filosto S. Anaemia in cancer: pathophysiology and treatment. *Cancer Treatment Reviews*. 2000. 26(4): 303–311.

NICE TA142. Anaemia (cancer-treatment induced) – erythropoietin (alfa and beta) and darbepoetin. May 2008.

Preston N, Hurlow A, Brine J, Bennett MI. Blood transfusions for anaemia in patients with advanced cancer. *Cochrane Database of Systematic Reviews*. 2012, Issue 2. Art No: CD009007. DOI: 10.1002/14651858.CD009007.pub2.

Tonia T, Mettler A, Robert N, Schwarzer G, Seidenfeld J, Weingart O, *et al*. Erythropoietin or darbepoetin for patients with cancer (review). *Cochrane Database for Systematic Reviews*. 2012. Issue 12. Art. No: CD003407. DOI: 10.1002/14651858.CD003407.pub5.

Anorexia and nutrition

Anorexia

- Loss of appetite (anorexia) is very common, particularly in patients with advanced disease or GI malignancy. The grading of anorexia is shown in Table 3.4.
- Subsequent weight loss is distressing for both patients and carers and can be the predominant feature of cachexia.

Table 3.4 CTCAE (V4.03) grading of anorexia.

Grade	Criteria
1	Loss of appetite without alteration of eating habits.
2	Oral intake altered without significant weight loss or malnutrition; oral nutritional supplements indicated.
3	Associated with significant weight loss or malnutrition (e.g. inadequate oral caloric and/or fluid intake); tube feeding or TPN indicated
4	Life-threatening consequences; urgent intervention indicated.
5	Death.

From the website of the National Cancer Institute (http://www.cancer.gov).

Cachexia

- *Definition*: a syndrome of ongoing loss of lean muscle mass which is not reversible using standard nutritional intervention and leads to a deterioration in function.
- Cachexia correlates with a reduction in performance status, lower tolerance of anti-cancer treatment, increased risk of complications and treatment delays and a reduction in overall survival.
- There are no predictive biochemical markers of cachexia, though CRP is recognised as an indicator of systemic inflammation.

Causes of reduced calorific intake

- Disseminated malignancy: can cause early satiety, dyspnoea, nausea, ascites and constipation.
- Dysphagia or physical GI obstruction.
- Anti-cancer and supportive treatments: can affect GI motility, lead to changes in taste and smell, mucositis or nausea/vomiting.
- Depression: can influence oral intake and exacerbate weight loss.

Management
General management

- Assess oral intake, weight loss and contributory symptoms and address potential reversible factors.
- Refer patients to a dietician. A multidisciplinary approach to nutrition is necessary for cachectic patients.
- Provide dietary counselling. A variety of low-volume, high-calorie oral supplements are available.
- Re-introduction of nutrition by any route after a period of malnutrition may result in refeeding syndrome.
  - Ingestion of a carbohydrate load can cause acute electrolyte shifts, resulting in clinically significant hypophosphatemia, hypokalaemia, hypocalcaemia, cardiac arrhythmias and systolic heart failure.

○ Patients may require close monitoring with twice daily blood tests and in-patient electrolyte replacement until feeding is re-established.

Management: artificial nutrition

- *Patients with refractory cachexia*:
  ○ Parenteral nutrition in terminally ill patients has not been shown to improve survival or symptom control.
  ○ A subset of patients may derive some benefit, for example prevention of delirium, but these patients are yet to be identified.
  ○ Complications of artificial nutrition include sepsis and catheter complications.
  ○ ASCO guidelines recommend that artificial nutrition should only be considered in patients with a prognosis of at least a month.
- *Patients without a functional GI tract*:
  ○ For example patients with malignant bowel obstruction.
  ○ Consider parenteral or artificial nutrition – results in a better quality of life for patients with a performance status of ≤2 and a survival of >3 months.
- *Patients undergoing treatment*:
  ○ Feeding via an artificial route may be considered in certain clinical situations (e.g. radical chemoradiotherapy in head and neck cancer, chemotherapy in oesophageal cancer) to help patients tolerate therapy.
  ○ A systematic review of different artificial feeding routes during head and neck cancer treatment found no difference in weight between NG and PEG fed patients six months following treatment. Due to limited evidence, a preferred feeding route was not recommended.

Management: pharmacological interventions

- *Corticosteroids*: corticosteroids (e.g. methylprednisolone 32–125 mg daily, prednisolone 10 mg daily or dexamethasone 3–8 mg daily) can be beneficial, although usually only for a short number of weeks.
- *Megestrol acetate*: may lead to improvements in appetite and weight but has mixed effects on quality of life and other symptoms.
- *Medroxyprogesterone acetate*: some evidence of improvement in appetite and quality of life.

Other relevant sections of this book

- Chapter 3, sections on bowel obstruction, dysphagia, mucositis, nausea and vomiting
- Chapter 9, section on enteral feeding tubes

References

Argiles JM, Lopez-Soriano FJ, Busquets S. Mechanisms and treatment of cancer cachexia *Nutrition, Metabolism & Cardiovascular Diseases*. 2012. 23(Suppl. 1): S19–24.

Dav R, Dalal S, Bruera E. Is there a role for parenteral nutrition or hydration at the end of life? *Current Opinion in Supportive and Palliative Care*. 2012. 6(3): 365–70.

Dolan EA. Malignant bowel obstruction: a review of current treatment strategies. *American Journal of Hospice and Palliative Medicine.* 2011. 28(8): 576–82.

Dy SM, Lorenz KA, Naeim A, Sanati H, Walling A, Asch SM. Evidence-based recommendations for cancer fatigue, anorexia, depression, and dyspnea. *Journal of Clinical Oncology.* 2008. 26(23): 3886–95.

Fearon K, Strasser F, Anker SD, Bosaeus I, Bruera E, Fainsinger RL, *et al.* Definition and classification of cancer cachexia: an international consensus. *Lancet Oncology.* 2011. 12(5): 489–95.

Marinella MA. Refeeding syndrome: an important aspect of supportive oncology. *Journal of Supportive Oncology.* 2009. 7(1): 11–6.

Nugent B, Lewis S, O'Sullivan JM. Enteral feeding methods for nutritional management in patients with head and neck cancers being treated with radiotherapy and/or chemotherapy. *Cochrane Database Systematic Reviews.* 2010. 17(3): CD007904.

Yavuzsen T, Davis MP, Walsh D, LeGrand S, Lagman R. Systematic review of the treatment of cancer- associated anorexia and weight loss. *Journal of Clinical Oncology.* 23(33): 8500–8511, 2005.

Ascites

Ascites is defined as the abnormal accumulation of intraperitoneal fluid. The grading of ascites is shown in Table 3.5. Of cancer patients with ascites, 95% have measurable metastatic disease and 90% have peritoneal disease. The presence of ascites is a poor prognostic factor associated with survival of a few months (except in ovarian cancer).

Symptoms/signs and causes

- *Symptoms/signs*: pain, abdominal distension, anorexia, nausea, vomiting, lower limb oedema, dyspnoea, altered body image.
- *Causes*:
  - Most commonly associated with ovarian cancer. Also associated with pancreaticobiliary, gastric, oesophageal and breast cancer.
  - Portal hypertension, splenomegaly or chronic liver impairment may contribute to transudative ascites.
  - Inferior vena cava obstruction or compression may also contribute to the development of ascites.

Table 3.5 CTCAE (V4.03) grading of ascites.

Grade	Criteria
1	Asymptomatic; clinical or diagnostic observations only; intervention not indicated.
2	Symptomatic; medical intervention indicated.
3	Severe symptoms; invasive intervention indicated.
4	Life-threatening consequences; urgent operative intervention indicated.
5	Death.

From the website of the National Cancer Institute (http://www.cancer.gov).

Management

There is currently no clear professional guidance on the management of malignant ascites.

Pharmacological interventions

Use of diuretics

- Serum albumin – ascites gradient (SAAG):
  - SAAG = serum albumin – ascites albumin.
  - Response to diuretics is seen in patients with a SAAG of > 1.1 g/dL or evidence of portal hypertension, but not in those with a SAAG of < 1.1 g/dL.
- Start spironolactone at a dose of 50–100 mg daily, with a dose increase every 3–7 days up to a maximum of 400 mg daily as required. Consider adding in 40 mg of furosemide if renal function is still satisfactory. Monitor electrolytes.

Other interventions

- *Therapeutic paracentesis and permanent peritoneal catheters*:
  - There are no randomised trials comparing paracentesis with diuretics in malignant ascites.
  - Patients who have significant symptoms (grade 3) or do not respond to medical treatment should be considered for therapeutic paracentesis. Paracentesis results in temporary relief of symptoms for 90% of patients.
  - Recurrence of ascites following paracentesis has driven the development of permanent peritoneal catheter drainage systems (e.g. PleurX® drains).
- *Peritoneo-venous shunts*:
  - Allows drainage from the peritoneal cavity into a large vein using tubing with a uni-directional valve.
  - *Contraindications include*: renal failure, cardiac failure, loculated ascites, portal hypertension and coagulopathy.
  - Haematogenous metastases due to the shunt and tumour growth along the shunt tract have been reported.
  - Studies have shown a much better outcome with shunts in ovarian and breast cancer and a poor outcome in GI cancer; therefore most literature advises against use in patients with ascites secondary to GI cancer.

Other management approaches

- *Intraperitoneal chemotherapy*:
  - Intraperitoneal chemotherapy prior to ascitic drainage has been attempted for control of peritoneal metastases and prevention of ascites reaccummulation.
  - A range of chemotherapeutics have been evaluated (with varying success), including cisplatin, 5-FU, carboplatin, etoposide, doxorubicin, paclitaxel and methotrexate.
  - This is not in routine UK clinical practice but used as a treatment option in the USA following optimal debulking surgery in ovarian cancer.
- *Hyperthermic intraperitoneal chemotherapy (HIPEC)*:
  - Activity of some chemotherapeutics (e.g. cisplatin, carboplatin, doxorubicin and mitomycin C) is enhanced in a hyperthermic medium at 40–43°C.

○ Best suited to patients with a good performance status and potentially resectable peritoneal disease. Optimal duration, dose and temperature are as yet unknown.

○ Studies with small numbers of patients have shown control of ascites and potential tolerability, but experience is limited to specialist centres.

○ Further trials are needed to evaluate the use of surgery followed by HIPEC.

Future agents

* *Catumaxomab*:
  ○ A CD3 and Epithelial Cell Adhesion Molecule (EpCAM) monoclonal antibody.
  ○ Trials in patients with EpCAM positive tumours and malignant ascites have shown encouraging results with a significantly delayed time to paracentesis. A randomised Phase IIIb study is in process.

* *Octreotide*:
  Small case series have suggested that octreotide may also control ascites and a Phase III placebo-controlled trial is in process.

Other relevant sections of this book

Chapter 9, section on ascitic drains (paracentesis)

References

Barni S, Cabiddu M, Ghilardi M, Petrelli F. A novel perspective for an orphan problem: old and new drugs for the medical management of malignant ascites. *Critical Reviews in Oncology/Hematology*. 2011. 79(2): 144–53.

Becker G, Daniel Galandib D, Blum HE. Malignant ascites: systematic review and guideline for treatment. *European Journal of Cancer*. 2006. 42(5): 589–97.

Courtney A, Nemcek AA, Jr., Rosenberg S, Tutton S, Darcy M, Gordon G. Prospective evaluation of the PleurX catheter when used to treat recurrent ascites associated with malignancy. Journal of vascular and interventional radiology. *Journal of Vascular and Interventional Radiology*. 2008. 19(12): 1723–31.

Keen A, Fitzgerald D, Bryant A, Dickinson HO. Management of drainage for malignant ascites in gynaecological cancer. *Cochrane Database of Systematic Reviews*. 2010. 20(1): CD007794.

White J, Carolan-Rees G. PleurX peritoneal catheter drainage system for vacuum-assisted drainage of treatment-resistant, recurrent malignant ascites: a NICE Medical Technology Guidance. *Applied Health Economics and Health Policy*. 2012. 10(5): 299–308.

Bone metastases and osteoporosis

Bone metastases

* Bone metastases are very common, particularly in patients with breast, prostate or lung cancer. The most common site of metastasis is the axial skeleton.
* Metastases may be predominantly osteolytic (e.g. in lung cancer), predominantly osteoblastic (e.g. in prostate cancer) or both osteolytic and osteoblastic.

Symptoms, signs and complications
- Pain and decreased mobility.
- Spinal cord compression.
- Bone marrow infiltration, which can cause anaemia or pancytopenia due to impairment of bone marrow synthetic function.
- Pathological fractures (more common in the femur or proximal parts of other long bones).
- Cranial nerve abnormalities (secondary to base of skull metastases).
- Hypercalcaemia.
- Increased retention of calcium in the bones can also cause hypocalcaemia, leading to secondary hyperparathyroidism and further bone loss.

Investigations
- Solitary lesions (especially lytic lesions) should be thoroughly investigated as they may not represent a bone metastasis. If there is doubt about the diagnosis, a biopsy should be considered.
- ALP may be raised (but may be normal).
- *Plain X-rays*: have a low sensitivity, particularly for small or early lesions.
- *Isotope bone scans*:
    - Detect osteoblastic activity, which causes an increase in tracer uptake. Can therefore miss purely osteolytic lesions.
    - Other causes of increased tracer uptake include: trauma, pelvic insufficiency fractures (e.g. secondary to pelvic radiotherapy or steroids), infection, osteoarthritis or inflammatory disease.
    - Systemic therapy can lead to increased tracer activity due to increased osteoblastic activity and care should be taken not to mistakenly interpret this as disease progression.
- *CT and MRI*: usually used to image specific body areas, rather than look for widespread metastatic disease. Have a high sensitivity and are also more specific than isotope bone scans, but it can still be difficult to determine whether vertebral fractures are due to osteoporosis or metastases.
- *PET scans*: not widely used, but can help to identify early bone metastases and assess response to treatment.

Management of bone metastases
General management
- Consider the patient's prognosis when deciding on the best treatment modality. Patients may live for years with bone metastases, for example approximately 25% of patients with bone metastases secondary to breast cancer are alive after five years.
- If there is a lesion in a long bone it is important to assess the risk of fracture and consider whether elective surgical intervention is indicated.
- Pain control can be problematic and often requires opioids, but NSAIDs can be particularly effective.

Radiotherapy

- Is effective in relieving pain in 60–80% of patients and results in complete pain relief in 20–30%. Also used for malignant cord compression as an oncological emergency.
- The onset of benefit is variable, ranging from a few days to weeks. Some patients have pain that is unresponsive to radiotherapy, whereas some have a long and durable response.
- There is debate about the most appropriate regime, but a systematic review has shown that 8 Gy as a single fraction is equivalent to fractionated regimes for palliation of pain.
- The spinal cord and other organs have a limited tolerance to radiotherapy, dependent on fraction size and total dose. Repeated fractions to the same area are not always possible.

Surgery

- May be indicated for cord compression, long bone fractures or for metastases at high risk of pathological fracture (e.g. lytic lesions, lesions causing functional pain, > 50% destruction of a single cortex of a long bone or avulsion of the lesser trochanter).
- Bones may not heal after pathological fractures (particularly secondary to lytic lesions). This leads to higher rates of fixation failure and the choice of procedure should reflect this (e.g. avoidance of sliding hip screws).
- Prophylactic internal fixation should usually be followed by radiotherapy to inhibit further tumour growth.

Radiopharmaceuticals

- Radionucleotides such as strontium-89 chloride, samarium-153, rhenium-186 or rhenium-188 localise to regions of high bone turnover and administer high local doses of radiation.
- Can be useful for the palliation of bone pain, particularly in patients with prostate cancer with diffuse multifocal disease.
- Pain relief usually starts within 1–3 weeks and lasts for 3–6 months.

Percutaneous vertebroplasty, kyphoplasty or cementoplasty

- Involves the injection of bone cement, usually into collapsed vertebral bodies, but can also be used in the scapula and ribs.
- Is effective at reducing pain and effects are seen more quickly than with radiotherapy. May also be used for prophylactic spinal fixation before significant vertebral collapse occurs.
- The procedure may be performed as a day case or involve an overnight stay in hospital.
- Complications are rare, but include cement PE and cord compression due to cement leakage into the spinal canal.

Bisphosphonates
- Can relieve bone pain, reduce the incidence and delay the onset of skeletal complications and may also have a role in preventing further bone metastases as well as have a direct apoptotic effect on cancer cells.
- Examples:
  - 4 mg of zoledronic acid IV in 100 ml of 0.9% saline over 15 minutes
  - 90 mg of pamidronate IV in 500 ml of 0.9% saline over two hours
  - 6 mg of ibandronate IV over 60 minutes every four weeks or ibandronate 50 mg PO OD
- *Side effects*: usually well tolerated but can cause flu-like symptoms, myalgia, arthralgia, nausea, peripheral oedema and osteonecrosis of the jaw. Consider calcium and vitamin D supplementation.
- Bisphosphonates are renally cleared and can cause a rise in creatinine. Renal function should therefore be monitored throughout treatment and the bisphosphonate dose reduced or withheld according to local protocols if there is deterioration in renal function. Ibandronate does not affect renal function.
- The optimal duration of treatment is unknown. In the absence of toxicities, treatment should be reviewed after 1–2 years and the benefits balanced with the increased risk of osteonecrosis of the jaw.

Systemic therapy and new therapies
- Appropriate endocrine therapy or chemotherapy may help to relieve pain.
- Denosumab inhibits osteoclast formation and activation and may be used for the prevention of skeletal events in patients with bone metastases from solid tumours.

Osteoporosis
- *Definition*: a disorder characterised by reduced bone mass, resulting in increased incidence of fractures.
- Diagnosed by DEXA scans, which report T scores. T scores indicate the difference in bone mineral density (BMD) as a standard deviation in comparison to the mean of the average young adult population:
  - T score ≥ -1.0 = normal bone density
  - T score of -1.0 to -2.5 = low bone mass/osteopenia
  - T score ≤ -2.5 = osteoporosis

Risk factors
- Aromatase inhibitors (e.g. letrozole, anastrozole). Note that this does not apply to tamoxifen, which has a beneficial effect on bone density.
- Androgen deprivation therapy.
- Early menopause – this can occur as a result of chemotherapy. Drugs such as goserelin (Zoladex®) cause an artificial menopause.
- Steroids.
- Other drugs, for example PPIs, certain antidepressants.

- Lifestyle factors, for example smoking, excess alcohol and inadequate exercise.
- Vitamin D deficiency and/or low calcium intake.
- Prior non-traumatic fracture or a family history of fracture.
- Body weight <70 kg.

Management

- *Calculate fracture risk*: the FRAX algorithm (available at www.shef.ac.uk/FRAX) is a risk assessment tool that provides an estimate of the ten-year probability of hip and major osteoporotic fracture by combining BMD measurements and clinical factors.
- *General advice*: calcium-rich diet, maintain an adequate intake of vitamin D (calcium and vitamin D supplements may be indicated), regular weight-bearing exercise and smoking cessation.
- *Monitoring*: consider repeat DEXA scans every two years in patients with an increased risk of fracture to monitor the impact of cancer treatment on bone mass.
- *Treatment*: consider therapeutic intervention in patients with a BMD of <−2.0. The mainstay of treatment is oral bisphosphonates, for example alendronate 10 mg OD or 70 mg once a week (with water on an empty stomach) or risedronate 5 mg OD.

Other relevant sections of this book

- Chapter 2, sections on hypercalcaemia, spinal cord compression
- Chapter 3, sections on dental disorders
- Chapter 6, section on endocrine therapy
- Chapter 8, section on pain management

References

Gralow JR, Biermann JS, Farooki A, Fornier MN, Gagel RF, Kumar RN, *et al*. NCCN Task Force Report: bone health in cancer care. *Journal of the National Comprehensive Cancer Network*. 2009. 7(Suppl. 3): S1–32; quiz S3–5.

Oliver TB, Bhat R, Kellet CF, Adamson DJ. Diagnosis and management of bone metastases. *JournaL Royal College of Physicians, Edinburgh*. 2011. 41(4): 330–8.

Selvaggi G, Scagliotti GV. Management of bone metastases in cancer: a review. *Critical Reviews in Oncology/Hematology*. 2005. 56(3): 365–78.

Bowel obstruction

Bowel obstruction most commonly occurs in patients with metastatic gynaecological, bowel or stomach cancer. However, it can occur in patients with metastatic cancer from almost any diagnosis, including lung cancer, breast cancer and malignant melanoma. The grading of bowel obstruction is shown in Table 3.6.

Table 3.6 CTCAE (V4.03) grading of GI obstruction.

Grade	Criteria
1	Asymptomatic; clinical or diagnostic observations only; intervention not required.
2	Symptomatic; altered GI function.
3	Hospitalisation indicated; elective operative intervention indicated; disabling.
4	Life-threatening consequences; urgent operative intervention indicated.
5	Death.

From the website of the National Cancer Institute (http://www.cancer.gov).

Obstruction can be divided into:
- Malignancy related (small or large bowel): the average prognosis is 80 days, but this is significantly improved if systemic treatment is appropriately administered after the acute episode has resolved.
- Non-malignancy related, for example secondary to adhesions, hernia(s) or post-operative complications.

Symptoms
These vary in onset and severity, but typically include:
- Bloating
- Abdominal pain
- Nausea and vomiting (faeculent vomiting is especially important)
- Constipation

Management
Management is dependent on the prognosis of the underlying cancer (e.g. curative versus palliative), performance status and the severity of the obstruction. Initial management involves stabilising the patient, managing symptoms and determining the site(s) of obstruction and whether the obstruction is partial or complete.

General management includes:
- Bloods – FBC, U&E, LFT, bone profile, coagulation, group and save.
- AXR and erect CXR – often initially undertaken to assess GI lumen diameter and presence of air below the diaphragm to rule out perforation.
- IV fluids – ensure electrolytes are replaced.
- NG tube may relieve nausea and vomiting and can reduce the pressure within the GI tract to further aid decompression in conservative treatment.
- Continuous subcutaneous syringe driver – anti-emetic (cyclizine 100–150 mg/24 hours) and analgesia.
- NBM/oral sips only.
- Radiology: CT abdomen/pelvis.
- Surgical referral after discussion with senior.

Specific management for obstruction:

- Conservative:
  - Dexamethasone IV/SC 6–16 mg may be useful in relieving obstruction.
  - Octreotide syringe driver – 300–900 mcg/24 hours to reduce gastric/GI secretions and thereby reduce the volume of vomit.
  - Metoclopramide (30–60 mg/24 hours) may be added to the syringe driver in place of cyclizine, but be wary of colic – if colic occurs stop metoclopramide.
  - Hysocine butylbromide (30–60 mg/24 hours) is useful for controlling colic and is most effective through a syringe driver.
  - In partial obstruction, softening laxatives may be useful. Low residue diets are better tolerated than high-fibre.
  - A venting gastrostomy may be placed to relieve nausea and vomiting in patients with indolent disease where the obstruction cannot be reversed.
- Intraluminal stent – requires a single site of obstruction only, not suitable in the majority of cases with small bowel obstruction.
- Surgical resection:
  - Needs senior discussion and careful patient selection – multiple points of obstruction are often not amenable to surgery, whereas single points of obstruction may be more appropriate.
  - Options include resection and intestinal bypassing.
  - The improvement in symptoms and outcomes is debatable and is usually dependent on the underlying primary, with a re-obstruction rate of up to 50%.
- Systemic therapy – for a carefully selected subgroup of patients, for example some cases of sub-acute obstruction in gynaecological cancer.
- TPN – typically used where therapy is being instigated to reverse the obstruction, for example surgery or chemotherapy. May be considered in patients treated with symptom relief alone where the natural history of disease is fairly indolent.

References

Chakraborty A, Selby D, Gardiner K, Myers J, Moravan V, Wright F Malignant bowel obstruction: natural history of a heterogeneous patient population followed prospectively over two years. *Journal of Pain and Symptom Management.* 2011. 41(2): 412–420.

Feuer DDJ, Broadley KE. Corticosteroids for the resolution of malignant bowel obstruction in advanced gynaecological and gastrointestinal cancer. *Cochrane Database of Systematic Reviews* 1999, Issue 3. Art. No.: CD001219.

Feuer DDJ, Broadley KE. Surgery for the resolution of symptoms in malignant bowel obstruction in advanced gynaecological and gastrointestinal cancer. *Cochrane Database of Systematic Reviews* 2000, Issue 3. Art No: CD002764.

Breathlessness

Breathlessness or dyspnoea is reported in more than 50% of patients with cancer. The grading of dyspnoea is shown in Table 3.7. It is a poor prognostic factor in patients with advanced disease.

Table 3.7 CTCAE (V4.03) grading of dyspnoea.

Grade	Criteria
1	Shortness of breath with moderate exertion.
2	Shortness of breath with minimal exertion; limiting instrumental ADL.
3	Shortness of breath at rest; limiting self-care ADL.
4	Life-threatening consequences; urgent intervention indicated.
5	Death.

From the website of the National Cancer Institute (http://www.cancer.gov).

Symptoms and signs
- Three subjectively different symptoms may be reported:
  - *Air hunger*: the patient feels that they need to breathe but cannot increase ventilation.
  - *Chest tightness*: the patient is unable to ventilate adequately and their chest feels constricted.
  - *Effort of breathing*: breathing causes fatigue and physical discomfort.
- Associated symptoms/signs include: chest pain, cough, fatigue, fever, peripheral oedema, wheeze, stridor and crepitations.

Causes
- Cardiopulmonary disease requiring increased respiratory effort:
  - Pulmonary or pleural disease
  - Pleural or pericardial effusion – consider cardiac tamponade in patients with previously asymptomatic pericardial effusions detected on imaging
  - SVCO
  - Infection
  - Pneumonitis (drug and radiation induced)
  - Lymphangitis
  - Obstructive lung disease
- Ventilation/perfusion mismatch:
  - PE
  - Pulmonary oedema
  - Anaemia
  - Pulmonary hypertension
- Systemic causes:
  - Fatigue
  - Respiratory muscle weakness
  - Sepsis
  - Metabolic acidosis
  - Abdominal distension, for example due to ascites, hepatomegaly or constipation

Management
General management
- Treat associated symptoms (e.g. pain, anxiety and depression), as dyspnoea can be a manifestation of wider issues.
- Cool air across the nose, mouth and face (e.g. from an electric fan) has been shown to improve the sensation of breathlessness.
- Opioids can relieve dyspnoea and 'breakthrough' doses of opioid are recommended.
- There is little evidence for the use of supplemental oxygen in cancer patients.
- Consider a trial of salbutamol (inhaled via a spacer or nebulised) if there is an element of bronchoconstriction.
- Treat reversible underlying causes:
  - Consider the risks/benefits of blood transfusion and erythropoesis stimulating agents in anaemic patients.
  - Early antibiotics for chest infection or sepsis of unknown source (follow local guidelines if the patient is at risk of neutropenic sepsis). Consider atypical infections, including fungal infection if there have been prolonged periods of neutropenia.
  - Appropriate management of abdominal symptoms, for example drainage of ascites, management of bowel obstruction.
  - Consider metabolic acidosis as a cause of dyspnoea. Repeated or prolonged steroid use may cause diabetes and ketoacidosis.
- Consider airway obstruction, SVCO, PE and pericardial effusion and treat as appropriate.

Lymphangitis
- Lymphangitic carcinomatosis or spread of cancer within the pulmonary lymphatic system can cause severe dyspnoea.
- Can occur in several types of cancer including lung, pancreas, colon, breast and cervical cancer.
- *Investigations*:
  - CXR or HRCT chest may detect abnormalities but in some cases imaging is not diagnostic.
  - The gold standard for diagnosis is detection of tumour microemboli in the pulmonary vasculature.
- *Management*: can be rapidly fatal, no proven treatments except for control of the underlying malignancy. Consider a one-week trial of steroids (e.g. dexamethasone 4–8 mg mane), and stop if there is no improvement.

Pleural effusion
- Exudative malignant pleural effusions can cause recurrent severe dyspnoea.
- Chest drains or thoracocentesis can relieve symptoms, but risks such as pneumothorax and pain need to be considered.

- Recurrent effusions in patients with an adequate performance status who do not have a very limited prognosis may require more definitive management (e.g. pleurodesis or insertion of an indwelling pleural catheter).
  - Thorascopic pleurodesis is more effective than tube thoracostomy or chest tube administration of sclerosing agents.
  - Permanent indwelling pleural catheters have a similar efficacy to pleurodesis and may also be useful for the management of effusions post pleurodesis.

Pneumonitis

- *Causes*:
  - Chemotherapeutic agents: for example bleomycin, gemcitabine and paclitaxel.
  - Targeted drugs: for example mTOR inhibitors (e.g. everolimus) and tyrosine kinase inhibitors.
  - Anti-lymphocyte antibodies: for example rituximab, ofatumumab and alemtuzumab.
  - Radiotherapy (see Chapter 5, management of early respiratory toxicity section).
- *Risk factors*: older age, poor performance status, poor baseline lung function.
- *Symptoms*: low grade fever, dry cough and worsening dyspnoea.
- *Management*:
  - Refer for respiratory physician review.
  - Consider bronchoalveolar lavage if the patient has a fever or there is suspicion of an infective cause.
  - Patients starting mTOR inhibitors:
    - An HRCT chest is recommended at baseline (although this is not routinely performed in all trusts).
    - On development of symptoms, re-image promptly with HRCT chest.
  - Consider high dose oral prednisolone (0.75–1 mg/kg) or IV methylprednisolone (2–5 mg/kg/day in two divided doses) for severe pneumonitis.
  - Consider dose reduction or withdrawal of drug if symptoms are affecting ADLs.

Other relevant sections of this book

- Chapter 2, sections on central airway obstruction and stridor, superior vena cava obstruction
- Chapter 3, sections on anaemia, chest pain and other cardiac complications, thromboembolism
- Chapter 9, section on chest drains and pleurodesis

References

Albiges L, Chamming's F, Duclos B, Stern M, Motzer RJ, Ravaud A, Camus P. Incidence and management of mTOR inhibitor-associated pneumonitis in patients with metastatic renal cell carcinoma. *Annals of Oncology*. 2012. 23(8): 1943–1953.

Berkey FJ. Managing the adverse effects of radiation therapy. *American Family Physician*. 2010. 15; 82(4): 381–8, 394.

Bertolaccini L, Viti A, Gorla A, Terzi A. Home-management of malignant pleural effusion with an indwelling pleural catheter: ten years experience. *European Journal of Surgical Oncology.* 2012. 38(12):1161–4.

Cachia E, Ahmedzai SH. Breathlessness in cancer patients. *European Journal of Cancer.* 2008. 44(8): 1116–1123.

Demmy TL, Gu L, Burkhalter JE, Toloza EM, D'Amico TA, Sutherland S, *et al.* Cancer and Leukemia Group B Optimal management of malignant pleural effusions (results of CALGB 30102). *Journal of the National Comprehensive Cancer Network.* 2012. 10(8): 975–82.

Dy SM, Lorenz KA, Naeim A, Sanati H, Walling A, Asch SM. Evidence-based recommendations for cancer fatigue, anorexia, depression, and dyspnea. *Journal of Clinical Oncology.* 2008. 26(23): 3886–95.

Guddatia AK, Marakb CP. Pulmonary lymphangitic carcinomatosis due to renal cell carcinoma. *Case Reports in Oncology.* 2012. 5(2) 246–252.

Kamal AH, Maguire JM, Wheeler JL, Currow DC, Abernethy AP. Dyspnea review for the palliative care professional: assessment, burdens, and etiologies. *Journal of Palliative Medicine.* 2011. 14(10): 1167–72.

Chest pain and other cardiac complications

Chest pain, heart failure and arrhythmias have multiple aetiologies that may be related to cancer or its treatment, and the CTCAE grading is dependent on the underlying cause. The common aetiologies and cancer specific details are discussed here. However, the treatment algorithms are akin to general medical patients and therefore specific details of the management of conditions such as arrhythmias and MI are not discussed in detail. Patients at high risk for cardiovascular disease should have a baseline ECG at the start of systemic treatment.

Chest pain

The usual medical causes of chest pain, such as MI or ischaemia, remain prevalent in the cancer population and should be excluded.

Causes
- Intrathoracic
  - Cardiac – MI/ischaemia, pericarditis, palpitations
  - Pulmonary – PE, pneumonia, pleurisy, tumour
  - Bone – bone metastasis +/– fracture
  - Thyroid – rarely painful
- Extrathoracic
  - Referred pain – spinal metastasis
  - Subcutaneous metastases
  - Surgical wounds, lines and tubes
- Treatment related

Direct toxicity of treatment, for example radiotherapy, myocardial ischaemia secondary to chemotherapy (see below).

Ischaemia

- Anti-metabolites (e.g. 5-FU, capecitabine), have been associated with cardiac events. This is thought to be due to coronary arteritis or coronary artery spasm.
  - Cardiac events (e.g. chest pain) typically occurs within 2–5 days of starting treatment. The rate may be as high as 7.5%, especially in patients with prior coronary artery disease or patients treated with a combination of capecitabine and oxaliplatin.
  - Chest pain and vasospasm may not be associated with a rise in troponin.
- Bevacizumab is associated with an increased risk of arterial thromboembolic events, including MI.
- Other causes of MI/ischaemia include: paclitaxel, docetaxel, cisplatin, interleukin-2, vinca alkaloids, sorafenib and erlotinib.

Investigations and management

- Detailed history of cancer, pain and related symptoms (e.g. SOB, cough, haemoptysis).
- Cardiac sounding chest pain should be treated as acute coronary syndrome until proved otherwise.
- Bloods, including FBC, U&E, LFT, coagulation, bone profile, troponin (if cardiac sounding chest pain).
- ECG.
- CXR.
- Consider: CT thorax, CTPA, bone scan for non-cardiac chest pain.
- Further management depends on the underlying cause.
- Senior review should take place prior to recommencement of any systemic therapy after a coronary event to assess whether to halt treatment altogether.

Arrhythmias

Cardiac arrhythmias are common in cancer patients. They may be transient and/ or asymptomatic and therefore may not require further management. However, symptomatic patients require acute assessment.

Arrhythmias due to direct tumour involvement are uncommon. Underlying cardiac disease is common and may be aggravated by chemotherapeutic agents or electrolyte disturbances. However, arrhythmias can also develop in patients with no existing cardiac history.

Causes

- Chemotherapy-related:
  - Paclitaxel and docetaxel: asymptomatic bradyarrhythmias, bradycardia-related syncope, heart block and ventricular arrhythmias
  - Anthracyclines: SVT, AF and QT prolongation
  - Thalidomide: bradyarrhythmias
  - Ifosfamide
  - Cisplatin
  - Interferon

- Other drugs, for example β-blockers, tricyclic antidepressants, digoxin
- Radiotherapy
- Comorbidities, for example coronary artery disease, heart failure, valve disease
- Concomitant conditions:
  - Electrolyte disturbances
  - Abnormalities in thyroid function, for example secondary to tyrosine kinase inhibitors
  - Sepsis
  - Pulmonary hypertension, for example secondary to PE

Management

Symptoms warranting immediate action:
- Syncope
- Confusion
- Haemodynamic compromise
- Myocardial ischaemia

If any of the above symptoms are present the acute/arrest team should be alerted. The patient should be assessed and treated as per Resuscitation Council guidelines: DC cardioversion/chemical cardioversion.

In the absence of unstable symptoms, the management includes:
- Bloods and IV access
- 12 lead ECG – check for broad or narrow complex tachycardia
- Discussion with a senior/on-call cardiologist

Narrow complex tachycardia:
- Regular complexes – use vagal manoeuvres, such as blowing into a 10 ml syringe. If no benefit use adenosine with ECG monitoring.
- Irregular complexes – most likely atrial fibrillation. Treatment may include β-blockers, diltiazem, digoxin and amiodarone.

Broad complex tachycardia:
- May be regular or irregular
- Should be discussed with a specialist

QT prolongation

- Increasingly associated with an expanding list of drugs. It is associated with the ventricular arrhythmia torsades de pointes and can lead to sudden death.
- Can be caused by many medications and care should be taken not to combine agents that can lead to QT prolongation. The list is not exhaustive but includes:
  - Antibiotics: erythromycin, clarithromycin, fluconazole
  - Psychotropics: haloperidol, chlorpromazine
  - Antiemetics: domperidone, ondansetron
  - Cardiac medications: sotalol, amiodarone, procainamide
  - Anti-cancer drugs: vemurafenib, vandetanib, dasatinib
- Identification of QT prolongation should lead to removal of the offending drug and careful monitoring.

Pericardial effusions and pericarditis

Pericardial effusions

- Pericardial effusions are most commonly associated with metastatic disease or as a complication of radiotherapy, but can also be caused by drugs (e.g. imatinib, all-*trans* retinoic acid). It may have an insidious onset or leave the patient in-extremis.
- *Symptoms and signs*: SOB, chest tightness, palpitations, tachycardia or tachypnoea, hypoxia, left and/or right sided heart failure.
- *Assessment*: thorough clinical examination, CXR and CT thorax.
- *Management*: refer to cardiology. Consider pericardial drainage, pericardial window (thoracic surgery) or systemic therapy (if good performance status and responsive cancer).

Pericarditis/myocarditis

- Causes include: cyclophosphamide, cytarabine, radiotherapy, malignancy, infections (viral, bacterial or fungal; e.g. Coxsackie, varicella, Epstein-Barr, TB), uraemia, MI, malignancy (especially bronchial and breast cancer, Hodgkin's disease and melanoma).
- *Symptoms and signs*: central chest pain worse on inspiration/lying flat (relieved by sitting forward), pericardial friction rub.
- *Assessment*: ECG may show saddle-shaped ST segments.
- *Management*: treat cause, analgesia (e.g. ibuprofen if no contraindications).

Heart failure

A reduction in LV ejection fraction (LVEF) can occur due to cardiotoxic anticancer therapy. It may involve a reduction in LVEF without symptoms or lead to symptoms of congestive heart failure. This may be reversible or irreversible.

Causes

- Anthracyclines (e.g. doxorubicin, epirubicin), mitoxantrone, alkylating agents (e.g. cyclophosphamide, ifosfamide), trastuzumab, lapatinib and VEGF-inhibitors, for example sunitinib (associated with 10% rate of 10% reduction in LVEF, which corrects on withdrawal of treatment). Usually a cumulative effect.
- Risk factors: prior cardiovascular disease, increasing age, combinations of two or more cardiotoxic agents or radiotherapy, cumulative dose. The use of dextrazoxane may reduce anthracycline-related toxicity.
- Onset:
  - Early onset (1–2% of patients) – chronic, progressive condition occurring within a year of infusion
  - Late onset (1–5% of patients) – may have a time lag of 10–20 years from infusion

Investigations and management

- Echo or MUGA scans will determine the extent of reduction in LVEF. Patients on regimes involving cardiotoxic agents (e.g. trastuzumab) should have regular monitoring of LVEF in accordance with local protocols.

- Investigations to exclude other causes of heart failure (e.g. MI, ischaemia).
- Asymptomatic patients should be treated dependent on drop in LVEF and other toxicities if LVEF is above 40%.
- Symptomatic patients – stop the offending drug.
- ACE-inhibitors (e.g. ramipril, started at 1.25 mg OD) and β-blockers can improve LVEF.
- Refer to cardiology if symptoms are severe or persist.

Radiation-related cardiac injury

Radiation-related cardiac injury is a late toxicity of treatment and is therefore most commonly described in those who have undergone curative treatment at a young age. Most published literature describes radiation-related cardiac injury in patients treated for early breast cancer and Hodgkin's disease, and showed an increased risk of myocardial ischaemia after radiotherapy. However, the patients analysed underwent less sophisticated radiotherapy techniques than those used today.

Risk factors include:
- Younger age at exposure
- Dose > 30–35 Gy
- Dose per fraction > 2 Gy
- Cytotoxic, endocrine or trastuzumab therapy
- Cardiac risk factors, for example hypertension, smoking, diabetes, dyslipidaemias

Radiation may damage coronary arteries, cardiac muscle, heart valves and pericardium leading to:
- Premature coronary artery disease secondary to arteritis – apparent 10–15 years after radiotherapy.
- Acute pericarditis with associated pericardial effusion. The effusion may be asymptomatic. Apparent 6–12 months after radiotherapy.
- Myocarditis and cardiac failure.
- Stenosis or regurgitation of the mitral and aortic valves.
- Arrhythmias secondary to fibrosis of the electrical conductive system.

Management
- There are no specific follow-up or surveillance protocols currently in place.
- Each complication is treated as any non-radiation related cardiac disorder.

Other cardiac complications
- Bulsulfan can cause endomyocardial fibrosis and cardiac tamponade.
- Radiotherapy to the thorax can lead to damage to the pericardium, myocardium, valves and coronary vessels.

References

Bovelli D, Plataniotis G, Roila F. Cardiotoxicity of chemotherapeutic agents and radiotherapy-related heart disease : ESMO Clinical Practice Guidelines. *Annals of Oncology*. 2010. 21(Suppl. 5); v277–82.

Curigliano G, Cardinale D, Suter T, Plataniotis G, de Azambuja E, Sandri MT, *et al.* Cardiovascular toxicity induced by chemotherapy, targeted agents and radiotherapy: ESMO Clinical Practice Guidelines. *Annals of Oncology.* 2012. 23 (7): vii155–66.

Ewer MS, Ewer SM, Suter T. Cardiac complications. In: Hong WK, Bast RC, Hait WN, Kufe DW, Pollock RE, Weichselbaum RR, *et al. Cancer Medicine,* eighth edition. People's Medical Publishing House: Shelton, CT. 2010.

Monsuez J-J. Detection and prevention of cardiac complications of cancer chemotherapy. *Archives of Cardiovascular Disease.* 2012. 105(6–7): 593–604.

Retter AS. Pericardial disease in the oncology patient. *Heart Disease.* 2006. 4(6): 387–91.

Resuscitation Council (UK). *Advanced Life Support,* sixth edition. Resuscitation Council: London. 2011.

Yeh ET, Tong AT, Lenihan DJ, Yusuf SW, Swafford J, Champion C, *et al.* Cardiovascular complications of cancer therapy: diagnosis, pathogenesis, and management. *Circulation.* 2004. 109(25): 3122–31.

Confusion and decreased conscious level

Delirium and confusion

Delirium has been reported in up to 85% of terminal cancer patients. Although it may be reversible in up to 50% of patients, it is often poorly diagnosed and therefore mismanaged. Delirium is associated with a poor prognosis, longer hospital stay, increased risk of hospital-acquired complications, distress for patients (and their families) and interferes with assessment of symptoms by impairing communication.

Definitions
* *Confusion*: difficulty in thinking coherently, clearly or at normal speed.
* *Delirium*: the acute disruption of attention and cognition, resulting in confusion and disorientation, but without permanent changes in the brain. May be hyperactive, hypoactive or a mixed picture.

Clinical features
The grading of confusion is shown in Table 3.8 and the grading of delirium is broadly similar. There is a constellation of clinical features that may lead to a diagnosis of delirium, which include:
* Reduction in consciousness or ability of patient to focus or shift attention.
* Not accountable by an underlying dementia condition.
* Short evolution of symptoms (hours to days) and variable during the day.
* Cause can be accountable to a medical condition/factor.
* Other symptoms include agitation, disorientation, lethargy, emotional instability, poor memory, hallucinations and disturbance of the sleep-wake cycle.

Causes of confusion and delirium
There are multiple factors which can cause confusion or precipitate delirium. Older patients and patients with multiple comorbidities/polypharmacy have an increased risk of delirium. The main causes to consider are listed below:
* Electrolyte abnormalities or endocrine causes (e.g. hyper/hypoglycaemia).
* Liver or renal failure, MI.

Table 3.8 CTCAE (V4.03) grading of confusion.

Grade	Criteria
1	Mild disorientation.
2	Moderate disorientation; limiting instrumental ADL.
3	Severe disorientation; limiting self-care ADL.
4	Life-threatening consequences; urgent intervention indicated.
5	Death.

From the website of the National Cancer Institute (http://www.cancer.gov).

- Hypoxia (e.g. secondary to pneumonia, PE, LVF or pneumonitis).
- Pain and discomfort, including urinary retention, faecal impaction.
- Inflammation or infection, including meningitis/encephalitis.
- Dehydration or nutritional:
  - Malnutrition, low albumin, Wernicke's encephalopathy
  - Alcohol withdrawal
- Medication: for example, benzodiazepines, antidepressants, opioids, steroids, anticholinergics, dopaminergics, metoclopramide, H2 receptor blockers and cytotoxics (e.g. vincristine).
- Post-ictal state.
- Intracranial causes:
  - Brain metastases/cerebral oedema/haemorrhage/hydrocephalus
  - Cranial surgery or irradiation
  - Cerebral infarction/ischaemia
  - Leptomeningeal disease
  - Progressive multifocal leukoencephalopathy (PML) – immunosuppressed patients (e.g. patients on rituximab) can develop PML secondary to JC virus infection
- Acute encephalopathy: most commonly caused by methotrexate or ifosfamide (see section below on ifosfamide-induced encephalopathy), but can also be caused by paclitaxel, 5-FU, interferon, etoposide, cytosine arabinoside or interleukin-2.
- Recent major surgery.
- Dementia, depression or other psychiatric illnesses.
- Pre-terminal event.

Management
- Assess patients for the presence and severity of confusion. The abbreviated mental test (AMT) shown in Table 3.9 may be helpful but has significant limitations.
- Diagnose and treat any underlying cause, including the withdrawal of any causative medications.
- *Environmental interventions*:
  - Place the patient in a quiet side room in a low stimulation environment.

Table 3.9 Abbreviated mental test.

Question	Score
What is your age?	1
What is the time?	1
Give the patient an address and ask them to repeat it at the end of the test (e.g. 42 West Street)	1
What year is it?	1
Where are we?	1
Recognition of 2 people	1
What is your date of birth?	1
When was WW1?	1
Who is the current monarch?	1
Count backwards from 20	1

Reproduced from Hodkinson HM. Evaluation of a mental test score for assessment of mental impairment in the elderly. *Age and Ageing*. 1972. 1(4): 233–8. (STM opt-out, with permission of Oxford University Press.)

- ○ Explore the possibility of a family member sitting with the patient as reassurance, consider 1:1 nursing and communicate clearly and simply.
- ○ A well-lit environment is preferable as the dark worsens disorientation and confusion (as seen in the phenomena of 'sun downing'). Minimise disruption of patients' normal sleep-wake cycle.
- *Medication*:
  - ○ Caution is needed and a short-acting benzodiazepine should be used in the first instance (e.g. lorazepam). Discussion with liaison psychiatry or an on-call psychiatrist may be helpful.
  - ○ Consider haloperidol 0.5–2 mg every 2–4 hours as needed, with titration to higher doses if patient remains agitated. Parenteral doses are about twice as potent as oral doses.
  - ○ Atypical antipsychotics, for example olanzapine, risperidone, may be used following specialist advice. One of the common side effects of olanzapine is sedation, which may be helpful for agitated patients.
  - ○ Palliative sedation (e.g. with midazolam) may be indicated if a patient has refractory delirium and has a prognosis of hours or days, but it is important to discuss this with patients' families.

Ifosfamide-induced encephalopathy

- Affects up to 50% of patients treated with oral ifosfamide.
- *Symptoms*: somnolence, agitation, confusion, hallucinations, coma, death (rare), disorientation, seizures, personality changes, cerebellar signs, extrapyramidal symptoms, urinary incontinence, decreased level of arousal.

- Starts between 12 to 146 hours after the start of administration, usually spontaneously reverses within 48–72 hours of discontinuing ifosfamide.
- *Risk factors*: more common if oral administration, short infusion time, high dose, poor performance status, renal failure, female, low serum albumin, concomitant cisplatin, brain irradiation, hepatic insufficiency, advanced age, disease confined to the pelvis.
- *Investigations*: brain MRI/CT and biochemistry are usually normal but EEG may be altered in up to 65% of patients.
- *Treatment and prophylaxis*:
  - Refer to local protocols regarding the use of methylene blue
  - Usually self-limiting
  - Consider admission, minimise other medication with other sedating agents
  - Consider a brief course of haloperidol if main features are agitation and hallucinations

Cognitive changes
- Several reviews and meta-analyses have concluded that there is evidence for cognitive changes in oncology patients, but there are methodological problems with many of the published studies.
- *Main changes include*: reduced concentration, verbal and visual memory and processing speed.
- *Cause*: not yet established, may be related to anxiety, depression, fatigue, the cancer itself or its treatment.
- *Treatment*: no specific evidence-based treatment, anecdotal evidence for brain games (e.g. puzzles, Sudoku).

Decreased conscious level
- *Assess*:
  - Airway, breathing, circulation.
  - Neurological status: neurological examination, CTCAE grading and GCS (see Tables 3.10 and 3.11).
  - Likely cause (e.g. any of the causes of confusion, shock, trauma, hypothermia). Check BM.

Table 3.10 CTCAE (V4.03) grading of depressed level of consciousness.

Grade	Criteria
1	Decreased level of alertness.
2	Sedation; slow response to stimuli; limiting instrumental ADL.
3	Difficult to rouse.
4	Life-threatening consequences.
5	Death.

From the website of the National Cancer Institute (http://www.cancer.gov).

Table 3.11 Glasgow Coma Scale (GCS).

	Best response	Score
Eye opening	Spontaneous eye opening.	4
	Eye opening in response to speech (in response to any speech or shout).	3
	Eye opening in response to pain.	2
	No eye opening.	1
Verbal response	Orientated (knows where he/she is and why, the year, season and month).	5
	Confused conversation (responds in a conversational manner but there is some disorientation and confusion).	4
	Inappropriate speech (random or exclamatory articulated speech, but no conversational exchange).	3
	Incomprehensible speech (moaning but no words).	2
	None.	1
Motor response	Obeys commands (patient does simple things you ask).	6
	Localising response to pain (purposeful movements towards changing painful stimuli).	5
	Withdraws to pain (pulls limb away from painful stimulus).	4
	Flexor response to pain (stimulus causes abnormal flexion of limbs).	3
	Extensor posturing to pain (stimulus causes limb extension).	2
	No response to pain.	1
Maximum score		15

Reprinted from *Lancet*, 2 (7872), Teasdale G, Jennett B, Assessment of coma and impaired consciousness. A practical scale, 81–4, 1974, with permission from Elsevier.

- *Management*:
  - ○ Control any seizures.
  - ○ Treat likely cause.
  - ○ Review if escalation to HDU/ITU is appropriate (and ensure family are fully informed).

References

Breitbart W, Alici Y. Evidence-based treatment of delirium in patients with cancer. *Journal of Clinical Oncology*. 2012. 30(11): 1206–14.

Hodkinson HM. Evaluation of a mental test score for assessment of mental impairment in the elderly. *Age and Ageing.* 1972. 1(4): 233–8.

Kang JH, Shin SH, Bruera E. Comprehensive approaches to managing delirium in patients with advanced cancer. *Cancer Treatment Reviews.* 2013. 39(1): 105–12.

Nicolao P, Giometto B. Neurological toxicity of ifosfamide. *Oncology.* 2003. 65(Suppl. 2): 11–6.

Pelgrims J, De Vos F, Van den Brande J, Schrijvers D, Prove A, Vermorken JB. Methylene blue in the treatment and prevention of ifosfamide-induced encephalopathy: report of 12 cases and a review of the literature. *British Journal of Cancer.* 2000. 82(2): 291–4.

Teasdale G, Jennett B. Assessment of coma and impaired consciousness. *A practical scale. Lancet.* 1974. 2(7872): 81–4.

Vardy J, Wefel JS, Ahles T, Tannock IF, Schagen SB. Cancer and cancer-therapy related cognitive dysfunction: an international perspective from the Venice cognitive workshop. *Annals of Oncology.* 2008. 19(4): 623–9.

Constipation

Constipation is defined as difficulty in defecation. It may lead to infrequent stools, difficulty passing stools or incomplete defecation. It is estimated that 80% of those with a cancer diagnosis will experience some degree of constipation. Faecal impaction (or obstipation) is the retention of faeces to the point where spontaneous resolution is unlikely. The grading of constipation is shown in Table 3.12.

Causes

Functional constipation is chronic constipation without a known cause. Secondary constipation is a result of medication or a medical condition. The most important differential diagnosis is bowel obstruction. However, once this has been ruled out, the following causes should be considered:

- Medication: for example chemotherapy, anti-emetics, opioids, iron or calcium supplements
- Cancer: for example pelvic/rectal masses, hypercalcaemia
- Lifestyle: dietary fibre, dehydration, lack of exercise
- Neurological: for example metastatic spinal cord compression, nerve damage from pelvic surgery/cancer, Parkinson's disease/syndrome, multiple sclerosis

Table 3.12 CTCAE (V4.03) grading of constipation.

Grade	Criteria
1	Occasional or intermittent symptoms; occasional use of stool softeners, laxatives, dietary modification, or enema.
2	Persistent symptoms, with regular use of laxative or enemas; limiting instrumental ADL.
3	Obstipation with manual evacuation indicated; limiting self-care ADL.
4	Life-threatening consequences; urgent intervention indicated.
5	Death.

From the website of the National Cancer Institute (http://www.cancer.gov).

- Depression and anxiety
- Other conditions:
  - Hypothyroidism
  - Diabetes
  - Anal fissure, haemorrhoids – may be a result of constipation, but may also exacerbate condition

Symptoms

- Early symptoms include: difficult stool and pain, less than three bowel movements per week, bloating.
- More severe symptoms include: abdominal distension, overflow diarrhoea, anorexia, nausea and vomiting.

Management

Early/mild constipation:

- Identify and modify exacerbating factors (e.g. medication).
- Lifestyle advice, increase mobility, encourage oral fluids.
- Use of laxatives:
  - Especially important with continuous opiate use.
  - NICE recommend a combination of stimulant and softening laxative (such as senna and lactulose).

Severe constipation:

- History and examination (including PR if appropriate – not in patients with platelets < 20 or neutrophils < 0.5) to exclude bowel obstruction.
- Bloods, including FBC, U&E, LFT, bone profile.
- AXR.
- Withhold or modify exacerbating medications.
- If not obstructed:
  - Titrate oral laxative
    - Regular use of laxative as above. Starting with stimulant and softener such as senna and docusate, with some evidence for efficacy of adding lactulose as well. Co-danthramer may also be effective, but is recommended only in palliative patients.
    - Addition/substitution for Movicol® regularly starting with one sachet BD, titrating to two sachets TDS.
  - If ineffective:
    - High stool (not palpable on PR) – consider eight sachets of Movicol® in one litre of fluid over six hours.
    - Low stool (palpable on PR):
      - Glycerol suppository or mini-enema (e.g. docusate).
      - Then phosphate enema. Enemas may need to be repeated in severe cases.
- If constipation remains after trying the above: take specialist advice.
- Although manual evacuation is on the CTC criteria it is not commonly used in practice without undertaking the above steps and first taking specialist advice.

References

Cancer Research UK. Constipation. Available from: http://www.cancerresearchuk.org/cancer-help/coping-with-cancer/coping-physically/bowel/ (accessed 1 January 2014).

National Institute for Health and Care Excellence. *Palliative Cancer Care – Constipation*. Available from: http://cks.nice.org.uk/ (accessed 1 January 2014).

National Institute for Health and Care Excellence. Constipation. Available from: http://cks.nice.org.uk/ (accessed 1 January 2014).

Dental disorders

General dental advice
- Poor oral health is associated with an increase in the incidence and severity of oral complications. Patients should be advised to brush their teeth, gums and tongue gently after every meal and at bedtime, to avoid alcohol mouthwashes and to use saline or sodium bicarbonate rinses.
- Advise patients to see their dentist and have any oral problems such as periodontal disease, pulpal infections, dental caries and poorly fitting dentures treated prior to starting oncology treatment if possible. Ideally, oral surgery should be completed at least 7–10 days before starting myelosuppressive therapy or 14 days prior to radiotherapy.
- Consider the use of prophylactic antibiotics if dental procedures need to be performed in patients with central venous catheters *in situ*.
- If dental procedures need to be performed during chemotherapy then check the patient's FBC and clotting:
  - If platelets < 75 1 x 10^9/L or abnormal clotting: postpone dental surgery if possible or consider platelet transfusion/correcting clotting abnormalities.
  - If neutrophils < 1 x 10^9/L: postpone dental work if possible or give prophylactic IV antibiotics.
  - If neutrophils $1–2.1$ x 10^9/L: consider prophylactic antibiotics.

Osteonecrosis of the jaw
- *Definition*: a disorder characterised by a necrotic process occurring in the bones of the jaw. See Table 3.13 for the grading of osteonecrosis.
- Causes include treatment with bisphosphonates, denosumab and radiotherapy.
- *Symptoms and signs*: an area of exposed, non-healing bone in the maxillofacial region for at least eight weeks (within the treatment area if the patient received radiotherapy), pain, altered/decreased sensation, inflammation, secondary infection, tooth mobility and fistula formation.

Post-radiotherapy osteonecrosis (PRON)
- The incidence of PRON ranges from 2.6 to 22% of patients receiving radical radiotherapy to the jaw, with the mandible being more commonly affected than the maxilla.

Table 3.13 CTCAE (V4.03) grading of osteonecrosis.

Grade	Criteria
1	Asymptomatic; clinical or diagnostic observations only; intervention not indicated.
2	Symptomatic; medical intervention indicated (e.g. topical agents); limiting instrumental ADL.
3	Severe symptoms; limiting self-care ADL; elective operative intervention indicated.
4	Life-threatening consequences, urgent intervention indicated.
5	Death.

From the website of the National Cancer Institute (http://www.cancer.gov).

- *Risk factors*: tooth extraction/dental trauma, oral infection, high radiotherapy dose or large volume of tissue irradiated.
- *Prevention strategies*: all patients receiving head and neck radiotherapy should have a thorough pre-treatment dental assessment. If possible, questionable teeth should be extracted at least 14 days (preferably at least 21 days) prior to radiotherapy and dental extraction during radiotherapy should be avoided.

Bisphosphonate-related osteonecrosis (BRON)
- Occurs in approximately 5 out of every 100 patients who receive bisphosphonates; 65% of cases affect the mandible, 26% the maxilla and 9% both sites.
- *Risk factors*:
  - Use of potent bisphosphonates: pamidronate is 10 times and zoledronic acid 10,000 times more potent than clodronate. The mean time of onsent of BRON is 6 years with pamidronate but only 18 months with zoledronic acid.
  - IV rather than oral bisphosphonates.
  - Longer duration of bisphosphonate treatment.
  - Dental procedures (60% of cases are preceded by a dental procedure).
  - Co-existent inflammatory dental disease.
  - Possibly also associated with poor oral hygiene.
  - Patients with bony prominences with thin overlying mucosa.
- Patients should have a dental review prior to starting long-term bisphosphonate therapy.
- Bisphosphonates should be stopped prior to elective dental procedures. However, there is no clear evidence regarding the most appropriate timeframe, so follow local guidelines. Suggestions include stopping treatment a minimum of 4–12 weeks prior to dental procedures and waiting for a further 4–12 weeks after dental work is completed prior to restarting bisphosphonate therapy.

Management of PRON or BRON
- Refer patients with suspected PRON or BRON to a specialist dentist/maxillofacial surgeon.

- An X-ray (orthopantomogram) or CT may be helpful to confirm the diagnosis, revealing osseous sclerosis or a 'ground glass' appearance, but symptoms may predate radiographic changes by weeks or months.
- Discontinue the use of tobacco and alcohol.
- Analgesia.
- Chlorhexidine rinses 2–3 times a day.
- Topical antibiotics (e.g. tetracycline) for PRON; consider oral antibiotics for BRON if evidence of infection (some experts also recommend the chronic use of antibiotics such as penicillin, cephalexin or a first-generation fluoroquinolone).
- Hyperbaric oxygen therapy for PRON (if available).
- Consider stopping bisphosphonate treatment.
- Surgical management may include:
  - Debridement/resection of affected areas.
  - Removal of symptomatic teeth (this is unlikely to exacerbate the condition).
  - Removal of bone sequestra (as long as this does not expose unaffected areas of bone).
  - Advanced lesions may require reconstruction.

References

National Cancer Institute. PDQ® Oral Complications of Chemotherapy and Head/Neck Radiation 2012. Available from: http://cancer.gov/cancertopics/pdq/supportivecare/oral-complications/HealthProfessional (accessed 1 January 2014).

National Institute of Dental and Craniofacial Research. *Dental Provider's Oncology Pocket Guide: Prevention and Management of Oral Complications*. 2009. Available from: http://www.nidcr.nih.gov/OralHealth/Topics/CancerTreatment/ReferenceGuideforOncologyPatients.htm (accessed 1 January 2014).

Sciubba J, Epstein J. Bisphosphonate-related osteonecrosis of the jaw. In: Davies N, Epstein J, (eds). *Oral Complications of Cancer and its Management*. Oxford University Press: Oxford. 2010. pp. 151–63.

Spijkervet F, Vissink A. Post-radiation osteonecrosis (osteoradionecrosis) of the jaw. In: Davies A, Epstein J, (eds). *Oral Complications of Cancer and its Management*. Oxford University Press: Oxford. 2010. pp. 117–22.

Diarrhoea

Diarrhoea is defined as a disorder characterised by frequent and watery bowel movements. The grading of diarrhoea is shown in Table 3.14.

Symptoms and signs
- *History*: frequency, volume, character (e.g. bloody, watery) and duration of diarrhoea, presence of nocturnal diarrhoea, associated symptoms (e.g. vomiting, pain), oral intake, any contact with other people with diarrhoea and recent

Table 3.14 CTCAE (V4.03) grading of diarrhoea.

Grade	Criteria
1	Increase of <4 stools daily over baseline. Mild increase in colostomy output as compared with baseline.
2	Increase of 4–6 stools daily over baseline. IV fluids indicated <24 hours. Moderate increase in colostomy output compared with baseline. Not interfering with ADL.
3	Increase of ≥7 stools daily over baseline. Incontinence, IV fluids ≥24 hours, hospitalisation. Severe increase in colostomy output compared with baseline. Interfering with ADL.
4	Life threatening consequences (e.g. haemodynamic collapse).
5	Death.

From the website of the National Cancer Institute (http://www.cancer.gov).

antibiotic use. Review any past medical history which might indicate the likely cause of the diarrhoea.

- *Signs*: dehydration, abdominal tenderness/guarding, fever.

Differential diagnoses and their management
Infective diarrhoea
- Send stool cultures (including for ova, amoeba, parasites and strongyloides if recent steroid use).
- *Clostridium difficile* associated colitis can occur even if there is no recent antibiotic use, particularly in patients receiving dose-dense regimes of paclitaxel. Treat according to local guidelines, for example mild cases: metronidazole 500 mg TDS for 10–14 days, severe cases: vancomycin 125 mg QDS for 10–14 days.

Chemotherapy-induced diarrhoea (CID)
- Can be life-threatening due to dehydration, electrolyte imbalances and renal failure.
- *Risk factors*: female, older age, performance status ≥2, bowel tumour, associated bowel pathology, concomitant radiotherapy.
- *Commonest causes*: fluoropyrimidines (e.g. capecitabine, 5-FU – especially bolus 5-FU) and irinotecan.
- *Other causes include*: cisplatin, docetaxel, paclitaxel, oxaliplatin, cyclophosphamide, methotrexate, pemetrexed, cabazitaxel, bortezomib, lapatinib, erlotinib, gefitinib, sorafenib, sunitinib, imatinib, everolimus, temsirolimus, ipilimumab and cetuximab.
- Severe diarrhoea and mucositis in the first cycle of 5-FU or capecitabine may be due to DPD deficiency (DPD is an enzyme involved in the metabolism of 5-FU to inactive metabolites).
- Irinotecan-induced diarrhoea can be 'early' or 'late'.
  - *Early*: occurs during or within hours of drug administration. Associated with lacrimation, cramping and rhinitis. Relieved by atropine 0.25 mg SC.

- *Late*: median time of onset of six days with the three-weekly schedule and eleven days with the weekly schedule.
- Ipilimumab is used in advanced melanoma and can cause severe, life-threatening enterocolitis (seek specialist advice):
  - If grade 3–4, stop ipilimumab permanently and give high dose corticosteroids (if no bowel perforation), for example 2 mg/kg/day IV methylprednisolone.
  - If moderate enterocolitis, withhold ipilimumab, give anti-diarrhoeal medication and start steroids, for examle PO prednisolone 1 mg/kg if diarrhoea persists for > 1 week.
  - Consider colonoscopy if ≥ grade 2.

Guidelines for the management of chemotherapy-induced diarrhoea

1 Uncomplicated grade 1–2 diarrhoea:
  (a) Dietary advice:
    (i) Avoid: milk/dairy products, alcohol, spicy foods, high fat and high fibre foods, caffeine-containing products, some fruit juices (e.g. orange or prune juice), sorbitol containing products (e.g. sugar free gum).
    (ii) Recommend: oral rehydration (8–10 large glasses a day) with fluids containing water, salt and sugar (e.g. broth, non-carbonated soft drinks). Frequent small meals (BRAT diet – bananas, rice, apples, toast, plain pasta).
  (b) Loperamide: initial 4 mg dose then 2 mg every four hours or after every loose stool. Stop when diarrhoea free for 12 hours.
  (c) Hold cytotoxic if diarrhoea grade 2 until symptoms resolve.
  (d) If not resolved after 12–24 hours:
    (i) Stool sample
    (ii) Increase loperamide to 2 mg 2 hourly (max 24 mg daily)
    (iii) Start oral antibiotics, for example ciprofloxacin 500 mg BD
    (iv) Consider codeine phosphate 30–60 mg QDS
  (e) If diarrhoea hasn't resolved after 24–48 hours but no adverse features:
    (i) Clinical review, bloods, send stool culture, refer to dietician
    (ii) Stop loperamide and consider second line agents, for example:
      - Octreotide (a synthetic long-acting somatostatin analogue). Start at 100–150 mcg SC TDS, may need to increase up to 500 mcg TDS. Side effects: bloating, cramping, flatulence, fat malabsorption, hypoglycaemia and hypersensitivity-like reactions
      - Budesonide CR capsules 9 mg OD PO.
2 Complicated diarrhoea (grade 3–4 or grade 1–2 with adverse features, for example fever, sepsis, neutropenia, nausea or vomiting ≥ grade 2, decreased performance status, dehydration, cramping, frank bleeding):
  (a) Admit to hospital for IV fluids, electrolyte replacement, stool culture.
  (b) Start octreotide at 100–150 μg SC TDS or 25–50 μg/hr IV (may need to increase up to 500 μg TDS).
  (c) Discontinue cytotoxic drugs and consider dose reduction for the next cycle (refer to local policy).
  (d) Antibiotics, for example ciprofloxacin 500 mg BD.

Neutropaenic enterocolitis/typhilitis

- Life threatening, commonest in neutropaenic patients with haematological malignancies.
- Caecum is almost always affected but can extend into ascending colon and terminal ileum. Typhilitis occurs in ileocaecal region only.
- *Symptoms/signs*: fever, abdominal pain (usually right lower quadrant), watery or bloody diarrhoea. Mimics appendicitis but presence of lower GI bleeding suggests typhilitis.
- *Investigations*:
  - AXR and CT (more sensitive) may show bowel wall thickening and a fluid-filled, dilated caecum. Perforation or abscess formation can occur.
  - Colonoscopy is relatively contraindicated due to the risk of perforation but flexible sigmoidoscopy can be performed if necessary to exclude other causes such as pseudomembranous colitis.
- *Management*:
Conservative:
  - IV fluids, bowel rest, NG suction.
  - Broad spectrum antibiotics (polymicrobial infection is common and bacteraemia or fungaemia can occur). Add fluconazole or amphotericin B if neutropenic with protracted fever (> 72 hours) despite antibiotics.
  - Nutritional and blood product support.
  - Avoid anticholinergics, opiates and anti-diarrhoeal agents as they may worsen ileus.
  - Consider GCSF.
- Consider surgery (usually a two-stage right hemicolectomy) if evidence of peritonitis, persistent GI bleeding (despite correcting coagulopathies), perforation or clinical deterioration.

Ischaemic colitis

- Similar presentation to that of neutropenic entercolitis (although patient may not be neutropenic).
- Can rarely occur with docetaxel, usually 4–10 days post administration.

Small bowel bacterial overgrowth

- *Causes include*: short bowel syndrome, strictures, chronic pancreatitis, decreased gut motility (e.g. secondary to drugs, diabetes, radiation enteritis), resection of the ileocaecal valve.
- Leads to malabsorption of fats, vitamin B12 and bile salts. Can lead to systemic sepsis
- *Diagnosis*: breath test. Jejunal aspirate is the gold standard but is more invasive.
- *Management*:
  - Treat underlying cause if possible.
  - Avoid drugs which decrease gut motility (e.g. narcotics).

- o Prokinetics may be helpful (e.g. metoclopramide, domperidone).
- o Advise avoidance of high carbohydrate foods as they can cause sudden osmotic fluid losses and increase bacterial proliferation. Suggest avoiding lactose-containing foods as lactase deficiency is common. Probiotics may be helpful.
- o Give a seven-day course of antibiotics, for example rifaximin 1200 mg/day, norfloxacin 400 mg BD, co-amoxiclav 625 mg TDS, metronidazole 250 mg TDS.

Pancreatic insufficiency
- Consider in patients with pancreatic or biliary malignancy.
- *Diagnosis*: measure faecal elastase.
- *Management*:
  - o Advise a low fat diet and start exogenous pancreatic enzymes, for example Creon® 10,000 capsules (1–2 capsules with each meal, dose increased as required).
  - o Give H2 receptor antagonists or PPIs along with the enzymes to reduce inactivation by gastric acid.

Bile acid diarrhoea
- Caused by excess bile acids in the colon.
- *Causes include*: ileal resection, cholecystectomy, pancreatic insufficiency and small intestinal bacterial overgrowth.
- *Diagnosis*: the best diagnostic test is the SeHCAT test (selenium-labelled bile acid administration, then a whole body scan or gamma camera after seven days) but this is often not available. If no tests are available, consider an empirical trial of a bile acid sequestrant (e.g. colestyramine).
- *Management*:
  - o Most patients will respond to colestyramine (dosing regimen is not fully established but the BNF suggests starting at 4 g daily, increased by 4 g at weekly intervals to 12–24 g daily in 1–4 divided doses as required). Colestyramine is difficult to tolerate due to its taste and texture and can cause nausea, cramps and constipation.
  - o Colesevelem is an alternative which is better tolerated (but currently unlicensed for diarrhoea) at a dose of 1.25–3.75 g/day.

Other causes include:
- Radiotherapy (see Chapter 5, management of early lower gastrointestinal toxicity section).
- Constipation and overflow diarrhoea.
- Hyperthyroidism.
- Inflammatory bowel conditions.
- Medications (including pro-motility drugs, PPIs, antacids with magnesium, antibiotics, colchicine, potassium supplements, theophylline, NSAIDs, bulk laxatives and stool softeners).
- Subacute bowel obstruction.

Other relevant sections of this book
Chapter 5, section on lower gastrointestinal side effects

References

Benson AB, 3rd, Ajani JA, Catalano RB, Engelking C, Kornblau SM, Martenson JA, Jr., *et al.* Recommended guidelines for the treatment of cancer treatment-induced diarrhea. *Journal of Clinical Oncology.* 2004. 22(14): 2918–26.

Bristol-Myers Squibb. Immune-mediated adverse reactions management guide. Available from: http://www.yervoy.co.uk/Images/1233_Clean%20copy%20irAR%20UKIPA0006_ v11_MECH.pdf (accessed 1 January 2014).

Quigley EM, Quera R. Small intestinal bacterial overgrowth: roles of antibiotics, prebiotics, and probiotics. *Gastroenterology.* 2006. 130(2 Suppl. 1): S78–90.

Sinicrope FA, Levin B. Gastrointestinal complications. In: Bast RJ, Kufe D, Pollock R, Weichselbaum R, Holland J, Frei E (eds). *Holland-Frei Cancer Medicine,* fifth edition. BC Decker: Hamilton. 2000.

Stein A, Voigt W, Jordan K. Chemotherapy-induced diarrhea: pathophysiology, frequency and guideline-based management. *Therapeutic Advances in Medical Oncology.* 2010. 2(1): 51–63.

Walters JR, Pattni SS. Managing bile acid diarrhoea. *Therapeutic Advances in Gastroenterology.* 2010. 3(6): 349–57.

Dysphagia

Dysphagia is defined as the difficult passage of food from the mouth to the stomach during one or more of the three phases of normal swallowing (i.e. oral, pharyngeal, oesophageal). The grading of dysphagia is shown in Table 3.15.

Symptoms and signs
- The patient may indicate the level of obstruction (e.g. oropharyngeal versus oesophageal) or report difficulty coordinating the swallowing movement (which is suggestive of a neurological cause).
- Establish if both solids and liquids are equally affected:
  - Solids affected first – usually an oesophageal cause.
  - Liquids affected first – usually a pharyngeal cause.
  - Both solids and liquids from the start – suggestive of a motility disorder.
- Assess symptom duration:
  - Intermittent symptoms may be due to oesophageal spasm.
  - Constant, progressive symptoms are suggestive of a malignant stricture.
- Associated symptoms/signs:
  - Oropharyngeal dysphagia is often associated with difficulty initiating swallowing, nasal regurgitation, coughing and choking.
  - Painful swallowing may be due to malignancy, oesophagitis, achalasia or oesophageal spasm.
  - Dysphagia can cause malnutrition, dehydration, cachexia and weight loss.
  - Effects on quality of life: for example frustration, anxiety and depression.

Table 3.15 CTCAE (V4.03) grading of dysphagia.

Grade	Criteria
1	Symptomatic, able to eat regular diet.
2	Symptomatic and altered eating/swallowing.
3	Severely altered eating/swallowing; tube feeding or TPN or hospitalisation indicated.
4	Life-threatening consequences, urgent intervention indicated.
5	Death.

From the website of the National Cancer Institute (http://www.cancer.gov)

Causes
- *Tumours*: for example oral, pharyngeal, oesophageal, gastric, intrathoracic disease (e.g. lung cancer, lymphoma) and some brain tumours.
- *Radiation*: head and neck radiotherapy and thoracic radiotherapy can cause oedema, strictures and/or nerve and tissue damage.
- *Surgery*: for example head and neck surgery, oesophagectomy.
- *Infections*: for example oesophageal candidiasis.
- *Non-malignant causes*: for example motility disorders, neurological disorders.

Investigations
- OGD is usually the investigation of choice, but barium swallow can also be helpful (particularly for motility disorders).
- CT chest/abdomen/pelvis can show external compression.
- ENT review if head and neck cancer.

Management
General management
- Refer all patients to a dietician, who can advise on appropriate supplements.
- Advise patients to eat small, frequent meals that are high in protein and energy and to sit upright after eating.
- Consider referral to SALT if the patient is coughing or choking when eating/drinking to assess risk of aspiration, which food consistencies are best tolerated and provide advice regarding swallowing techniques.
- Consider if further nutritional support is required (e.g. PEG feeding in patients with head and neck cancer undergoing radiotherapy). Patients undergoing head and neck radiotherapy may have had prophylactic placement of a RIG or PEG.

Management of oesophageal strictures
There are a variety of different techniques that can be used to relieve dysphagia due to oesophageal strictures and the choice of procedure depends on:
- Local availability.
- Need for rapid symptom relief (stenting provides the fastest relief of symptoms).
- Patient's prognosis (radiotherapy, laser therapy or PDT are more appropriate than stenting in patients with a longer life expectancy).

Palliative radiotherapy

- May involve external beam radiotherapy and/or brachytherapy (however, brachytherapy may not be available locally).
- *Effectiveness*:
  - Radiation oesophagitis can cause an initial worsening of dysphagia before subsequent improvement.
  - It takes a few weeks before symptoms improve.
  - Best results are seen in patients with mild dysphagia who are managing at least a semi-solid diet.
  - Brachytherapy is superior to stenting if patients live for longer than 20 weeks.
- *Side effects/complications include*: post-treatment strictures, formation of tracheo-oesophageal fistulae.

Oesophageal stenting

- Stents may be metal or plastic and may be partially or fully covered.
- *Effectiveness*:
  - More than 90% of self-expanding metal stents are successfully deployed and relieve dysphagia in up to 95% of patients. Self-expanding plastic stents are similar but can be repositioned or removed if needed and cause less chest pain.
  - Results in a rapid improvement in symptoms within days of stent insertion.
  - Symptoms recur in approximately 20% of patients by ten weeks due to tumour overgrowth, stent migration or blockage.

Laser therapy

- Uses a neodymium yttrium aluminum garnet (Nd:YAG) laser to vaporise malignant tissue to restore luminal patency.
- Usually involves 3–4 outpatient treatments, which are performed every other day.
- May be combined with radiotherapy, which prolongs the interval between treatments but leads to an increased risk of strictures and fistulae.
- *Effectiveness*:
  - Successfully relieves dysphagia in >90% of appropriately selected patients, that is, patients with exophytic tumours that are not infiltrating and not associated with tight strictures.
  - Can be used for tumours near the upper oesophageal sphincter, where stents are contraindicated.
  - Usually needs to be repeated every 4–6 weeks due to tumour regrowth.
  - Associated with lower mortality and better quality of life than stenting. Therefore, if available, laser (or PDT) therapy is recommended in some guidelines as the first-line treatment for patients with exophytic tumours.
- *Side effects/complications include*: perforation (occurs in <5% of patients).

Photodynamic therapy (PDT)

- Uses a photosensitising agent and a non-thermal laser to ablate tissue.
- Is technically easier to perform than Nd:YAG laser therapy.

- *Effectiveness*:
  - Post-treatment oesophagitis can lead to an initial worsening of dysphagia.
  - Can be used for tumours near the upper oesophageal sphincter, where stents are contraindicated.
  - More effective than Nd:YAG laser therapy and leads to longer responses.
  - Associated with lower mortality and better quality of life than stenting. Therefore, if available, PDT (or laser) therapy is recommended in some guidelines as the first-line treatment for patients with exophytic tumours.
- *Side effects/complications*: in comparison with Nd:YAG laser therapy, PDT is associated with more minor side effects such as photosensitivity, but fewer major complications (e.g. perforation).

Other techniques

- *Argon plasma coagulation*:
  - Not widely used but may be comparable to Nd:YAG laser therapy and PDT.
  - Can be used to control tumour regrowth in patients with stents.
- *Surgery*: not recommended due to the high mortality rate.
- *Chemotherapy*: can improve dysphagia and so may be appropriate for patients with a good performance status (but may lead to other chemotherapy-induced toxicities).
- *Oesophageal dilatation*:
  - May be used following surgery or radiotherapy to dilate recurrent benign or malignant strictures.
  - Leads to an immediate improvement in symptoms. However, dilatation is not usually recommended as the improvement only lasts for approximately two weeks and therefore repeat procedures are needed.
  - There is a small risk of oesophageal perforation.

Other relevant sections of this book

- Chapter 3, section on anorexia and nutrition
- Chapter 5, section on upper gastrointestinal side effects
- Chapter 9, section on oesophageal stents and dilatation

References

Hanna WC, Sudarshan M, Roberge D, David M, Waschke KA, Mayrand S, *et al*. What is the optimal management of dysphagia in metastatic esophageal cancer? *Current Oncology*. 2012. 19(2): e60–6.

Javle M, Ailawadhi S, Yang GY, Nwogu CE, Schiff MD, Nava HR. Palliation of malignant dysphagia in esophageal cancer: a literature-based review. *Journal of Supportive Oncology*. 2006. 4(8): 365–73, 79.

Malagelada J, Bazzoli F, Elewaut A, Fried M, Krabshuis J, Lindberg G, *et al*. World Gastroenterology Organisation practice guidelines: dysphagia 2007. Available from: http://www.worldgastroenterology.org/dysphagia.html (accessed 1 January 2014).

Scottish Intercollegiate Guidelines Network (SIGN). *Management of Oesophageal and Gastric Cancer*. A National Clinical Guideline no. 87. 2006. SIGN: Edinburgh. 2006. Available from: http://www.sign.ac.uk (accessed 1 January 2014).

Fatigue

Fatigue is defined as a disorder characterised by a state of generalised weakness with a pronounced inability to summon sufficient energy to accomplish daily activities. The grading of fatigue is shown in Table 3.16. Fatigue can be a significant side-effect of chemotherapy and radiotherapy and may influence treatment choice or patient adherence with treatment.

Overview
- Fatigue is reported by 60–90% of cancer patients, most often whilst undergoing chemotherapy.
- Symptoms may be cumulative, especially in patients on targeted treatments, where treatment may be for many months or even years.
- Fatigue can last months to years following completion of treatment and therefore is also an important consideration for cancer survivors; 33% of patients report fatigue five years after completion of treatment.
- Fatigue can be a very emotive area for patients and carers as expectations of both groups may conflict with actual symptoms; and fatigue can also have social and financial effects.

Management
Contributory factors
- Treat reversible causes of fatigue, for example anaemia, hypothyroidism, hypoadrenalism, malnutrition, alcohol/substance abuse, medication side effects or comorbidities.
- Treat other symptoms which may be contributing to the fatigue, for example pain, depression or anxiety.

Table 3.16 CTCAE (V4.03) grading of fatigue.

Grade	Criteria
1	Fatigue relieved by rest.
2	Fatigue not relieved by rest; limiting instrumental ADL.
3	Fatigue not relieved by rest; limiting self-care ADL.
4	—
5	—

From the website of the National Cancer Institute (http://www.cancer.gov).

Exercise
- A meta-analysis showed that aerobic exercise significantly reduced fatigue:
  - The effect is greater in patients post treatment than in patients on treatment.
  - The majority of studies to date have been in breast cancer patients. Significant benefit was seen in breast and prostate cancer patients but not in patients with haemotological malignancies.
- Exercise may have a palliative effect for patients on treatment and aids recuperation in those post treatment.
- The evidence is conflicting as to whether exercise significantly improves anxiety or depression.
- The most effective type and duration of exercise is currently unclear and needs prospective evaluation.

Psychosocial interventions
- Education about fatigue, coping techniques and activity management (balance between activity and rest) significantly improves fatigue.
- Psychotherapy and cognitive behavioural therapy can also significantly improve fatigue.
- However, the majority of Phase III trials of psychosocial interventions have been performed in breast cancer patients and the effect of the intervention on fatigue was often not sustained during follow-up.

Pharmacological interventions
- Psychostimulants:
  - *Methylphenidate*: initial trials suggested a possible beneficial effect, but this was not confirmed in a Phase III randomised controlled trial.
  - *Modafenil*:
    - Dose: in one trial, patients were started on 100 mg daily of modafenil and this was increased to 200 mg daily after three days.
    - Has shown some benefit in clinical trials in patients with severe baseline fatigue, but not in mild or moderate fatigue.
  - *Dexamphetamine*: trials have shown no significant effect on fatigue.
- Antidepressants
A placebo-controlled trial with paroxetine showed no improvement in fatigue. Bupropion may alleviate symptoms of fatigue but this needs prospective evaluation.
- Steroids
Studies with medroxyprogesterone acetate and megestrol acetate have not shown a significant effect on fatigue.
- Erythropoesis stimulating agents:
  - In anaemic patients on chemotherapy, both erythropoietin and darbopoetin showed a significant improvement in cancer-related fatigue compared to placebo or standard care.
  - However, trials of erythropoesis stimulating agents in cancer patients have also shown a significant risk of death and thrombovascular events.

- Supplements:
  - Trials have not shown any evidence that ginseng, L-carnitine and co-enzyme Q10 help with cancer-related fatigue.
  - Guarana may significantly improve fatigue but these effects may be due to caffeine.

Other relevant sections of this book
Chapter 3, sections on anaemia, psychiatric disorders

References

Auret KA, Schug SA, Bremner AP, Bulsara M. A randomized, double-blind, placebo-controlled trial assessing the impact of dexamphetamine on fatigue in patients with advanced cancer. *Journal Pain Symptom Management.* 2009. 37(4): 613–21.

Cramp F, Byron-Daniel J. Exercise for the management of cancer-related fatigue in adults *Cochrane Database of Systematic Reviews.* 2012. 11: CD006145.

Goedendorp MM, Gielissen MFM, Verhagen CAHHVM, Bleijenberg G. Psychosocial interventions for reducing fatigue during cancer treatment in adults. *Cochrane Database of Systematic Reviews.* 2009. Issue 1. Art. No.: CD006953.

Jean-Pierre P, Morrow GR, Roscoe JA, Heckler C, Mohile S, Janelsins M, *et al.* A phase 3 randomized, placebo-controlled, double-blind, clinical trial of the effect of modafinil on cancer-related fatigue among 631 patients receiving chemotherapy: a University of Rochester Cancer Center Community Clinical Oncology Program Research base study. *Cancer.* 2010. 116(14): 3513–20.

Minton O, Richardson A, Sharpe M, Hotopf M, Stone P. Drug therapy for the management of cancer-related fatigue. *Cochrane Database of Systematic Reviews.* 2010. Issue 7 (7): CD006704.

Pachman DR, Barton DL, Swetz KM, Loprinzi CL. Troublesome symptoms in cancer survivors: fatigue, insomnia, neuropathy, and pain. *Journal of Clinical Oncology.* 2012. 30(30): 3687–96.

Puetz TW, Herring MP. Differential effects of exercise on cancer-related fatigue during and following treatment: a meta-analysis. *American Journal of Preventative Medicine.* 2012. 43(2): e1–24.

Fertility and pregnancy

Fertility

- Infertility is defined as inability to conceive after one year of intercourse without contraception. The grading of oligospermia is shown in Table 3.17 and the grading of irregular menstruation is shown in Table 3.18.
- Cancer treatments including surgery, chemotherapy and radiation can adversely affect fertility or predispose the patient to early gonadal failure.
- Surveys have shown increased risk of distress and poorer quality of life in cancer survivors that are infertile after treatment. There is also some evidence that patients would choose a treatment regimen with a lower risk of infertility even if it were not as efficacious.

Table 3.17 CTCAE (V4.03) grading of oligospermia.

Grade	Criteria
1	Sperm concentration >48 million/ml or motility >68%.
2	Sperm concentration 13–48 million/ml or motility 32–68%.
3	Sperm concentration <13 million/ml or motility <32%.
4	—
5	—

From the website of the National Cancer Institute (http://www.cancer.gov).

Table 3.18 CTCAE (V4.03) grading of irregular menstruation.

Grade	Criteria
1	Intermittent menses with skipped menses for no more than 1–3 months.
2	Intermittent menses with skipped menses for more than 4–6 months.
3	Persistent amenorrhoea for more than six months.
4	—
5	—

From the website of the National Cancer Institute (http://www.cancer.gov).

- Discussions with patients are required early in the treatment pathway to facilitate early referral to fertility specialists. Some methods of female fertility preservation may delay initiation of chemotherapy by up to six weeks.
- Female fertility may be compromised despite the return of regular menses as a decrease in ovulatory reserve may reduce the chances of conception and precipitate earlier ovarian failure.

Factors influencing fertility post treatment
- Chemotherapy agents used (see Tables 3.19 and 3.20)
- Location of radiation field
- Increasing age of patient
- Sex of patient
- Pre-treatment fertility
- Dose intensity (see Tables 3.19 and 3.20)
- Method of treatment administration
- Diagnosis

Possible causes of reduced pre-treatment fertility in male cancer patients
- Diagnosis, for example testicular cancer or Hodgkin's lymphoma
- Anatomical, for example retrograde ejaculation

Table 3.19 The impact of radiation therapy or systemic chemotherapy agents on spermatogenesis in patients with cancer.

Agent	Cumulative dose	Azoospermia	Additive effect with other chemotherapy drugs	Comments
Radiation				
Gonads	2.5 Gy/0.6 Gy	Permanent/temp	Yes	3–7 week courses worse than single dose, 0.15 Gy decrease count
Total body	8 Gy single	Permanent	Yes	
	12 Gy fract			
Chemotherapy				
Cyclophosphamide	19 gm/m^2	Yes		
Chlorambucil	1.4 g/m^2	Yes		
Cisplatin	500 mg/m^2	Yes		
Procarbazine	4 g/m^2	Yes		
Carboplatin	> 2 g/m^2	Likely		
Nitrosureas				
Busulfan	> 600 mg/kg	Likely		
Ifosfamide	> 30 g/m^2	Likely	+ cyclophosphamide	
Carmustine	1 g/m^2	Likely		
Lomustine	500 mg/m^2	Likely		
Nitrogen mustard		Unknown		Used with other highly gonadotoxic agents
Melphalan		Unknown		Same
Actinomycin D		Unknown		Same
Doxorubicin	770 mg/m^2	Temp oligo (alone)	Yes	Azoo in combo
Cytosine arabinoside	1 g/m^2	Temp oligo (alone)	Yes	Azoo in combo

Vinblastine	50 g/m^2	Temp oligo (alone)	Yes	Azoo in combo
Vincristine	8 g/m^2	Temp oligo (alone)	Yes	Azoo in combo; less toxic than vinblastine
Paclitaxel		Unknown		
Docetaxel		Unknown		
Gemcitabine		Unknown		
Trastuzumab		Unknown		
Irinotecan		Unknown		
Oxaliplatin		Unknown		

Abbreviations: Azoo = azoospermia; Combo = combination; Oligo = oligospermia; Temp = temporary.

Reproduced from *Cancer Treatment Reviews*, 30(2), Puscheck E, Philip PA, Jeyendran RS. Male fertility preservation and cancer treatment. 173–80, 2004, with permission from Elsevier.

Table 3.20 Risk of female gonadotoxicity of various antineoplastic agents.

	High risk (> 80%)	Intermediate risk	Low risk (< 20%)	Unknown risk
Single agents	Cyclophosphamide Bulsulfan Melphalan Chlorambucil Dacarbazine Procarbazine Ifosfamide Thiotepa Nitrogen mustard	Anthracyclines Cisplatin Carboplatin Ara-C	Methotrexate Bleomycin 5-fluorouracil Actinomycin-D Vinca alkaloids Mercaptopurine Etoposide Fludarabine	Taxanes Oxaliplatin Irinotecan Monoclonal antibodies Tyrosine kinase inhibitors
Combinations and radiation therapy	High-dose cyclophosphamide/busulfan and haematopoietic stem cell transplantation Ovarian irradiation CMF, CAF, FEC x6 in women >40years	CMF, CAF, FEC x6 in women 30–39years AC, EC x4 in women >40years	ABVD CMF, FEC, CAF x6 in women <30years CHOP, CVP Protocols for AML, ALL AC x4 in women <40years	

From Pentheroudakis G, Orecchia R, Hoekstra HJ, Pavlidis N. Cancer, fertility and pregnancy: ESMO Clinical Practice Guidelines for diagnosis, treatment and follow-up. *Annals of Oncology.* 2010 21 (Suppl. 5): v266–73. Reproduced with permission of Oxford University Press.

- Primary or secondary hormonal insufficiency
- Germ cell damage or depletion

Possible cause of reduced fertility in female cancer patients

- Diagnosis, for example endometrial or cervical cancer
- Anatomical changes to reproductive organs due to treatment, for example uterine fibrosis following pelvic radiotherapy or trachelectomy
- Hormonal imbalance
- Depletion of follicles or interruption of follicle maturation

Methods of fertility preservation

Various methods of fertility preservation are available. NICE guidance recommends that people diagnosed with cancer who are starting treatment that is likely to affect their fertility are offered gamete cryopreservation. This should be discussed in the setting of the diagnosis, treatment plan, prognosis and possible outcome of future fertility treatment. NICE recommend that cryopreserved sperm, oocytes and embryos are stored for an initial ten-year period.

Fertility preservation for men

- *Sperm cryopreservation*:
  - Sperm collected after masturbation, from testicular tissue (e.g. if unable to ejaculate due to sacral nerve dysfunction) or from post-masturbation urine sample.
  - Samples with poor motility or low sperm counts are acceptable as can use intracytoplasmic sperm injection for future *in vitro* fertilisation.
  - There is a potentially higher risk of genetic damage in sperm if this is collected after the start of chemotherapy.
- *Hormonal manipulation*: suppression of testosterone and the GnRH axis in men has not been shown to prevent azoospermia or enhance recovery post chemo-radiation and is therefore not recommended.
- *Testicular tissue cryopreservation and reimplantation*: experimental option for pre-pubertal boys, not routinely used in clinical practice.

Fertility preservation for women

- *Embryo cryopreservation*:
  - Requires 10–14 days of ovarian stimulation from beginning of menstrual cycle before oocyte collection (yield very low without FSH stimulation).
  - Need donor or partner sperm for fertilisation prior to freezing.
  - Letrozole or tamoxifen can be used to avoid oestrogen exposure.
- *Oocyte cryopreservation*:
  - No donor/partner sperm required.
  - Has 3–4 times lower success rate than embryo cryopreservation (2% of live births/thawed oocyte).

- *Hormonal manipulation*:
  - Use of LHRH analogues, for example goserelin 3.6 mg monthly for ovarian protection has only been retrospectively evaluated thus far, although prospective trials are in progress.
  - Studies so far have only reported on menses, not on longer-term fertility preservation.
- *Ovarian tissue cryopreservation and reimplantation*: investigational procedure. Concerns regarding possible reintroduction of malignant cells, though no cases reported as yet.
- *Gonadal shielding during radiation treatment*
- *Oophoropexy/ovarian transposition*:
  - Movement of ovaries away from radiation field to reduce exposure.
  - Laparoscopic procedure close to initiation of treatment to minimise procedure failure.
- *Fertility-preserving surgical procedures*: trachelectomy for early stage cervical cancer conserves the uterus, no evidence of increased risk of recurrence thus far.

Pregnancy following cancer treatment
- It is recommended that all patients wait at least 12 months following cancer treatment before childbearing and that those at risk of relapse avoid childbearing for two to three years.
- All pregnancies following cancer treatment should be considered high risk for perinatal complications and be monitored closely.
- Radiation to the uterus at doses greater than 20–30 Gy results in an increased risk of miscarriage.
- *Outcomes*: if fertility has been successfully preserved there should be no increased risk of functional defects or malignancy in offspring.

Cancer in pregnancy
It is estimated that 1 in 1000 cancers are diagnosed during pregnancy. The treatment strategy needs to be fully discussed with patient, family and a multidisciplinary team, including an obstetrician, neonatologist and psychologist and will depend on the diagnosis and stage of the cancer, the stage of pregnancy and the patient's wishes. There is no difference in survival in patients diagnosed with pregnancy-associated breast cancer, except in untreated patients. Metastases to the foetus are rare and are most commonly caused by metastatic melanoma.

Investigations
- Minimise ionising radiation if possible, for example CXR with abdominal shielding, ultrasound.
- Gadolinium contrast crosses the placenta and has been shown to be teratogenic in animal models and so MRI with contrast should be avoided.

General management

- Supportive medications should be prescribed with care during pregnancy.
- If the pregnancy is sustained, delivery should be after the 32nd–35th week and a suitable interval should ensure that there is no remaining chemotherapy-induced myelosuppression.
- The placentas of women with known or suspected metastatic melanoma should be reviewed by a histopathologist.
- Avoid breastfeeding on chemotherapy.

Oncology treatment

- Anti-cancer chemotherapeutics are teratogenic if used in the first trimester, but can be used from the second trimester onwards. There is an increased risk of foetal malformation, intrauterine death and premature labour.
- The safest compounds seem to be the taxanes, cisplatin, anthracyclines, 5-FU and the vinca alkaloids. There is no data on pemetrexed, oxaliplatin and gemcitabine or with targeted agents such as tyrosine kinase inhibitors.
- Foetal radiation exposure above 5–10 Gy is associated with an increased risk of developmental disorders and should be avoided until the post-partum period if possible.
- Anti-oestrogens such as tamoxifen should be avoided in pregnancy due to risk of teratogenicity.

References

Lee SJ, Schover LR, Partridge AH, Patrizio P, Wallace WH, Hagerty K, *et al.*, and American Society of Clinical Oncology. American Society of Clinical Oncology recommendations on fertility preservation in cancer patients. *Journal of Clinical Oncology.* 2006. 24(18): 2917–3.

Loren AW, Mangu PB, Beck LN, Brennan L, Magdalinski AJ, Partridge AH, *et al.* Fertility preservation for patients with cancer: American society of clinical oncology clinical practice guideline update. *Journal of Clinical Oncology.* 2013. 31(19): 2500–10.

Pentheroudakis G, Orecchia R, Hoekstra HJ, Pavlidis N. Cancer, fertility and pregnancy: ESMO Clinical Practice Guidelines for diagnosis, treatment and follow-up. *Annals of Oncology.* 2010. 21(Suppl. 5): v266–73.

Puscheck E, Philip PA, Jeyendran RS. Male fertility preservation and cancer treatment. *Cancer Treatment Reviews.* 2004. 30(2): 173–80.

Urriticoechea A, Arnedos M, Walsh G, Dowsett M, Smith IE. Ovarian protection with goserelin during adjuvant chemotherapy for pre-menopausal women with early breast cancer (EBC). *Breast Cancer Research and Treatment.* 2008. 110(3): 411–16.

Haematuria

Haematuria is the presence of microscopic or macroscopic blood in the urine. The grading of haematuria is shown in Table 3.21.

Table 3.21 CTCAE (V4.03) grading of haematuria.

Grade	Criteria
1	Asymptomatic; clinical or diagnostic observations only; intervention not indicated.
2	Symptomatic; urinary catheter or bladder irrigation indicated; limiting instrumental ADL.
3	Gross haematuria; transfusion, IV medications or hospitalisation indicated; elective endoscopic, radiologic or operative intervention indicated; limiting self-care ADL.
4	Life-threatening consequences; urgent radiologic or operative intervention indicated.
5	Death.

From the website of the National Cancer Institute (http://www.cancer.gov).

Causes
- Infection: UTI, pyelonephritis, TB.
- Cancer: RCC, TCC of the bladder or urethra, prostatic cancer, penile cancer.
- Anti-cancer drugs: for example cyclophosphamide, ifosfamide, tyrosine kinase inhibitors, intravesical chemotherapy/immunotherapy.
- Trauma: renal stone, instrumentation.
- Contamination: for example menses.
- Renal cause: for example embolism, glomerulonephritis, interstitial nephritis, IgA nephropathy.
- Haematological: sickle cell anaemia, coagulopathy, anti-coagulant medication.
- Vasculitis.

Symptoms
- Microscopic haematuria is diagnosed as the presence of 3+ red blood cells/high-power field on microscopy.
- Gross haematuria is evident to the naked eye. Blood in the urine may be visible with only 1 ml of blood in 1 litre of urine. It can be an alarming symptom which is often reported early.
- The presence of clots within the urine should be checked as this will change the management.

Investigations and management
General management:
- FBC, coagulation screen, U&E, LFT, bone profile
- Urine dipstick

Microscopic haematuria:
- Check for proteinuria/casts – if present, check for glomerulonephropathy.
- Check for infection – treat and recheck for haematuria.
- If neither of the above, proceed as per gross haematuria.

Gross/macroscopic haematuria:
- Send cytology.
- Imaging – consider USS KUB, IV pyelogram and/or CT abdomen/pelvis.

- Cystoscopy.
- Urinary catheter with irrigation may be required if gross haematuria with clots – these cases should also be discussed with an urologist.

Haemorrhagic cystitis
- Chemotherapy:
  - Most commonly associated with cyclophosphamide and ifosfamide.
  - It is dose dependent, occurring in up to 40% of patients treated with high-dose cyclophosphamide and around 5% of patients treated at lower doses.
  - The causative agent is the hepatic metabolite acrolein, which is directly toxic to the bladder mucosa leading to necrosis and haemorrhage. MESNA is co-administered with high-dose cyclophosphamide. This binds to acrolein reducing its toxicity without affecting the cytotoxic effects of cyclophosphamide itself.
  - Specific protocols are in place for haematuria during cyclophosphamide treatment.
- External beam radiotherapy and brachytherapy, for example to the cervix, GU tract or rectum:
  - May occur acutely post treatment or as a late complication from six months to many years after treatment.
  - There is less evidence for treating haemorrhagic cystitis secondary to radiotherapy but hyperbaric oxygen has been shown to be beneficial.

References

Abdi E. Urological symptoms and side effects of treatment. In: Oliver IN. *The MASCC Textbook of Cancer Supportive Care and Survivorship*. New York: Springer. 2011. pp. 281–300.
BMJ. Haematuria. Best Practice. July 2013. Available from: http://bestpractice.bmj.com/best-practice/monograph/316.html (accessed 1 January 2014).

Hearing loss

- May occur as a result of cancer treatment and can be permanent, partially or completely reversible. The grading of hearing loss is shown in Table 3.22.
- High frequencies are the most commonly affected, resulting in impairment of speech discrimination.
- Symptoms do not always correlate with audiological tests, with some patients having audiological evidence of impaired hearing but no symptoms, and vice versa.
- May be associated with tinnitus, which can interfere with sleep and concentration and cause strong emotional reactions.

Causes
- Chemotherapy drugs:
  - Cisplatin: causes bilateral, progressive, high-tone hearing loss, which can occur after the first dose.

Table 3.22 CTCAE (V4.03) grading of hearing loss.

Grade	Criteria
1	Subjective change in hearing in the absence of documented hearing loss. If in a monitoring programme: threshold shift of 15–25 dB averaged at two contiguous test frequencies in at least one ear.
2	Hearing loss but hearing aid or intervention not indicated, limiting instrumental ADL. If in a monitoring programme: threshold shift of > 25 dB averaged at two contiguous test frequencies in at least one ear.
3	Hearing loss with hearing aid or intervention indicated, limiting self-care ADL. If in a monitoring programme: threshold shift of 15–25 dB averaged at three contiguous test frequencies in at least one ear, therapeutic intervention indicated.
4	Decrease in hearing to profound bilateral loss (absolute threshold > 80 dB), non-serviceable hearing.
5	—

From the website of the National Cancer Institute (http://www.cancer.gov).

- ○ Carboplatin (much less common than cisplatin).
- ○ Vincristine.
- Other ototoxic drugs, for example gentamicin (particularly in combination with ototoxic chemotherapy).
- Otitis media.
- Radiotherapy:
  - ○ Can cause sensorineural hearing loss if the ear is included in the radiation field.
  - ○ Hearing loss may be worse if cisplatin is used concurrently.
  - ○ Early hearing loss occurs during or shortly after radiation and may improve within one year, but late toxicity causing further hearing loss can occur months or years after radiotherapy.

Risk factors
- Dose and schedule of cisplatin: for example increased toxicity with a two weekly schedule, doses > 60 mg/m², high cumulative doses (e.g. > 600 mg/m²).
- History of noise exposure.
- Pre-treatment sensorineural ear damage.
- Renal impairment.
- Radiation dose.
- May be more severe in older patients.

Audiological testing
- If a patient is at risk of ototoxicity, consider if audiological monitoring is required for early detection of toxicity.
- Refer for audiological testing if there any concerns about possible ototoxicity and consider changing the chemotherapy regime.

- Audiological testing may involve ultra-high frequency audiometry and evoked otoacoustic emission testing, which can identify ototoxic damage earlier than pure tone threshold testing.

References

American Academy of Audiology. Clinical Practice Guidelines Ototoxicity Monitoring 2009. Available from: http://www.audiology.org/resources/documentlibrary/Pages/Ototoxicity-Monitoring.aspx (accessed 1 January 2014).

Bokemeyer C, Berger CC, Hartmann JT, Kollmannsberger C, Schmoll HJ, Kuczyk MA, *et al.* Analysis of risk factors for cisplatin-induced ototoxicity in patients with testicular cancer. *British Journal of Cancer.* 1998. 77(8): 1355–62.

Dille MF, Konrad-Martin D, Gallun F, Helt WJ, Gordon JS, Reavis KM, *et al.* Tinnitus onset rates from chemotherapeutic agents and ototoxic antibiotics: results of a large prospective study. *Journal of the American Academy of Audiology.* 2010. 21(6): 409–17.

Low WK, Toh ST, Wee J, Fook-Chong SM, Wang DY. Sensorineural hearing loss after radiotherapy and chemoradiotherapy: a single, blinded, randomized study. *Journal of Clinical Oncology.* 2006. 24(12): 1904–9.

Hiccups

Hiccups are a sudden contraction of the diaphragm and intercostal muscles followed by glottis closure almost immediately afterwards. Episodes may last up to 48 hours. Beyond this is termed persistent hiccups. An episode lasting longer than one month is termed intractable hiccups. See Table 3.23 for the grading of hiccups.

Pathophysiology

- The reason for hiccups is debated and the mechanism is complex. There is a greater tendency for men to be affected. In around 80% of cases only a unilateral diaphragm is affected.
- Hiccups often commence during inspiration and are inhibited by elevations in pCO_2. This is the basis of breath holding as a therapeutic measure.

Table 3.23 CTCAE (V4.03) grading of hiccups.

Grade	Criteria
1	Mild symptoms; intervention not indicated.
2	Moderate symptoms; medical intervention indicated; limiting instrumental ADL.
3	Severe symptoms; interfering with sleep; limiting self-care ADL.
4	—
5	—

From the website of the National Cancer Institute (http://www.cancer.gov).

Causes

- Directly related to the cancer: for example oesophagogastric, colon, pancreatic, hepatoma, liver metastasis, lung cancer, thoracic or abdominal lymphoma, renal cancer.
- Metabolic disturbance: for example hyponatraemia, hypokalaemia, hypocalcaemia, renal failure, uraemia.
- Drug-induced:
  - Antibiotics
  - Corticosteroids
  - Opioids
  - Chemotherapy (particularly in men): cisplatin, carboplatin, cyclophosphamide, docetaxel, etoposide, gemcitabine, irinotecan, paclitaxel, vinorelbine
- CNS pathology: for example stroke, haemorrhage, encephalitis, brain abscess.
- Thoracic pathology: for example pneumonia, pleural effusion, mechanical ventilation.
- GI pathology: for example gastric distension/outlet obstruction, small bowel. obstruction, inflammation, ulcer, pancreatitis, ascites, subdiaphragmatic abscess.
- Psychogenic.

Investigations

- Investigations should be targeted to the possible cause. The temporal relationship to drugs and chemotherapy may be helpful.
- Blood tests – U&E, calcium.
- CXR and further radiological investigation dependent on history (e.g. CT head/neck/thorax).

Treatment

1 Episodes lasting less than 48 hours:
   (a) No specific remedy is usually required and hiccups often resolve spontaneously.
   (b) Hiccups may follow acute gastric distension, therefore avoidance of rapid food intake/carbonated drinks may help.
   (c) Case series have recommended various folk remedies, but no non-pharmacologic manoeuvre has been demonstrated as superior to any other.
   (d) A rise in pCO_2 has been shown to reduce hiccups, for example through manoeuvres such as breath-holding or breathing into a paper bag.
2 Persistent or intractable hiccups
   A Cochrane review in 2013 found a lack of good evidence for pharmacological or non-pharmacological treatments. The following treatments have been tried, but it is important to balance their likely activity against possible side effects.
   (a) Pharmacological treatment:
       (i) Metoclopramide 10 mg TDS
       (ii) Baclofen 5 mg TDS
       (iii) Amitriptyline or gabapentin (titrated as for neuropathic pain)

    (iv) Calcium-channel blockers, for example nifedipine 5 mg PRN or 5–20 mg TDS (risk of hypotension)

    (v) Haloperidol 1.5 mg TDS or 3 mg nocte

    (vi) Midazolam (as part of end of life care)

(b) Phrenic nerve blockade:

This is rarely undertaken but may provide symptom relief in carefully selected cases.

References

Becker DE. Nausea, vomiting, and hiccups: A review of mechanism and treatment. *Anesthesia Progress*. 2010. 57: 150–157.

Marinella MA. Diagnosis and management of hiccups in the patient with advanced cancer. *The Journal of Supportive Oncology*. 2009. 7: 122–7.

Moretto EN, Wee B, Wiffen PJ, Murchison AG. Interventions for treating persistent and intractable hiccups in adults. *Cochrane Database of Systematic Reviews*. 2013. Issue 1. Art. No: CD008768.

Hyperglycaemia and hypoglycaemia

Diabetes and cancer

Diabetic patients may have diabetic complications (e.g. renal impairment, neuropathy) that impact on their cancer treatment. Management of diabetic oncology patients can be challenging and referral to a diabetes specialist may be required.

General principles of management

1 Consider the patient's prognosis:

    (a) The importance of tight glycaemic control is different for a patient undergoing curative treatment in comparison to patients receiving palliative treatment. However, both hyper and hypoglycaemia can impair patients' quality of life.

    (b) For patients with advanced cancer:

        (i) Aim to keep glucose between 6–15 mmol/L.

        (ii) Remember to explain and reassure patients regarding the new targets for their glucose control.

        (iii) For patients with a prognosis of more than one year: consider evening basal insulin in combination with daytime oral hypoglycaemic agents.

    (c) For patients with a prognosis of months:

        (i) Insulin alone is simpler than a combination of tablets and insulin.

        (ii) Use the simplest insulin regime possible as carers are likely to be increasingly involved in giving insulin.

        (iii) Use 75% of the total previous dose if switching from a twice daily to a once daily regime.

2 Consider whether the patient has Type 1 or Type 2 diabetes. Without insulin, Type 1 diabetics will develop diabetic ketoacidosis (DKA) and die if this is untreated. Type 2 diabetics may enter a hyperosmolar, non-ketotic state.

3 Review medication, particularly:

   (a) The dose of metformin if renal function deteriorates.

   (b) The use of sulphonylureas if liver function deteriorates or the patient is only managing small meals.

4 Diet:

   (a) Avoidance of sugary foods is often impractical when food choices are limited.

   (b) If the patient is unwell: advise sipping sugar-free liquids regularly (aim for 100 ml/hour) and frequent small meals of easily digested foods (e.g. soup, milky drinks) if unable to eat their usual meals.

PET scans

- Usually use the glucose analogue FDG as a tracer. FDG accumulation in tissue is proportional to the amount of glucose utilised and scan results can therefore be affected by glycaemic control.
- Inform radiology if a patient is diabetic and follow local guidelines.
- Patients have their glucose checked prior to having the scan. Guidelines vary, but in general, if plasma glucose is <7 mmol/l (120 mg/dl) the PET scan can go ahead. If ≥7–11 mmol/L (depending on local protocol) then either reschedule the PET or consider giving short acting insulin (note that insulin must not be given unless the interval between giving insulin and administering FDG is >4 hours).

Hyperglycaemia

Hyperglycaemia is defined as an elevated concentration of blood sugar. The grading of hyperglycaemia is shown in Table 3.24.

Symptoms and causes

- *Symptoms*: dry mouth, polyuria, polydipsia, blurred vision, lethargy and recurrent infections.

Table 3.24 CTCAE (V4.03) grading of hyperglycaemia.

Grade	Criteria
1	Fasting glucose value >ULN – 160 mg/dL; Fasting glucose value >ULN – 8.9 mmol/L.
2	Fasting glucose value >160–250 mg/dL; Fasting glucose value >8.9–13.9 mmol/L.
3	> 250–500 mg/dL; > 13.9–27.8 mmol/L; hospitalisation indicated.
4	> 500 mg/dL; > 27.8 mmol/L; life-threatening consequences.
5	Death.

ULN = upper limit of normal.
From the website of the National Cancer Institute (http://www.cancer.gov).

- *Causes include*:
  - TPN, NG or PEG feeding or IV fluids
  - Steroids
  - Acute illness/sepsis in diabetic patients
  - Inability to take regular diabetes medication
  - Drugs, for example PI3K inhibitors

Management
- Check urinary ketones:
  - If positive:
    - Consider if performing an ABG and managing the patient as for early DKA is appropriate.
    - If patients are relatively well, consider continuing their usual insulin regime and adding in an additional 10% of their current total average daily insulin dose as short acting insulin every two hours with monitoring of their ketone levels. If ketones do not improve then admit for rehydration and insulin.
  - If negative, give short-acting insulin (e.g. 5–10 units of Actrapid®) every 6–8 hours based on glucose concentrations.
- *Due to NG/PEG feeding or TPN*: consider basal insulin.
- *Steroid-induced*:
  - Review the indication for steroid treatment and the dose.
  - Screen patients for diabetes before starting steroids and monitor their glucose levels.
  - Short courses of steroids (< 3 days) may only require closer glucose monitoring. Review anti-glycaemic therapy if a longer course of steroids is planned and consider referral to a diabetes specialist.
  - Patients who were on insulin before starting steroids will usually require both basal and prandial insulin and an increase in their insulin dose.
  - Once daily steroids:
    - Tend to cause a late afternoon/early evening rise in blood sugar.
    - Consider a morning sulphonylurea (e.g. gliclazide) or isophane insulin (e.g. Insulatard®).
  - Twice daily steroids: consider insulin glargine once daily (in the morning).

Hypoglycaemia
Hypoglycaemia is defined as a low concentration of blood sugar. The grading of hypoglycaemia is shown in Table 3.25.

Symptoms and causes
- *Symptoms*: odd behaviour, confusion/reduced consciousness, blurred vision, seizures, sweating, tachycardia, hunger, headache and trembling.
- *Causes include*: poor oral intake or vomiting in diabetic patients, oral hypoglycaemic drugs, insulin, liver failure, insulinoma, phaeochromocytoma, hepatoma and haematological malignancies (rare).

Table 3.25 CTCAE (V4.03) grading of hypoglycaemia.

Grade	Criteria
1	< LLN – 55 mg/dL; < LLN – 3.0 mmol/L.
2	< 55–40 mg/dL; < 3.0–2.2 mmol/L.
3	< 40–30 mg/dL; < 2.2–1.7 mmol/L.
4	< 30 mg/dL; < 1.7 mmol/L; life-threatening consequences; seizures.
5	Death.

LLN = lower limit of normal.
From the website of the National Cancer Institute (http://www.cancer.gov).

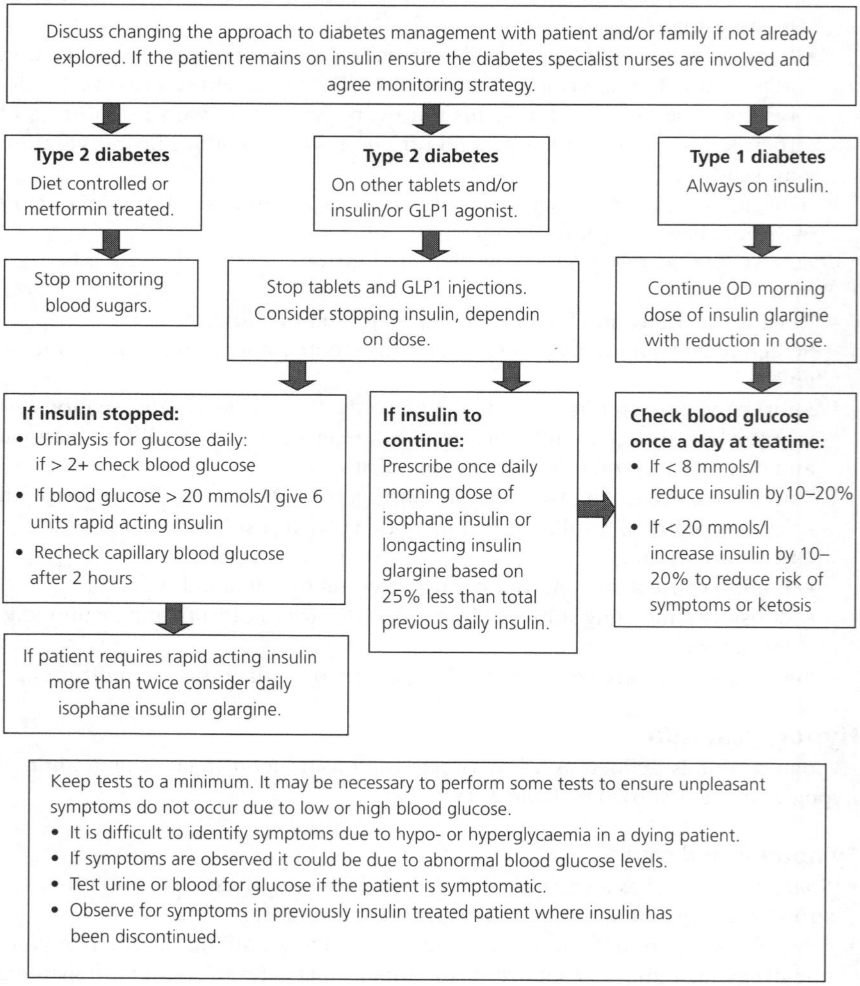

Discuss changing the approach to diabetes management with patient and/or family if not already explored. If the patient remains on insulin ensure the diabetes specialist nurses are involved and agree monitoring strategy.

Type 2 diabetes
Diet controlled or metformin treated.

Type 2 diabetes
On other tablets and/or insulin/or GLP1 agonist.

Type 1 diabetes
Always on insulin.

Stop monitoring blood sugars.

Stop tablets and GLP1 injections. Consider stopping insulin, dependin on dose.

Continue OD morning dose of insulin glargine with reduction in dose.

If insulin stopped:
- Urinalysis for glucose daily: if > 2+ check blood glucose
- If blood glucose > 20 mmols/l give 6 units rapid acting insulin
- Recheck capillary blood glucose after 2 hours

If insulin to continue:
Prescribe once daily morning dose of isophane insulin or longacting insulin glargine based on 25% less than total previous daily insulin.

Check blood glucose once a day at teatime:
- If < 8 mmols/l reduce insulin by 10–20%
- If < 20 mmols/l increase insulin by 10–20% to reduce risk of symptoms or ketosis

If patient requires rapid acting insulin more than twice consider daily isophane insulin or glargine.

Keep tests to a minimum. It may be necessary to perform some tests to ensure unpleasant symptoms do not occur due to low or high blood glucose.
- It is difficult to identify symptoms due to hypo- or hyperglycaemia in a dying patient.
- If symptoms are observed it could be due to abnormal blood glucose levels.
- Test urine or blood for glucose if the patient is symptomatic.
- Observe for symptoms in previously insulin treated patient where insulin has been discontinued.

Figure 3.1 Flowchart for the management of diabetes at the end of life. Adapted with permission from Diabetes UK. End of Life Diabetes Care: a Strategy Document Commissioned by Diabetes UK. 2012. Reproduced with permission of Diabetes UK.

Management
- If patient is alert and well, give one or more of the following:
  - Sweet drink
  - Glucotabs
  - Dextrose tablets
- Patients on PEG feeds: stop the feed and give 100 ml of a sweet drink via the PEG.
- If patient unwell/unresponsive:
  - 50–100 ml 50% IV dextrose fast followed by 50 ml normal saline flush or glucagon 1 mg IM or SC. Glucagon may not be effective in patients with liver disease.
  - Give sweet drinks when patient conscious.
- Monitor blood sugars, review drug chart and adjust medication as appropriate.
- If the patient has overdosed on a long-acting insulin or oral hypoglycaemic agent, consider a 10% dextrose drip (adjust the rate according to blood glucose).

End-of-life care
Although fine glycaemic control is not appropriate in patients in their last days to weeks of life, do not ignore symptomatic hyper or hypoglycaemia. Individual hospitals may have their own guidelines. An example pathway is shown in Figure 3.1.

References

Boellaard R, O'Doherty MJ, Weber WA, Mottaghy FM, Lonsdale MN, Stroobants SG, *et al*. FDG PET and PET/CT: EANM procedure guidelines for tumour PET imaging: version 1.0. *European Journal of Nuclear Medicine and Molecular Imaging*. 2010. 37(1): 181–200.

Diabetes UK. *End of Life Diabetes Care*. A Strategy Document Commissioned by Diabetes UK. 2012.

Morganstein MD, Tan S, Gore M, MD Feher MD. Prevalence of diabetes in patients admitted to a cancer hospital. *British Journal of Diabetes & Vascular Disease*. 2012. 12: 178–80.

Poulson J. The management of diabetes in patients with advanced cancer. *Journal of Pain and Symptom Management*. 1997. 13(6): 339–46.

Psarakis H. Clinical challenges in caring for patients with diabetes and cancer. *Diabetes Spectrum*. 2006. 19(3): 157–62.

Hypertension and hypotension

Hypertension
Hypertension is defined as a pathological increase in blood pressure (BP) or a repeated elevation in BP to > 140/90 mmHg. The grading of hypertension is shown in Table 3.26.

Hypertension is the most frequent comorbid condition that directly affects patients' prognosis and is a risk factor for chemotherapy-induced cardiotoxicity,

Table 3.26 CTCAE (V4.03) grading of hypertension.

Grade	Criteria
1	Pre-hypertension (systolic BP 120–139 mmHg or diastolic BP 80–89 mmHg).
2	Stage 1 hypertension (systolic BP 140–159 mmHg or diastolic BP 90–99 mmHg); medical intervention indicated; recurrent or persistent ($\geq$ 24 hrs); symptomatic increase by > 20 mmHg (diastolic) or to > 140/90 mmHg if previously within normal limits; monotherapy indicated.
3	Stage 2 hypertension (systolic BP $\geq$ 160 mmHg or diastolic BP $\geq$ 100 mmHg); medical intervention indicated; more than one drug or more intensive therapy than previously used indicated.
4	Life-threatening consequences (e.g. malignant hypertension, transient or permanent neurologic deficit, hypertensive crisis); urgent intervention indicated.
5	Death.

From the website of the National Cancer Institute (http://www.cancer.gov).

stroke, heart failure, MI and chronic kidney disease. In addition, poorly controlled BP can result in potentially beneficial anti-angiogenic drugs being discontinued.

Causes
- Drugs:
  - Anti-angiogenic drugs: for example bevacizumab, sunitinib, sorafenib, pazopanib.
  - Chemotherapy drugs: for example cyclophosphamide, cisplatin, vincristine, paclitaxel.
  - Endocrine therapies: for example anastrozole, exemestane, letrozole.
- Phaeochromocytoma.
- Cushing's syndrome.
- Other causes: e.g. essential hypertension, renal disease, endocrine disorders, irradiation to kidneys in childhood.

General management
- Perform a cardiovascular risk assessment (e.g. assess for diabetes, renal disease, cardiovascular disease and other cardiovascular risk factors).
- Identify and treat patients with pre-existing hypertension before starting anti-angiogenic drugs.
- Target BP should correspond to guidelines:
  - 130/80 mmHg in patients with diabetes or kidney disease
  - 140/90 mmHg in other patients
- Many patients are anxious about coming to hospital/chemotherapy and may have 'white-coat hypertension'. If BP in clinic is > 140/90 mmHg consider ambulatory BP monitoring or home BP monitoring to confirm the diagnosis.

If using home BP measurements, BP should be taken twice daily (in the morning and evening) for at least 4–7 days.
- Patients with hypertension should usually be referred to their GP for management. If BP control remains difficult then consider referral to a specialist.
- Actively monitor BP during anti-angiogenic treatment, particularly during the first cycle, which is when most of the rise in BP is expected to occur, for example systolic BP can rise by 29 mmHg and diastolic BP by 27 mmHg during the first cycle.
- Check local protocols for guidelines regarding cut-off limits for BP above which anti-angiogenic agents should be withheld or discontinued.

NICE guidelines for the treatment of hypertension
- *Step 1*:
  - If < 55 years old: start an ACE inhibitor or angiotensin II receptor blocker.
  - If the patient is a black person of African or Caribbean family origin or is > 55 years old: start a calcium channel blocker (or thiazide-like diuretic if unable to tolerate a calcium channel blocker or evidence of heart failure).
- *Step 2*: add in a calcium channel blocker or an ACE inhibitor/angiotensin II receptor blocker.
- *Step 3*: add in a thiazide-like diuretic.
- *Step 4*: consider further adding in a further diuretic (e.g. low-dose spironolactone), an α-blocker or a β-blocker.

Hypotension
Hypotension is defined as a blood pressure which is below the normal expected for an individual in a given environment. The grading of hypotension is shown in Table 3.27.

Causes
- Drugs:
  - Monoclonal antibodies such as cetuximab, rituximab and alemtuzumab cause cytokine release, which can lead to hypotension (particularly within the first few hours of infusion).
  - Other oncology drugs that cause hypotension include: etoposide, paclitaxel, interferon-α and all-*trans* retinoic acid.
  - Some drugs, such as interleukin-2, can cause capillary leak syndrome. This leads to hypotension due to the extravasation of plasma proteins and fluid into the extravascular space and, if severe, can be fatal.
  - Non-oncology medication such as β-blockers and some antidepressants.
- Anaphylaxis
- Dehydration
- Anaemia
- Sepsis
- Haemorrhage
- PE

Table 3.27 CTCAE (V4.03) grading of hypotension.

Grade	Criteria
1	Asymptomatic, intervention not indicated.
2	Non-urgent medical intervention indicated.
3	Medical intervention or hospitalisation indicated.
4	Life-threatening and urgent intervention indicated.
5	Death.

From the website of the National Cancer Institute (http://www.cancer.gov).

- Adrenal disorders (including metastatic disease, steroid use)
- Cardiac arrhythmias, MI, cardiogenic shock
- Carcinoid crisis
- Comorbidities, e.g. autonomic disorders such as diabetes mellitus or Parkinson's disease

Management
- Carefully monitor BP in patients at risk of hypotension (e.g. patients receiving alemtuzumab), particularly those with pre-existing cardiac disease.
- Assess the severity of hypotension.
- Consider IV fluids.
- Treat the cause (if known).
- Manage any acutely unwell patient as per standard practice.

References

electronic Medicines Compendium. SPC Proleukin2011.. Available from: http://www.medicines.org.uk/emc/medicine/19322/SPC/proleukin/ (accessed 1 January 2014).

Jain M, Townsend RR. Chemotherapy agents and hypertension: a focus on angiogenesis blockade. *Current Hypertension Reports.* 2007. 9(4): 320–8.

Maitland ML, Bakris GL, Black HR, Chen HX, Durand JB, Elliott WJ, *et al.* Initial assessment, surveillance, and management of blood pressure in patients receiving vascular endothelial growth factor signaling pathway inhibitors. *Journal of the National Cancer Institute.* 2010. 102(9): 596–604.

Mouhayar E, Salahudeen A. Hypertension in cancer patients. *Texas Heart Institute Journal:* from the Texas Heart Institute of St Luke's Episcopal Hospital, Texas Children's Hospital. 2011. 38(3): 263–5.

National Institute for Health and Care Excellence (NICE). *Hypertension: Clinical Management of Primary Hypertension in Adults* (CG127). National Institute for Health and Care Excellence: London. 2011.

Yeh ET, Tong AT, Lenihan DJ, Yusuf SW, Swafford J, Champion C, *et al.* Cardiovascular complications of cancer therapy: diagnosis, pathogenesis, and management. *Circulation.* 2004. 109(25): 3122–31.

Lymphoedema

Lymphoedema is defined as the accumulation of fluid containing proteins and other elements in the tissue spaces, resulting in swelling. It is a chronic and incurable condition. The grading of lymphoedema is shown in Table 3.28.

Symptoms and signs
- Can occur in the limbs, head, neck, trunk or genital areas and cause fibrosis of the venous and lymphatic systems.
- Can cause pain, tightness, paraesthesiae, swelling, reduced range of movement and heaviness of the affected areas.
- Skin changes include: hyperkeratosis, blisters, papillomatosis (warty growths due to fibrosis of overdilated lymphatics), leakage of lymph fluid through the skin surface and recurrent skin infections.
- Patients with severe lymphoedema may rarely develop lymphangiosarcoma.

Causes
The causes are not fully understood but may result from a disturbance in fluid balance and a reduced immunological response. This may be secondary to damage to the lymphatic system, lymph node metastases, infiltrative carcinoma or pressure from large tumours.

Factors which may increase the risk of lymphoedema
- Surgery:
  - Lymphoedema may be more likely to occur after mastectomy than after breast-conserving surgery.
  - The greater the number of lymph nodes removed, the higher the risk of lymphoedema. The use of sentinel lymph node biopsies has led to a decrease in the incidence of lymphoedema, but it still affects approximately 28% of patients who have had an axillary dissection.
  - Lymphoedema can occur years after surgery, but the risk is highest in the first three years.

Table 3.28 CTCAE (V4.03) grading of lymphoedema.

Grade	Criteria
1	Trace thickening or faint discolouration.
2	Marked discolouration; leathery skin texture; papillary formation; limiting instrumental ADL.
3	Severe symptoms, limiting self-care ADL.
4	—
5	—

From the website of the National Cancer Institute (http://www.cancer.gov).

- Post-operative complications, including wound infections and seromas.
- Radiotherapy to the axilla, breast, chest wall or groin (particularly following surgery).
- Infections, burns and/or puncture wounds.
- BMI > 30.

Diagnosis
- Lymphoedema is usually diagnosed clinically, based on the history and clinical signs.
- The differential diagnosis includes axillary vein thrombosis and infection. It is also important to consider tumour involvement of the axilla or brachial plexus.

General advice for lymphoedema prevention and management
- Try to avoid using the 'at risk' or lymphoedematous arm for venepuncture, cannulation and BP measurements if possible:
  ○ There is little clear evidence that these procedures cause lymphoedema, but on the other hand there is no evidence that they do not.
  ○ If there is an urgent, life-saving need to administer IV fluids, blood products or drugs then this must take preference over the small risk of lymphoedema.
  ○ Drug absorption is unpredictable in lymphoedematous arms.
  ○ There is no evidence that the use of a tourniquet for < 10 minutes (e.g. during carpal tunnel surgery) triggers lymphoedema but it can led to a short-term increase in lymphoedema.
  ○ BP measurements may be inaccurate in lymphoedematous arms.
- Treat any infections promptly.
- Encourage:
  ○ Maintenance of ideal body weight.
  ○ Good skin care to reduce the risk of infection.
  ○ Exercise.
- Refer the patient to a lymphoedema team.
- Consider a referral for psychological support as lymphoedema can lead to anxiety and depression (particularly in younger women) and also affect patients' employment and self-image.

Treatment
- Infections in lymphoedematous areas are a serious complication and should be treated promptly with antibiotics:
  ○ Causative organisms are often streptococcal (or, more rarely, staphylcoccal), therefore consider using a penicillin, cephalosporin or macrolide.
  ○ Consider prophylactic antibiotics for patients with recurrent infections.
- Complex decongestive therapy (CDT) is a combination of skin care, exercise, compression bandaging and manual lymphatic drainage (MLD):
  ○ Compression garments (e.g. sleeves/stockings) or bandages (if the limb is a difficult size or shape for a compression garment) should be worn unless

there are contraindications to their use. They need to be replaced every 3–6 months to ensure a good fit.

- ○ MLD is a type of massage carried out by a trained therapist. It uses hand movements to stimulate lymph drainage and move lymph away from areas where it has collected. Patients can be taught a simpler version.
- Diuretics are not used as they lead to an increase in protein concentration and therefore result in an increase in swelling, inflammation and fibrosis.
- Low-level laser therapy may be effective.
- Surgery is rarely performed but may be used to debulk tissue or divert lymphatic drainage.
- Chemotherapy: lymphoedema may be due to relapsed disease that can respond to chemotherapy (e.g. lower limb lymphoedema in ovarian cancer).
- Much of the evidence for the prevention and management of lymphoedema is anecdotal and so further trials are needed to establish a stronger evidence base.

References

Bennett Britton TM, Purushotham AD. Understanding breast cancer-related lymphoedema. *The Surgeon.* 2009. 7(2): 120–4.

Clinical Resource Efficiency Support Team (CREST). Guidelines for the diagnosis, assessment and management of lymphoedema 2008. Available from: http://www.gain-ni.org/index.php/audits/guidelines (accessed 1 January 2014).

Harris SR, Hugi MR, Olivotto IA, Levine M. Clinical practice guidelines for the care and treatment of breast cancer: 11. Lymphedema. *Canadian Medical Association Journal (Journal de l'Association médicale canadienne).* 2001. 164(2): 191–9.

Paskett ED, Dean JA, Oliveri JM, Harrop JP. Cancer-related lymphedema risk factors, diagnosis, treatment, and impact: a review. *Journal of Clinical Oncology.* 2012. 30(30): 3726–33.

The Royal College of Anaesthetists. Breast Cancer Related Lymphoedema – information for doctors on patients with lymphoedema 2009. Available from: http://www.rcoa.ac.uk/document-store/breast-cancer-related-lymphoedema-%E2%80%93-information-doctors (accessed 1 January 2014).

Mucositis

Mucositis

- *Definition*: inflammatory and/or ulcerative lesions of the oral and/or GI tract, usually caused by cancer therapies.
- One of the most common toxicities of treatment. See Table 3.29 for the grading of mucositis.
- Typically starts 7–10 days after high-dose cancer treatment and, if uncomplicated, heals within 2–4 weeks of stopping treatment.

Risk factors

- *Age*: more common in younger patients
- Radiotherapy or chemoradiotherapy for head and neck cancers (severe mucositis occurs in approximately 85% of patients)

Table 3.29 CTCAE (V4.03) grading of mucositis.

Grade	Criteria
1	Asymptomatic or mild symptoms; intervention not indicated.
2	Moderate pain; not interfering with oral intake; modified diet indicated.
3	Severe pain; interfering with oral intake.
4	Life-threatening consequences; urgent intervention indicated.
5	Death.

From the website of the National Cancer Institute (http://www.cancer.gov).

- Chemotherapy, particularly:
  - Regimes containing 5-FU, capecitabine, methotrexate or doxorubicin
  - Induction chemotherapy for acute leukaemia
  - Conditioning regimes for patients undergoing haematopoietic stem cell transplants
- Targeted agents, for example sunitinib, sorafenib and mTOR inhibitors (e.g. everolimus, temsirolimus)
- Combinations of therapies (e.g. chemotherapy plus radiotherapy)
- Smoking and alcohol intake
- Pre-existing poor oral hygiene, dental or periodontal disease
- Patients who had mucositis during their first cycle of treatment

Symptoms and consequences of mucositis
- Decreased saliva, change in taste (including causing a metallic taste) and difficulty speaking.
- Pain (which can be severe).
- Difficulty eating, drinking and swallowing. This may lead to weight loss, malnutrition and fatigue. Patients may require enteral nutritional support, for example via a gastrostomy, particularly if they are receiving chemoradiotherapy for head and neck cancer.
- Increased risk of infection, which can be local (e.g. Candida, Herpes simplex) or result in systemic sepsis. The mouth is a common source of bacteraemia in neutropaenic patients.
- Bleeding, diarrhoea and electrolyte abnormalities.
- Treatment delays/dose reductions.

Signs
- The first sign is mucosal erythema, which is often associated with a burning sensation.
- This is followed by the formation of solitary, elevated, white, slightly painful patches which develop into multiple shallow ulcers. These may be covered by a pseudomembrane which is laden with bacteria and the ulcers may subsequently coalesce into large painful areas.

- Often the hard palate, dorsal tongue and gingiva are spared. This can help to distinguish treatment-induced mucositis from candidiasis or viral infections.

General advice

- Optimise dentition prior to treatment. A pre-treatment dental assessment is necessary for all patients with head and neck cancers undergoing radiotherapy.
- Avoid acidic, spicy, sharp, salty, dry foods and hot drinks.
- Advise patients undergoing radiotherapy to stop smoking as smoking can increase the duration and severity of mucosal reactions (as well as worsen the patient's outcome).
- Good dental hygiene:
  - Use a soft toothbrush (not a foam toothbrush) and replace it regularly.
  - Careful dental flossing.
  - Clean teeth four times a day (after each meal and at bedtime).
  - Clean dentures after each meal and soak overnight.
  - Avoid alcohol-containing mouthwashes.
  - Saline mouthwashes 4–6 times a day: for example ¼ to ½ a teaspoon of salt in a cup of warm water.

Prevention

- Oral cryotherapy (e.g. ice chips in the mouth for approximately 30 minutes) can be used in patients receiving bolus 5-FU, edatrexate or high dose melphalan.
- Ranitidine or omeprazole can help to prevent epigastric pain following 5-FU, cyclophosphamide or methotrexate.
- Palifermin (keratinocyte growth factor 1) may be used (if available) in haematology patients for three days pre-conditioning and three days post transplant.
- Low-level laser therapy may be available in some centres prior to stem cell transplants.

Suggested general principles of treatment

Most oncology departments have local guidelines for the management of mucositis (see below for an example). The efficacy of many available treatments is currently unproven. See Chapter 5 for further advice regarding the treatment of radiotherapy-induced mucositis.

First-line: bland mouthwashes (e.g. saline or sodium bicarbonate).

Second-line options:

- Dispersible co-codamol 30/500 (2 tablets QDS).
- Soluble aspirin (especially for radiotherapy-induced mucositis). Use 300 mg up to four times a day as a mouthwash, gargle (do not swallow) if any oropharyngeal pain. Not recommended for haematology patients.
- Difflam® spray 4–8 sprays every 1.5–3 hours (may sting).
- 1% topical lidocaine gel (QDS). Provides pain relief but needs frequent administration.
- Bonjela® – up to every three hours.
- Mucaine equivalent (antacid and oxetacaine) 10 ml QDS before meals.

- Hydrocortisone 2.5 mg buccal tablets – useful for patients with a single ulcerated area. Allow tablet to dissolve in contact with the ulcer four times daily.
- Sucralfate 5 ml QDS (efficacy unproven).

Third-line:

- Opiate-based analgesia (patient-controlled analgesia with opiates is particularly recommended for transplant patients).
- Mucosal coating agents, for example Gelclair®, Orabase®, provide a physical barrier over mucosal surfaces and therefore shield oral lesions from food, liquid and saliva. Their efficacy is currently unproven but some patients report that they find them helpful.
- Also consider water-soluble lubricating agents including artificial saliva if the patient has a dry mouth.

Current guidelines do *not* recommend the routine use of:

- Antibacterial lozenges
- Glutamine
- Chlorhexidine

Neutropenic ulcers

- Neutropenic ulcers are related to low neutrophil counts and can be multiple, painful and variable in size (often large). They frequently affect the gingivae, tongue, palate and tonsils.
- Increasing the patient's neutrophil count by the administration of GCSF is associated with an improvement in the ulceration.

Herpes simplex virus-1 (HSV-1) associated mucositis

- Reactivation of HSV-1 occurs in 50–90% of patients receiving high-dose chemotherapy or bone marrow transplantation.
- HSV-1 associated mucositis tends to be more severe and longer in duration.
- Consider HSV infection in patients with painful ulcers or vesicles and swab for culture.
- *Treatment*: aciclovir 200–400 mg PO five times daily, usually for five days (longer if new lesions appear during treatment or if healing incomplete).
- Consider prophylaxis with aciclovir 200–400 mg PO QDS for high-risk patients (e.g. patients with acute leukaemia).

Oral candidiasis

- Commonly occurs in patients receiving cancer treatments and causes a burning sensation and taste changes.
- *Candida albicans* is the commonest organism, but *Candida tropicalis* and *Candida glabrata* are also found in a significant number of patients and are more likely to lead to systemic infection.
- Different presentations of oral candidiasis:
  - Pseudomembraneous candidiasis: common and causes thick, white, curd-like pseudomembranes overlying an erythematous mucosa.
  - Erythematous candidiasis: causes intensely red, inflamed areas of mucosa, often underneath dentures or occurring after antibiotic therapy.

- ○ Angular chelitis: causes erythema and fissuring of the angles of the lips.
- ○ Chronic hyperplastic keratitis: this is rare but results in hyperkeratotic white patches.
- • *Treatment*:
  - ○ In general, topical agents are preferred to systemic agents due to their side effect profiles and potential for drug interactions.
  - ○ Topical nystatin is commonly used (100,000 units QDS after food, usually for seven days) but has variable efficacy due to its short contact time with the affected areas.
  - ○ Fluconazole 50 mg OD for 7–14 days is effective at preventing oral fungal infection and reducing oral fungal colonisation.

Other relevant sections of this book

Chapter 5, section on management of early head and neck toxicity

References

Keefe DM, Schubert MM, Elting LS, Sonis ST, Epstein JB, Raber-Durlacher JE, *et al.* Updated clinical practice guidelines for the prevention and treatment of mucositis. *Cancer.* 2007. 109(5): 820–31.

Lalla RV, Latortue MC, Hong CH, Ariyawardana A, D'Amato-Palumbo S, Fischer DJ, *et al.* A systematic review of oral fungal infections in patients receiving cancer therapy. *Supportive Care in Cancer.* 2010. 18(8): 985–92.

Peterson DE, Bensadoun RJ, Roila F. Management of oral and gastrointestinal mucositis: ESMO Clinical Practice Guidelines. *Annals of Oncology.* 2010. 21(Suppl. 5): v261–5.

Redding SW. Role of herpes simplex virus reactivation in chemotherapy-induced oral mucositis. *NCI Monographs.* 1990(9): 103–5.

Sonis S, Treister N. Oral mucositis. In: Davies A, Epstein J (eds). *Oral Complications of Cancer and its Management.* Oxford University Press: Oxford. 2010.

Watters AL, Epstein JB, Agulnik M. Oral complications of targeted cancer therapies: a narrative literature review. *Oral Oncology.* 2011. 47(6): 441–8.

Nausea and vomiting

Nausea and/or vomiting are common problems in oncology, affecting up to 70% of patients with advanced cancer. It is important to remember that there may be multiple causes of an individual patient's symptoms. The grading of nausea is shown in Table 3.30 and the grading of vomiting in Table 3.31.

Symptoms and signs
- • Nausea is often associated with autonomic symptoms such as cold sweats and tachycardia. This can be more distressing for patients than vomiting without nausea.
- • Other associated symptoms include constipation, diarrhoea and pain.
- • Signs include dehydration, abdominal distension or tenderness, an abdominal mass, abnormal or absent bowel sounds.

Table 3.30 CTCAE (V4.03) grading of nausea.

Grade	Criteria
1	Loss of appetite without alteration in eating habits.
2	Oral intake decreased without significant weight loss, dehydration or malnutrition.
3	Inadequate oral caloric or fluid intake; tube feeding, TPN, or hospitalisation indicated.
4	—
5	—

From the website of the National Cancer Institute (http://www.cancer.gov).

Table 3.31 CTCAE (V4.03) grading of vomiting.

Grade	Criteria
1	1–2 episodes (separated by 5 minutes) in 24 hours.
2	3–5 episodes (separated by 5 minutes) in 24 hours.
3	≥ 6 episodes (separated by 5 minutes) in 24 hours; tube feeding, TPN or hospitalisation indicated.
4	Life-threatening consequences; urgent intervention indicated.
5	Death.

From the website of the National Cancer Institute (http://www.cancer.gov).

- *Assess*: timing of symptoms, particularly in relation to meals/drugs (delayed nausea/vomiting refers to symptoms occurring > 24 hours after chemotherapy), amount of vomit, presence of haematemesis/coffee-ground vomit, oral intake.

Causes
1 Gastrointestinal:
   (a) Bowel obstruction, paralytic ileus
   (b) Pyloric stenosis
   (c) Delayed gastric emptying, for example due to ascites, hepatomegaly, autonomic dysfunction, opioids and other drugs
   (d) Gastroenteritis
   (e) Acute pancreatitis
2 Neurological/psychiatric:
   (a) Raised intracranial pressure
   (b) Vestibular disorders
   (c) Other CNS causes: for example migraine, brainstem lesions
   (d) Anticipatory nausea/vomiting:
      (i) Occurs in up to 20% of patients by the time of their fourth cycle of treatment.

(ii) Risk factors: < 50 years, anxiety, expectation of nausea and vomiting, susceptibility to motion sickness, vomiting after previous chemotherapy.

(iii) Can be relieved by benzodiazepines, for example lorazepam 0.5 mg PRN.

(e) Psychiatric disorders

3 Metabolic/endocrine abnormalities

For example, hypercalcaemia, hyponatraemia, diabetic ketoacidosis, Addison's disease, uraemia.

4 Medication:

(a) Anti-cancer drugs:

(i) Highly emetic drugs include: cisplatin, cyclophosphamide.

(ii) Moderately emetic drugs include: carboplatin, oxaliplatin, doxorubicin, epirubicin, irinotecan, ifosfamide, bendamustine.

(iii) Mildly emetic drugs include: paclitaxel, docetaxel, etoposide, pemetrexed, 5-FU, capecitabine, gemcitabine, lapatinib, sunitinib, everolimus, trastuzumab.

(b) Other drugs: for example antibiotics, opiates, digoxin, antifungals.

5 Radiotherapy:

(a) The risk of nausea and/or vomiting depends on the dose, fractionation, irradiated volume, radiotherapy technique, whether the patient received concurrent or recent chemotherapy and the site irradiated.

(b) Common sites for nausea and vomiting induced by radiotherapy are total body irradiation, cranial and upper abdominal tumours (e.g. pancreas and lower oeseophagus (see Chapter 5 for more details).

6 Other causes:

(a) Infections: for example UTIs

(b) Pregnancy

(c) Alcohol

Managment

- Investigate and treat the underlying cause if possible.
- Advise patients to eat small, frequent low fat meals (if not in bowel obstruction).
- Anti-emetics:
  ○ Most effective when used prophylactically. Local guidelines for prophylactic anti-emetics for chemotherapy and radiotherapy should be followed. Most chemotherapy prescription proformas include the recommended anti-emetics for that specific chemotherapy regime.
  ○ Consider the most appropriate route of administration – IV or SC medication may be required.
  ○ The most appropriate anti-emetic depends on the underlying cause of the patient's symptoms and potential side effects of the anti-emetic (see Table 3.32).
  ○ Prokinetic drugs (e.g. metoclopramide) are potentially antagonised by anticholinergic drugs (e.g. cyclizine) and therefore these should not be combined.

Table 3.32 Overview of commonly used anti-emetics.

Anti-emetic	Dose	Cause of nausea/vomiting	Side effects
Aprepitant	PO: 125 mg on day 1, 80 mg on days 2 and 3.	Prophylaxis of chemotherapy-induced nausea and vomiting.	Diarrhoea, dyspepsia, constipation, headache, dizziness, hiccups.
Cyclizine	PO/IM/IV: 50 mg TDS. SC infusion: 150 mg/24 hours.	Intestinal obstruction with colic (add hyoscine butylbromide 60 mg SC over 24 hours). Raised intracranial pressure. Vestibular causes.	Anticholinergic symptoms, for example dry mouth, urinary retention. Risk of arrhythmias and hypotension in patients with heart disease/rhythm disturbance.
Dexamethasone	PO: 4–16 mg.	Raised intracranial pressure. Prophylaxis for chemotherapy-induced nausea and vomiting.	Increased blood glucose, oesophageal ulceration, dyspepsia, candidiasis, insomnia, muscle weakness.
Domperidone	PO: 10–20 mg TDS. PR: 60 mg BD.	Impaired gastric emptying.	QT prolongation. Less likely to cause extrapyramidal side effects than metoclopramide.
Haloperidol	PO: 1.5–5 mg nocte/BD (max. 5–10 mg/day). SC infusion: 2.5–10 mg/24 hours.	Drugs. Metabolic abnormalities. Abdominal radiotherapy.	Extrapyramidal side effects. QT prolongation, arrhythmias. Use with caution in patients with severe hepatic impairment.
Levomepromazine	PO or SC: 6.25–25 mg nocte (titrated to 12.5–25 mg BD if necessary). SC infusion: 5–25 mg/24 hours.	Raised intracranial pressure. Uraemia. Drugs. Other causes. Often used as second line therapy when other drugs have failed.	Sedation and anticholinergic symptoms. Risk of arrhythmias and hypotension in patients with heart disease/rhythm disturbance. Can worsen extrapyramidal side effects of drugs, such as antidepressants.

Metoclopramide	PO/IV/IM: 10–20 mg TDS. SC infusion: 30–100 mg/24 hours.	Impaired gastric emptying. Intestinal obstruction (without colic).	Restlessness, drowsiness, fatigue, can cause worsening colic (therefore do not use in bowel obstruction)
Ondansetron	PO/IM/IV: 4–8 mg stat then 8 mg BD. PR: 16 mg OD.	Abdominal radiotherapy. Chemotherapy-induced. Second line therapy for chemical causes.	Can worsen extrapyramidal side effects of drugs such as antidepressants. Constipation, headache, flushing, rectal irritation from suppositories. QT prolongation.
Prochlorperazine	PO: 5–10 mg TDS/QDS. IM: 12.5 mg stat.	Labyrinthine disorders.	Confusion, extrapyramidal and anti-cholinergic symptoms.

○ Remember to consider if dose reductions are required in patients with renal or hepatic impairment.
○ If the patient is still vomiting after optimal anti-emetic therapy, consider adding in lorazepam or high dose IV metoclopramide.
○ Review the need for anti-emetics if the underlying cause has been resolved.

Other relevant sections
• Chapter 2, sections on hypercalcaemia, raised intracranial pressure
• Chapter 3, section on bowel obstruction

References

Basch E, Prestrud AA, Hesketh PJ, Kris MG, Feyer PC, Somerfield MR, *et al*. Antiemetics: American Society of Clinical Oncology clinical practice guideline update. *Journal of Clinical Oncology*. 2011. 29(31): 4189–98.
Glare P, Miller J, Nikolova T, Tickoo R. Treating nausea and vomiting in palliative care: a review. *Clinical Interventions in Aging*. 2011. 6: 243–59.
Harris DG. Nausea and vomiting in advanced cancer. *British Medical Bulletin*. 2010. 96: 175–85.
Roila F, Herrstedt J, Aapro M, Gralla RJ, Einhorn LH, Ballatori E, *et al*. Guideline update for MASCC and ESMO in the prevention of chemotherapy and radiotherapy-induced nausea and vomiting: results of the Perugia consensus conference. *Annals of Oncology*. 2010. 21(Suppl. 5): v232–43.

Neuropathy

Neuropathy is defined as a disorder characterised by the inflammation or degeneration of nerves. Neuropathy can be sensory, motor or autonomic. The grading of neuropathy is shown in Table 3.33.

Symptoms and signs
• Peripheral sensory neuropathy: intermittent distal paraesthesiae and numbness which can persist for longer periods as the condition worsens. The numbness may become more proximal or may start to affect function.
• Peripheral motor neuropathy: distal weakness which can deteriorate, becoming more proximal and pronounced.
• Autonomic neuropathy: orthostatic hypotension, syncope, sweating, diarrhoea, constipation or ileus, impotence or urinary disturbances.

Causes
Neurotoxic chemotherapeutics
• Around 30–40% of patients report chemotherapy-induced peripheral neuropathy.
• Peripheral sensory neuropathy is a common dose-limiting toxicity of several chemotherapy agents, including taxanes, platinums, vinca alkaloids, thalidomide and proteasome inhibitors.

Table 3.33 CTCAE (V4.03) grading of neuropathy.

Grade	Dysaesthesia	Peripheral sensory neuropathy	Peripheral motor neuropathy
1	Mild sensory alteration.	Asymptomatic; loss of deep tendon reflexes or paraesthesiae.	Asymptomatic; clinical or diagnostic observations only; intervention not indicated.
2	Moderate sensory alteration; limiting instrumental ADL.	Moderate symptoms; limiting instrumental ADL.	Moderate symptoms; limiting instrumental ADL.
3	Severe sensory alteration; limiting self-care ADL.	Severe symptoms; limiting self-care ADL.	Severe symptoms; limiting self-care ADL; assistive device indicated.
4	—	Life-threatening consequences; urgent intervention indicated.	Life-threatening consequences; urgent intervention indicated.
5	—	Death.	Death.

From the website of the National Cancer Institute (http://www.cancer.gov).

- Onset and recovery is variable and can lead to dose modifications, reduced dose intensity and early cessation of treatment.
- *Risk factors*:
  ○ Pre-existing neuropathy (e.g. due to diabetes).
  ○ Poor nutritional status.
  ○ History of alcohol abuse.
  ○ Studies are underway to investigate genetic polymorphisms that may predispose to neuropathy.

Cisplatin
- Grade 2 neuropathy occurs in 6% of patients.
- Predominantly sensory with loss of vibration sense and paraesthesiae. Can also cause sensorineural hearing loss.
- Develops within three to six months of initiation of treatment and can worsen after treatment. Usually reversible.

Oxaliplatin
- Peripheral neuropathy occurs in 90% of patients.
- *Acute sensory neuropathy*:
  ○ Paraesthesiae, dysaesthesia and muscle cramps. Triggered by cold.
  ○ Pharyngolaryngeal dysaesthesia can occur, causing a feeling of difficulty in breathing.
  ○ *Chronic sensory neuropathy*: symptoms will have partly resolved in 80% of patients in 4–6 months and are likely to have completely resolved in 40–50% of patients by 6–8 months, but can be permanent in the remaining patients.

Taxanes
- Paclitaxel:
  - Painful sensory neuropathy occurs in 30% of patients.
  - Starts 24–72 hours post infusion and can last for up to seven days.
  - Affects proprioception, vibration sense and fine touch.
  - Can also develop a mild motor neuropathy with distal weakness.
- Docetaxel:
  - Peripheral neuropathy occurs less commonly than with paclitaxel.
  - Symptoms are milder than with paclitaxel and resolve spontaneously.

Vinca alkaloids (e.g. vincristine, vinorelbine and vinblastine)
- Painful sensory neuropathy. This is usually reversible on treatment cessation but can take several months.
- One third of patients also report autonomic dysfunction, and muscle weakness can develop in advanced neuropathy.

Bortezomib
- Painful peripheral sensory neuropathy; 10% also report autonomic neuropathy.
- Resolves in up to 75% of patients within six months.

Thalidomide
- Dose dependent cumulative sensory neuropathy occurs in 40% patients due to destruction of dorsal root ganglia.
- Causes significant paraesthesiae and loss of touch and pain sensation.
- Around 25% recover within six months.

Other causes
- Radiotherapy: radiotherapy can cause damage to nerves within the radiation field, for example brachial plexus injury is possible following lung radiotherapy
- Local tumour invasion, for example sciatic nerve or brachial plexus invasion
- Mechanical nerve compression, for example due to spondylolisthesis
- Infectious agents, for example Bell's palsy secondary to herpes zoster infection
- Diabetes
- Hypothyroidism
- Vitamin B12 or thiamine deficiency
- Chronic alcohol abuse
- Vasculitis
- Uraemia
- Exposure to heavy metal toxins

Management
- Advise patients to stop smoking, limit alcohol consumption and correct vitamin deficiencies.

- Meticulous foot care and early attention to wounds is important.
- Patients should not undertake activities that require full nervous function (e.g. assess if a patient with a peripheral lower limb sensory or motor neuropathy is safe to drive).
- Active and passive exercise can improve muscle strength and prevent wasting. Consider a physiotherapy referral for patients with a motor neuropathy.

Neuroprotective treatment
- *Calcium and magnesium infusions*:
  - Increasing extracellular calcium has been suggested as a neuroprotective strategy but this has not been proven to be effective.
- *Glutathione*:
  - May prevent accumulation of platinum compounds in the dorsal root ganglia.
  - Early studies with glutathione have shown promising effects on neuropathy caused by carboplatin, oxaliplatin and paclitaxel chemotherapy.
- *Dose modification*:
  - Can be seen as a strategy to enhance neuroprotection.
  - Alternative treatment regimens and dose reduction guidelines based on toxicity criteria can help limit the neuropathy. This, however, needs to be considered at the risk of less efficacious treatment.
  - One study showed that discontinuation and reintroduction of oxaliplatin based on toxicity criteria resulted in a decrease in neuropathy with the same response rate.

Pharmacological treatment
- Established chemotherapy-induced neuropathy and associated neuropathic pain is difficult to treat. Few trials have specifically evaluated chemotherapy induced neuropathic pain.
- Pregabalin has shown promise in early phase trials. It was increased to a target dose of 150 mg three times daily. Gabapentin, however, was not shown to be effective in Phase III studies.
- A systematic review of amitriptyline in chronic neuropathic pain has shown that there is no unbiased evidence of a positive effect and that effectiveness may be overestimated in current practice.
- Early studies suggest that serotonin and norepinephrine uptake inhibitors (SNRI) such as venlafaxine and duloxetine may reduce oxaliplatin-related neuropathy.

Neurostimulation
- Early data suggests that acupuncture may be useful.
- Scrambler therapy, an electrocutaneous nerve stimulation treatment may also help treat chemotherapy-induced neuropathy.
- Small studies have shown that transcutaneous electrical nerve stimulations (TENS) can have beneficial effects in patients with neuropathic pain secondary to diabetes.

References

Albers JW, Chaudhry V, Cavaletti G, Donehower RC. Interventions for preventing neuropathy caused by cisplatin and related compounds. *Cochrane Database of Systematic Reviews*. 2011. 16(2): CD005228.
Beijers AJ, Jongen JL, Vreugdenhil G. Chemotherapy-induced neurotoxicity: the value of neuroprotective strategies. *Netherlands Journal of Medicine*. 2012. 70(1): 18–25.
Moore RA, Derry S, Aldington D, Cole P, Wiffen PJ. Amitriptyline for neuropathic pain and fibromyalgia in adults. *Cochrane Database of Systematic Reviews*. 2012. 12: CD008242.
Pachman DR, Barton DL, Swetz KM, Loprinzi CL. Troublesome symptoms in cancer survivors: fatigue, insomnia, neuropathy, and pain. *Journal of Clinical Oncology*. 2012. 30(30): 3687–96.
Pieber K, Herceg M, Paternostro-Sluga T. Electrotherapy for the treatment of painful diabetic peripheral neuropathy: a review. *Journal of Rehabilitation Medicine*. 2010. 42(4): 289–95.
Smith EM, Pang H, Cirrincione C, Fleishman S, Paskett ED, Ahles T. *et al.*, and Alliance for Clinical Trials in Oncology Effect of duloxetine on pain, function, and quality of life among patients with chemotherapy-induced painful peripheral neuropathy: a randomized clinical trial. *Journal of the American Medical Association*. 2013. 309(13): 1359–67.

Neutropenia

Neutropenia is the reduction in neutrophils below the normal range. Moderate neutropenia is defined as a neutrophil count of 0.5–1.0 x10⁹/L and severe neutropenia is a count of <0.5 x10⁹/L. The grading of neutropenia is shown in Table 3.34.

Causes
In cancer patients, neutropenia is often an expected side effect of chemotherapy, chemo-radiotherapy or, less commonly, radiotherapy. It is particularly related to dose dense, dose intense or chemo-radiotherapy treatments. Some protocols are associated with higher rates of febrile neutropenia and have antibiotic prophylaxis or GCSF built into their regimens. It is important to ensure that these patients receive these components of their treatment.
* Causes of expected neutropenia:
  ○ Secondary to treatment (the commonest cause in patients receiving anti-cancer treatment).
  ○ Secondary to cancer: for example extensive bone marrow infiltration secondary to breast or prostate cancer.
* Causes of unexpected neutropenia:
  ○ congenital
    ▪ Rare
    ▪ Ethnic variation – particularly in patients of African descent
* Acquired:
  ○ Reduction in neutrophil production:
    ▪ Aplastic anaemia
    ▪ Vitamin B12, folate or iron deficiency

Table 3.34 CTCAE (V4.03) grading of neutropenia.

Grade	Criteria
1	< lower limit normal to $1.5 \times 10^9/L$
2	$< 1.5–1.0 \times 10^9/L$
3	$< 1.0–0.5 \times 10^9/L$
4	$< 0.5 \times 10^9/L$
5	—

From the website of the National Cancer Institute (http://www.cancer.gov).

- Chemical exposure (e.g. benzene)
- Medication (e.g. phenytoin, chloramphenicol)
- Alcohol abuse
- Autoimmune neutropenia
- Infections – EBV, hepatitis B or C, HIV, CMV, typhoid
○ Increased neutrophil turnover:
  - Hypersplenism
  - Acute bacterial infection
○ Unclear mechanism:
  - Medications, for example analgesics, anti-inflammatories, anticonvulsants, antibiotics, antihistamines, diuretics, hypoglycaemics, antidepressants
  - Thyroid dysfunction
  - Infections – malaria, toxoplasmosis

Management
- Patients with neutropenia may be clinically well and require no further intervention. They should receive clear information about contacting the unit/hospital if they become unwell and their neutrophil count should be checked at expected time points, for example prior to next cycle of treatment (although this is regimen dependent).
- Patients suspected to be neutropenic who are unwell or febrile should be managed as outlined in the section on febrile neutropenia in Chapter 2.

Management of unexpected neutropenia
- History and examination to determine possible aetiology
- FBC, U&E, folate, B12, iron, ferritin, LFT, TFTs, anti-nuclear and anti-DNA antibodies and rheumatoid factor.
- Most cases will resolve spontaneously, but approximately one third will be chronic or idiopathic.
- Discussion with the haematology team may be undertaken if the cause cannot be established and further systemic treatment is affected.

GCSF

* Stimulates the production of neutrophils and may reduce the duration of neutropenia.
* Can be used for peripheral stem cell or bone marrow transplantation, but these indications are not covered in this book.
* Long-acting and short-acting preparations are available. These should be given at least 24 hours after chemotherapy. In the acute setting, short-acting preparations are administered daily until recovery of the neutrophil count (protocols may state to stop on second day of recovery). Examples include:
  * *Long-acting*: pegfilgrastim 6 mg SC 24 hours after chemotherapy (one dose per cycle)
  * *Short-acting*: lenograstim 150 µg (19.2 MIU) per m² SC OD or filgrastim (preparations include: Neupogen® 5 µg/kg SC OD)
* Side effects include: musculoskeletal/bone pain, GI disturbances, headache, rash, interstitial pneumonia (rare).

Primary prophylaxis
* Recommended for regimes with a greater than 20% rate of febrile neutropenia.
* Guidelines recommend considering primary prophylaxis if: HIV positive, radiotherapy administered to >20% of bone marrow or over 65 years old and receiving intensive, curative regimes (e.g. CHOP).

Secondary prophylaxis
In patients who previously developed febrile neutropenia or neutropenia that resulted in a dose delay/dose reduction of curative treatment, consider GCSF to reduce the probability of life-threatening infection or further dose delays/reductions with the next cycle of treatment

Treatment of febrile neutropenia
* Not used for uncomplicated cases.
* Recommended in protracted febrile neutropenia (> 7 days), or those with severe sepsis, pneumonia or fungal infection.

Other relevant sections of this book
Chapter 2, section on febrile neutropenia

References

Crawford J, Caserta C and Roila F. Hematopoietic growth factors: ESMO clinical practice guidelines for the applications. *Annals of Oncology*. 2010. 21(Suppl. 5): v248–51.

Willacy H, Rull G. Neutropenic patients and neutropenic regimes. Patient.co.uk. Available from: http://www.patient.co.uk/doctor/neutropenic-patients-and-neutropenic-regimes (accessed 1 January 2014).

Proteinuria

Proteinuria is the presence of excessive protein within the urine. The grading of proteinuria is shown in Table 3.35.

Causes
- Chemotherapeutic agents, for example streptozocin
- Biological agents, for example VEGF-inhibitors (e.g. bevacizumab, sunitinib)
- UTI
- Hypertension
- Diabetes mellitus
- Multiple myeloma
- Systemic lupus erythematosis
- Nephritis/nephropathy (related to treatment/cancer or other condition such as amyloidosis)

Symptoms
Proteinuria itself is usually asymptomatic. Patients may describe 'frothy' urine in severe cases. Symptoms are dependent on the cause:
- Bone pain in myeloma
- Signs of infection with UTI
- Oedema – to ankles, sacrum or peri-orbital areas – especially in nephrotic syndrome

Investigations
- FBC, U&E, coagulation, albumin, lipid profile
- Urine dipstick and microscopy
- 24-hour urine protein collection
- USS KUB
- CT abdomen/pelvis

Table 3.35 CTCAE (V4.03) grading of proteinuria.

Grade	Criteria
1	1+ proteinuria. Urinary protein < 1.0 g/24 hours.
2	2+ or 3+ proteinuria. Urinary protein 1.0–3.4 g/24 hours.
3	4+ proteinuria. Urinary protein >= 3.5 g/24 hours.
4	Nephrotic syndrome: triad of urinary protein > 3–3.5 g/24 hours, hypoalbuminaemia (albumin < 25 g/L) and generalised oedema. Often with hyperlipidaemia.
5	—

From the website of the National Cancer Institute (http://www.cancer.gov).

Management
- Treat any possible underlying cause
- Refer to a renal physician – particularly if haematuria or casts
- Advise regarding adequate oral fluid intake
- Referral to dietician for 'renal diet'
- Consider risk of thromboembolism

Bevacizumab-related proteinuria
This affects around 33% of patients on bevacizumab and may lead to discontinuation of treatment in severe cases. The management is dependent on the level of proteinuria.

At baseline:
- Dipstick analysis should demonstrate no proteinuria or 1+ proteinuria.
- If dipstick demonstrates 2+ proteinuria – proceed to 24 hour urine protein (must be ≤2 g/24 hours).

Monitoring whilst on treatment:
- Grade 1: continue bevacizumab.
- Grade 2: continue bevacizumab; 24-hour urine collection within three days prior to next treatment.
  - 24-hour collection: ≤ 2 g/24 hours – proceed with bevacizumab. Revert to urine dipstick if <1 g/24 hours.
  - 24-hour collection: > 2 g/24 hours – hold bevacizumab and repeat urine collection 24 hours prior to next treatment.
- Grade 3: hold bevacizumab and check 24 hour urine protein. Restart if falls below 2 g/24 hours.
- Grade 4: discontinue bevacizumab.

References

BC Cancer Agency Cancer Management Guidelines. *Management Guidelines of Bevacizumab-Related Side Effects.* Available from: http://www.bccancer.bc.ca/NR/rdonlyres/6D39414F-EC1A-4BE2-9ACB-6DE017C9B4C4/19258/Managementforbevacizumabsideeffects_1 Dec06.pdf (accessed 1 January 2014).

Hull RP, Goldsmith DJA. Nephrotic syndrome in adults. *British Medical Journal.* 2008. 336(7654): 1185–9.

Kandula P, Agarwal R. Proteinuria and hypertension with tyrosine kinase inhibitors. *Kidney International.* 2011. 80(12): 1271–7.

Kelly RJ, Billemont B, Rixe O. Renal toxicity of targeted therapies. *Target Oncology.* 2009. 4(2): 121–3.

Pruritus

Pruritus is defined as an unpleasant cutaneous sensation that induces the desire to scratch. The grading of pruritus is shown in Table 3.36.

Table 3.36 CTCAE (V4.03) grading of pruritus.

Grade	Criteria
1	Mild or localised; topical intervention indicated.
2	Intense or widespread; skin changes from scratching (e.g. oedema, papulation, excoriations, lichenification, oozing/crusts); oral intervention indicated; limiting instrumental ADL.
3	Intense or widespread; constant; limiting self-care ADL or sleep; oral corticosteroid or immunosuppressive therapy indicated.
4	—
5	—

From the website of the National Cancer Institute (http://www.cancer.gov).

Assessment

- *History*: including whether the itch is generalised or localised as well as exacerbating factors, drug history and past medical history. Assess the impact on the patients' quality of life, for example. ability to sleep.
- *Examination*: including rashes, consequences of scratching (e.g. excoriation, secondary infection).

Causes

- Malignancy:
  - The onset of paraneoplastic pruritus may predate the diagnosis of cancer.
  - Pruritus is more common in haematological malignancies (e.g. lymphoma, leukaemia and myeloma) than solid tumours. However, many solid tumours, (e.g. breast, lung, colon, gastric, glioblastoma, carcinoid, melanoma) and metastatic skin infiltration can also cause pruritus.
  - Pruritus may be localised (e.g. scrotal itch with prostate cancer, vulval itch with cervical cancer) or generalised.
- Biliary or hepatic disease:
  - May be secondary to underlying malignancy or due to other causes.
  - Pruritus occurs in up to 80% of patients with cholestasis and tends to start with the palms and soles before becoming more generalised.
- Renal failure: may be secondary to the underlying malignancy or due to unrelated causes.
- Drugs:
  - Opioids.
  - Medications that can cause cholestasis, for example erythromycin, hormonal therapies.
  - Hypersensitivity reactions to treatment, for example platinum-based drugs, taxanes.
  - Interferon, interleukin-2.
  - GCSF.
  - Rash secondary to EGFR inhibitors (e.g. gefitinib, erlotinib, cetuximab, panitumumab).

- Radiotherapy: can cause skin dryness, resulting in pruritus.
- Other dermatological conditions: for example eczema, psoriasis.
- Insect bites or infections: including scabies, candida, HIV and syphilis.
- Endocrine disorders: e.g. thyroid disease, diabetes mellitus.
- Iron-deficiency anaemia.

Management
General management
- Treat the underlying cause if possible.
- Reduce the dose or discontinue any causative medication (if possible). Switching opioids may help with opioid-induced pruritus.
- Avoid any exacerbating factors, for example heat, frequent bathing, alcohol, spicy foods, tight clothing.
- Avoid soap and use soap substitutes (e.g. aqueous cream) instead.
- Tepid (rather than hot) showers or baths.

Topical therapies
- Topical emollients (e.g. aqueous cream) containing menthol (0.25–2%) or phenol (0.5–2%), applied several times a day can help to suppress the sensation of itch by inducing surface cooling.
- Capsaicin (0.025%) QDS may be effective, but can cause an initial burning sensation and so is more suitable for localised areas of pruritus.
- Lidocaine (2.5%) can also be used for localised pruritus, but can lead to skin sensitisation and there is a risk of toxicity (e.g. arrhythmias) if used in large quantities.
- Doxepin (5%) TDS-QDS to < 10% of the body surface may relieve itch (particularly in dermatitis) but can be sedating.
- Topical corticosteroids may be useful for localised areas.

Systemic therapies
- *Antihistamines*: for example hydroxyzine 10–50 mg BD or chlorpheniramine 4 mg TDS. Useful for pruritus due to allergy or urticaria, but there is little evidence for their use for pruritus due to other causes.
- *Antidepressants*: for example paroxetine 5–10 mg nocte can relieve pruritus due to cholestasis, uraemia, malignancy or opioids. Effects start within 24–48 hours but may wear off after 4–6 weeks. Mirtazapine 7.5–10 mg nocte is an alternative, but can be sedating.
- Cholestyramine 4–8 g daily in a suitable liquid can relieve itching due to cholestasis, but is unpalatable and difficult to tolerate.
- Ondansetron 8 mg OD or BD or granistron 1 mg OD may be useful for pruritus due to cholestasis, opioids or uraemia.
- Other antiemetics (e.g. aprepitant and levomepromazine) also have an antipruritic effect.
- Cimetidine 400–1200 mg/day is particularly useful in pruritus due to lymphoma.

- Corticosteroids, for example dexamethasone 4 mg OD.
- Rifampicin 75 mg OD to 150 mg BD can be used for pruritus due to cholestasis.
- NSAIDS can help relieve pruritus caused by cutaneous metastases (particularly in breast cancer).
- Oral opioid antagonists can relieve pruritus (particularly in cholestasis), but are usually not appropriate due to the need for opioids for pain relief or relief of breathlessness.
- Thalidomide can also relieve pruritus, particularly in renal failure.

UVB phototherapy
May help with pruritus secondary to uraemia, cholestasis and malignant skin infiltrations, but is usually not practical as treatment is often required three times a week.

Other relevant sections of this book
Chapter 3, section on rash

References

Chiang HC, Huang V, Cornelius LA. Cancer and itch. *Seminars in Cutaneous Medicine and Surgery*. 2011. 30(2): 107–12.

Lidstone V, Thorns A. Pruritus in cancer patients. *Cancer Treatment Reviews*. 2001. 27(5): 305–12. Epub 2 March 2002.

Seccareccia D, Gebara N. Pruritus in palliative care: Getting up to scratch. *Canadian Family Physician, Médecin de famille canadien*. 2011. 57(9): 1010–3, e316–9.

Twycross R, Greaves MW, Handwerker H, Jones EA, Libretto SE, Szepietowski JC, *et al.* Itch: scratching more than the surface. *Quarterly Journal of Medicine*. 2003. 96(1): 7–26.

Psychiatric disorders

Overview
Up to 50% of patients with cancer experience a form of psychological distress. This can range from anxiety and depression to psychotic disorders. There are also patients with pre-identified psychiatric disorders who go on to have a cancer diagnosis. Current literature suggests these patients do worse than their counterparts and require close liaison with their usual psychiatric team.

Adjustment disorder, depression and suicidal ideation
An adjustment disorder can be seen after a significant stressor and can manifest in low mood, anxiety, and emotional and behavioural change while adjusting to the change in circumstances. The treatment for this is principally supportive and may include psychological interventions. An adjustment disorder is usually expected to resolve within six months or with the removal of the stressor.

Depression should be suspected when there is anhedonia (inability to gain pleasure), feelings of worthlessness or excessive guilt, poor concentration, biological symptoms of depression (although difficult in cancer patients as overlap with illness or treatment side effects, e.g. weight loss, poor sleep, lack of energy, reduced libido) or if there are ruminations on self-harm or suicide.

If depression is suspected a referral to liaison psychiatry is recommended. Depression is not only common but is also debilitating and adversely effects outcome so its recognition and appropriate referral is of paramount importance.

Non-psychological causes of depression
- CNS: dementia, delirium, tumour, infection
- Metabolic: electrolyte disturbances, hypothyroidism, hypoadrenalism, B12/folate deficiency
- Anaemia
- Pain
- Drugs: tamoxifen, sedatives, corticosteroids, chemotherapies (e.g. bleomycin, vincristine, vinblastine, interferon, interleukin), androgen deprivation therapy.

Management strategies
- Pharmacological – good in severe depression, equal to psychological counselling in milder depression in non-cancer patients:
  - Consider drug-to-drug interactions (particularly between antidepressants and chemotherapy)
  - Start low and titrate dose over an initial four-week assessment period
- Psychological therapies – supportive psychotherapy and cognitive behavioural therapies are the two most commonly used. Often access is through cancer support units and charitable organisations.

Suicidal ideation
If the patient discloses thoughts of self-harm or suicide, or this is suspected, an urgent referral to psychiatric colleagues is warranted as physical illness increases the risk of completed suicide in individuals with depression.
- The suicide rate amongst cancer patients is twice that of the general population and is thought to be a slight underestimate.
- Suicidal ideation should be directly enquired about if there are concerns about depression and acted on if there is concern.
- Risk factors include: depression, loss of hope, pain, social isolation, advanced illness, pre-existing psychopathology, subjective loss of control and delirium.

Anxiety
Anxiety may affect 10–30% of cancer patients. It is characterised by feelings of apprehension of danger and dread, accompanied by restlessness, tension, tachycardia and/or dyspnoea unattached to a clearly identifiable source. The grading of anxiety is shown in Table 3.37. There is increasing recognition and support for

Table 3.37 CTCAE (V4.03) grading of anxiety.

Grade	Criteria
1	Mild symptoms, intervention not indicated.
2	Moderate symptoms, limiting instrumental ADL.
3	Severe symptoms; limiting self-care ADL; hospitalisation not indicated.
4	Life-threatening; hospitalisation indicated.
5	Death.

From the website of the National Cancer Institute (http://www.cancer.gov).

ongoing anxiety after cessation of treatment and follow-up in through survivorship programmes.

Causes

Anxiety can be classified into groups which include situational, existential and organic causes. Situational and existential causes are obviously very important to cancer patients.

Organic causes include:

- CNS tumours
- Carcinoid syndrome
- Pulmonary causes, for example hypoxia, bronchospasm and lymphangitis
- Endocrine causes, for example thyrotoxicosis, phaeochromocytoma, hyponatraemia, hypoglycaemia
- Cardiac causes, for example tachyarrhythmias
- Pain
- Delirium
- Medication related: antipsychotics, metoclopramide, flumazenil, antibiotics (e.g. isoniazid and ciprofloxacin), thyroxine, corticosteroids, theophylline
- Withdrawal states, for example benzodiazepine, alcohol or tobacco withdrawal
- Serotonergic syndrome: SSRIs or SNRIs

Symptoms

- Poor concentration, irritability, insomnia and physical symptoms such as tension, sweating, dry mouth and chest pain.
- Co-existing depression is frequent and should be treated.

Management

Patients may have a pre-existing panic disorder or generalised anxiety. If the patient is already known to community psychology or psychiatry teams, then close liaison is advised. Multidisciplinary team working is well recognised in anxiety management and will include multiple teams within the hospital, such as nursing staff, psychologists and specialist nurses, as well as community teams.

Patients without previously diagnosed anxiety disorder may require specific action depending on the severity of their anxiety.
- Identify and treat any organic cause.
- Review any exacerbating factors, for example high dose steroids.
- Self-help or educational material to reduce anxiety or enable independent support for symptom control may be sufficient for mild symptoms.
- Benzodiazepines (e.g. lorazepam), have been used to reduce symptoms. They should be used cautiously. Only short-term treatment is recommended (less than two weeks).
- Psychological support and behavioural management techniques should be considered for moderate symptoms or where educational material has not proven useful. Referral for consideration to a specialist oncology-psychology team is available in many areas.
- Further pharmacological treatment includes selective serotonin reuptake inhibitors (SSRIs). Expert advice should be considered to balance toxicities and drug interactions, for example withdrawal syndrome. SSRIs are also associated with increased suicidal tendency in patients less than 30 years old.

Psychosis

Psychosis is a serious mental illness associated with abnormality of thought and a loss of ability to differentiate between what is real and what is unreal. It is differentiated from delirium in that delirium usually has brief onset, and is associated with significant confusion and disorientation in time. Psychosis usually has an insidious onset and the patient usually presents in clear consciousness, that is to say they are usually orientated in time and place.

Psychosis may result from:
- A pre-existing psychiatric illness, such as schizophrenia or bipolar disorder.
- Medication, such as high-dose steroids (this includes doses commonly used within an oncology setting, although steroid-induced psychosis is relatively rare).
- Substance misuse and alcohol abuse.
- Physical conditions such as brain tumours or Parkinson's.

If psychosis is suspected, refer to liaison psychiatry and a joint approach will be required to manage the patient safely and appropriately. Antipsychotic medication should only be initiated on psychiatric advice, outside of extreme emergencies, as a full psychiatric assessment will be required to confirm the diagnosis prior to initiating treatment.

In patients with psychosis it can also be useful to employ environment interventions such as placing the patient in a side room, offering reassurance and using a 1:1 psychiatric nurse to support the patient if necessary.

Mental Capacity Act (2005)

This is important in consenting patients for treatment. It may also be needed more acutely if a patient is a risk to themselves or others and, for example, wants to be discharged. The capacity of the patient should be examined to ensure their decision-making ability remains intact. All patients are assumed to have capacity for a specific decision until found otherwise.

Capacity is assessed in two stages, ensuring all steps have been taken to allow the patient to make a decision (e.g. wearing glasses and hearing aids):

1 Presence of a condition that may impair the mind. If yes, proceed to 2.
2 Functional assessment regarding the specific decision at that point in time. Each of the following must be achieved:
   (a) Able to understand the information pertinent to the decision.
   (b) Retain the information long enough to enable a decision to be made.
   (c) Use and weigh up this information to make a decision (including the consequences of the decision or not making any decision).
   (d) Ability to communicate this decision.

In cases of delirium, for example, they may lack capacity and decisions can be made in the patient's best interests. The use of proportional restraint may be needed to ensure the patient's safety.

In cases regarding treatment decisions where the patient more permanently lacks capacity, they may have an appointed person with Lasting Power of Attorney (LPA). It should be ensured that this LPA covers the patient's healthcare decisions. If this is not present then an Independent Mental Capacity Advocate (IMCA) should be appointed.

In cases where the possible lack of capacity is contentious the treating team should liaise closely with the Liaison Psychiatry service to best determine the course of management with regards to decision making. Again, if capacity is found to be lacking an IMCA should be appointed.

Mental Health Act 1983

In known or suspected cases of a functional psychiatric disorder (not directly resulting from a physical cause such as delirium) the Mental Health Act 1983 may be used to allow a period of assessment and/or treatment in England and Wales.

The section of the act that can be used depends on whether the patient is an in-patient or outpatient:

- For in-patients, Section 5:2 allows the patient to be detained by a doctor for up to 72 hours to allow a formal Mental Health Act Assessment to take place. Advice on enacting the Mental Health Act and completing the 5:2 form should be obtained with advice from the on-call psychiatric service or liaison psychiatry team.
- For outpatients, including those patients seen in outpatient clinics, Section 2 applies for assessment and Section 3 for treatment. The psychiatric team and police should be informed for outpatients, who can then arrange for the patient to be taken to a place of safety.

Other relevant sections of this book

Chapter 3, section on confusion and decreased conscious level

References

Mental Capacity Act (2005). Available from: http://www.legislation.gov.uk/ukpga/2005/9/contents (accessed 1 January 2014).

Mental Health Act (1983). Available from: http://www.legislation.gov.uk/ukpga/2007/12/contents (accessed 1 January 2014).

National Institute for Health and Care Excellence. *Generalised Anxiety Disorder and Panic Disorder (with or without Agoraphobia) in Adults: Management in Primary, Secondary and Community Care* (CG113). London: National Institute for Health and Care Excellence: London. 2011.

NHS Choices. Psychosis. Available from: http://www.nhs.uk/Conditions/Psychosis/Pages/Introduction.aspx (accessed 1 January 2014).

Wein S, Sulkes A and Stemmer S. The oncologist's role in managing depression, anxiety and demoralization with advanced cancer. *Cancer Journal.* 2010. 16(5): 493–499.

Rash

Skin or nail changes are a common side effect of many anti-cancer therapies and can significantly affect patients' quality of life. The standard CTCAE grading (see Tables 3.38 and 3.39) do not always accurately reflect the severity of the rash, but none of the various other proposed grading systems are currently widely used.

General advice
- *Avoid*: hot water, heat exposure, excessive skin friction, tight clothes/shoes, traumatic activity (particularly in the first few weeks after starting treatment) and alcohol-based cosmetic products.
- *Recommend*: using suncream, paying careful attention to cuts/open areas to prevent infection, shoes with padded insoles to reduce the pressure on feet.

Table 3.38 CTCAE (V4.03) grading of hand-foot syndrome/palmar plantar erythrodysesthesia (PPE)/acral erythema.

Grade	Criteria
1	Minimal skin changes or dermatitis (e.g. erythema, oedema, or hyperkeratosis) without pain.
2	Skin changes (e.g. peeling, blisters, bleeding, oedema, or hyperkeratosis) with pain; limiting instrumental ADL.
3	Severe skin changes (e.g. peeling, blisters, bleeding, oedema, or hyperkeratosis) with pain; limiting self-care ADL.
4	—
5	—

From the website of the National Cancer Institute (http://www.cancer.gov).

Table 3.39 CTCAE (V4.03) grading of acneiform rash.

Grade	Criteria
1	Papules and/or pustules covering <10% BSA, which may or may not be associated with symptoms of pruritus or tenderness.
2	Papules and/or pustules covering 10–30% BSA, which may or may not be associated with symptoms of pruritus or tenderness; associated with psychosocial impact; limiting instrumental ADL.
3	Papules and/or pustules covering >30% BSA, which may or may not be associated with symptoms of pruritus or tenderness; limiting self-care ADL; associated with local superinfection with oral antibiotics indicated.
4	Papules and/or pustules covering any percentage BSA, which may or may not be associated with symptoms of pruritus or tenderness and are associated with extensive superinfection with IV antibiotics indicated; life-threatening consequences.
5	Death.

From the website of the National Cancer Institute (http://www.cancer.gov).

Hand-foot syndrome due to chemotherapy
Symptoms and signs
- Starts as a symmetrical tingling/burning sensation on the palms and/or soles followed by painful erythema, blistering, desquamation and extensive superficial exfoliation which can significantly impact on patients' ability to perform ADLs (see Figure 3.2).
- Hands are more commonly affected than feet.
- Rarely, a morbilliform eruption or faint erythema may also be seen on the scalp, neck, chest and extremities.
- Chronic PPE can result in the loss of fingerprints, which can be problematic (e.g. if travelling to the USA).

Causes
Capecitabine, 5-FU, docetaxel, cyclophosphamide, doxorubicin, vincristine, etoposide, cytarabine, vincristine, vinblastine and methotrexate.

Management
- The mainstay of management is dose reduction or temporary/permanent discontinuation of the causative drug. This usually leads to resolution of signs and symptoms within several days to weeks.
- Regular application of emollient creams, for example Udderly Smooth cream®.
- Cool packs on hands or bathing in cool water may relieve pain.
- Reduce friction (e.g. avoid using hand tools, pat rather than rub hands dry) and avoid rubber gloves.
- Pyridoxine was previously thought to be helpful but the benefit has not been proven in randomised controlled trials and is not currently recommended.

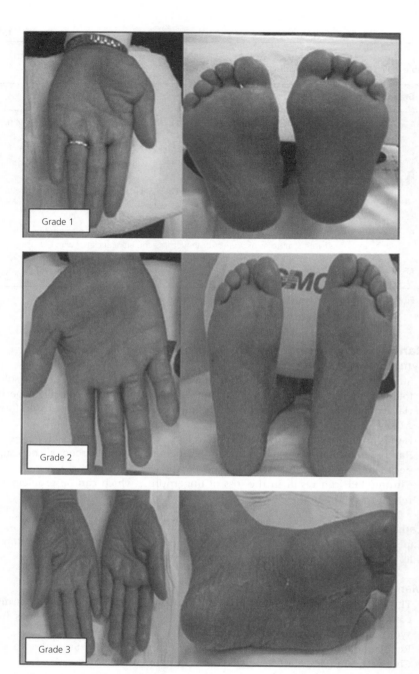

Figure 3.2 Hand foot syndrome secondary to capecitabine. Reproduced from Son HS, Lee WY, Lee WS, Yun SH, Chun HK. Compliance and effective management of the hand-foot syndrome in colon cancer patients receiving capecitabine as adjuvant chemotherapy. *Yonsei Medical Journal*. 2009. 50(6): 796–802 (open access article). To see a colour version of this figure, see Plate 3.2.

Hand-foot syndrome due to tyrosine kinase inhibitors (e.g. sorafenib, sunitinib)
Symptoms and signs
- Localised tender lesions (+/- blisters) with a peripheral halo of erythema form in pressure areas (e.g. fingertips, heels) or in flexures within 2–4 weeks of starting treatment.
- After several weeks painful, thickened or hyperkeratotic skin forms at the sites of the lesions, impairing function and weight-bearing.

Prevention
- Before starting treatment, examine the skin for existing hyperkeratotic areas/ calluses on soles/palms that may benefit from removal (e.g. by a pedicure).
- If the patient has evidence of abnormal weight-bearing, consider referral to an orthotist for an orthotic device.

Management
- Dose reduction or treatment discontinuation.
- Regular application of emollient creams.
- Consider topical keratolytics (e.g. 20–40% urea or 6% salicylic acid BD) for hyperkeratotic areas.
- If grade 2–3, consider clobetasol 0.05% ointment (Dermovate®) BD to erythematous areas, topical analgesics, for example 2% lidocaine and systemic analgesia (e.g. NSAIDs or codeine).

Acneiform rash
Symptoms and signs
- Papulopustular rash (usually in cosmetically sensitive areas, for example face, scalp, upper chest and back) (see Figure 3.3).
- Seborrheic dermatitis-like rash on the face.
- Pruritus, pain, burning sensation and irritation.
- Usually starts within 2–4 weeks of starting treatment, peaks around week 4–6 and then decreases in severity.
- May become infected (usually with *Staphylococcus aureus*), resulting in oozing and formation of yellowish crusts.
- Resolves within four weeks of stopping treatment, but post-inflammatory skin changes (e.g. hyperpigmentation and erythema) can persist for months or years.

Causes
- Very common in patients treated with EGFR inhibitors, for example erlotinib, gefitinib, cetuximab or panitumumab.
- Risk factors:
  - Erlotinib: non-smokers, fair skin, > 70 years
  - Cetuximab: male, < 70 years

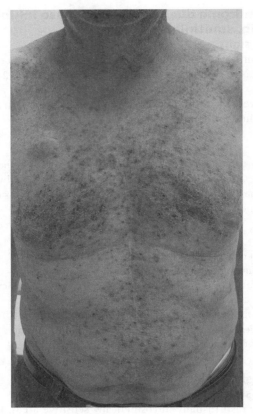

Figure 3.3 Panitumumab-related rash. Reproduced from Fabbrocini G, Cameli N, Romano MC, Mariano M, Panariello L, Bianca D, *et al*. Chemotherapy and skin reactions. *Journal of Experimental & Clinical Cancer Research*. 2012. 31: 50 (open access article). To see a colour version of this figure, see Plate 3.3.

Prevention/prophylaxis
- Regular application of moisturising cream (+/– moisturising aftershave).
- Hydrocortisone 1% cream BD.
- Doxycycline 100 mg PO BD (or minocycline 100 mg/day).

Management
- Regular application of emollients, for example Aveeno® oatmeal lotion.
- Topical antibiotics, for example clindamycin 1% gel BD.
- Oral tetracycline antibiotics, for example doxycycline 100 mg BD, have an anti-inflammatory as well as an antibacterial effect.
- Medium to high potency topical corticosteroids, for example hydrocortisone 1% OD/BD.
- Scalp lesions: erythromycin 2% lotion.

- May require dose delay or dose reduction if severe.
- If grade 3, consider oral corticosteroids (e.g. prednisolone 0.5 mg/kg) for up to ten days.
- For grade 3, highly symptomatic patients in whom other measures have failed: consider isotretinoin (0.3–0.5 mg/kg), IV corticosteroids, IV antibiotics, IV antihistamines and IV hydration.
- Development of the rash may correlate with response to EGFR inhibitor therapy and an increase in survival.

Skin cracking and fissuring
Symptoms and signs
- Often affects fingertips or palms and may be associated with nail changes or PPE (see Figure 3.4).
- Can be very painful and lead to an increased risk of infection.
- Usually occurs 30–60 days after starting treatment.

Causes
EGFR inhibitors, capecitabine, docetaxel and paclitaxel.

Management
- Cover fingertips to avoid friction, recommend protective footwear.
- Regular application of thick moisturising creams or zinc oxide creams.
- Liquid glues, for example LiquiBand® can be used to seal the cracks to relieve pain and help prevent infections.
- If superinfected, consider topical antibiotics, for example fusidic acid 2% cream or mupirocin 2% cream TDS.
- Steroid tape (Cordran® tape) and hydrocolloid dressings may help painful, erythematous areas.

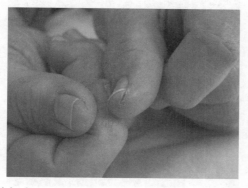

Figure 3.4 Fissures of the fingertips in a patient treated with taxanes. Reproduced from Fabbrocini G, Cameli N, Romano MC, Mariano M, Panariello L, Bianca D, *et al.* Chemotherapy and skin reactions. *Journal of Experimental & Clinical Cancer Research.* 2012. 31: 50. BioMed Central (open access article). To see a colour version of this figure, see Plate 3.4.

Nail changes
Symptoms and signs
- Paronychia – tender, oedematous, often purulent inflammation of the nail fold (see Figure 3.5).
- Periungual pyogenic granuloma-like lesions (which often bleed easily).
- Beau's lines, nail pitting or discolouration.
- Onycholysis (separation of the nail plate from the underlying nail bed).
- Onychodystrophy.
- Pain and functional limitation.
- Often starts on the big toe and may persist even after treatment is stopped.

Causes
EGFR inhibitors (usually starts after ≥ 2 months of treatment), docetaxel, paclitaxel, doxorubicin and epirubicin.

Management
- Paronychia can become superinfected – send a swab for culture to see if antibiotics (e.g. co-amoxiclav, cefalexin, clindamycin) are required.
- Antimicrobial soaks (e.g. dilute white vinegar in water) may help to prevent superinfection.
- Consider topical corticosteroid/antibiotic combinations, for example betamethasone valerate 0.1% plus fusidic acid 2% cream (Fucibet®).

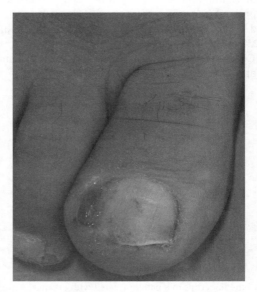

Figure 3.5 Paronychia in a patient treated with lapatinib. Reproduced from Fabbrocini G, Cameli N, Romano MC, Mariano M, Panariello L, Bianca D, *et al.* Chemotherapy and skin reactions. *Journal of Experimental & Clinical Cancer Research.* 2012. 31: 50. BioMed Central (open access article). To see a colour version of this figure, see Plate 3.5.

- Consider an oral tetracycline (e.g. doxycycline 100 mg BD).
- Consider electrocautery, silver nitrate or nail avulsion to eliminate excessive granulation tissue.

Xerosis (dry skin)
Signs and symptoms
- Dry, scaly, itchy skin (especially areas affected or previously affected by EGFR-inhibitor induced papulopustular rash).
- May also cause dryness of the vagina/perineum (causing discomfort on micturition).
- Usually starts approximately 30–60 days after starting treatment.

Causes
- Many drugs, but particularly EGFR inhibitors (especially gefitinib).
- Risk factors: age, pre-existing eczema, prior cytotoxic treatment.

Management
- Regular application of thick moisturising creams, for example urea, colloidal, oatmeal or petroleum-based creams.
- If severe, consider topical steroid creams, for example betamethasone dipropionate 0.05–1% cream (Diprosone®), clobetasone 0.05% cream (Eumovate®) or hydrocortisone butyrate 0.1% cream (Locoid®) thinly OD/BD.

Hyper or hypopigmentation
Signs and symptoms
- May affect the skin, hair, nails or mucous membranes.
- Can be localised or diffuse, with patterns corresponding to anatomic features or related to excoriation, dressings, ECG pads, etc.

Causes
A common side effect of many drugs, including bleomycin, doxorubicin, 5-FU, capecitabine, vinorelbine, ifosfamide, cisplatin, carboplatin, methotrexate, cyclophosphamide and docetaxel.

Management
Usually slowly disappears without treatment when chemotherapy is stopped. Pruritus may be relieved by oral antihistamines.

Radiation recall
This is when the administration of a chemotherapeutic agent results in erythema at a site that was previously irradiated or sunburnt (may have been weeks or months ago).
- Causes include: doxorubicin, gemcitabine, methotrexate, etoposide, doxorubicin, 5-FU, paclitaxel and docetaxel.
- Management: minimise sun exposure, good wound care, consider topical steroids.

Other skin toxicities

- *Raynaud's phenomenon*: for example due to bleomycin or cisplatin.
- *Scleroderma-like reactions*: for example due to bleomycin or docetaxel.
- *Hypersensitivity reactions*: any drugs but especially the platinums, monoclonal antibodies and antibiotic-based drugs.
- *Flushing*: for example due to bleomycin, 5-FU, cyclophosphamide, carboplatin, cisplatin, paclitaxel, docetaxel, tamoxifen or etoposide.
- *Photosensitivity*: for example due to vemurafenib, methotrexate, 5-FU, dacarbazine or vinblastine.
- *Keratoacanthomas and squamous cell carcinomas*: may appear 7–8 weeks after starting treatment with vemurafenib and are managed by excision.
- *Actinic keratoses and seborrhoeic keratoses*: for example due to 5-FU, cisplatin, cytarabine, docetaxel, doxorubicin or vincristine. May regress during therapy but if not then topical low-moderate potency steroids may help.
- *Neutrophilic eccrine hidradenitis*: for example due to cytarabine, bleomycin, doxorubicin or cyclophosphamide. Tender or asymptomatic red papules, plaques, pustules, macules or nodules on the face, ears and trunk, associated with fever. Usually heals without treatment, but systemic steroids, ibuprofen or dapsone may be beneficial.
- *Other toxicities include*: porphyrias, fixed drug eruptions and Stevens-Johnson syndrome.

Other relevant sections of this book

- Chapter 3, section on pruritus
- Chapter 5, section on skin toxicities

References

Corrie PG, Bulusu R, Wilson CB, Armstrong G, Bond S, Hardy R, *et al*. A randomised study evaluating the use of pyridoxine to avoid capecitabine dose modifications. *British Journal of Cancer*. 2012. 107(4): 585–7.

Fabbrocini G, Cameli N, Romano MC, Mariano M, Panariello L, Bianca D, *et al*. Chemotherapy and skin reactions. *Journal of Experimental & Clinical Cancer Research*. 2012. 31: 50.

Lacouture ME, Wu S, Robert C, Atkins MB, Kong HH, Guitart J, *et al*. Evolving strategies for the management of hand-foot skin reaction associated with the multitargeted kinase inhibitors sorafenib and sunitinib. *Oncologist*. 2008. 13(9): 1001–11.

Lacouture ME, Anadkat MJ, Bensadoun RJ, Bryce J, Chan A, Epstein JB, *et al*. Clinical practice guidelines for the prevention and treatment of EGFR inhibitor-associated dermatologic toxicities. *Supportive Care in Cancer*. 2011. 19(8): 1079–95.

Lassere Y, Hoff P. Management of hand-foot syndrome in patients treated with capecitabine (Xeloda). *European Journal of Oncology Nursing*. 2004; 8(Suppl. 1): S31–40.

Pinto C, Barone CA, Girolomoni G, Russi EG, Merlano MC, Ferrari D, *et al*. Management of skin toxicity associated with cetuximab treatment in combination with chemotherapy or radiotherapy. *Oncologist*. 2011. 16(2): 228–38.

Saif MW, Elfiky AA. Identifying and treating fluoropyrimidine-associated hand-and-foot syndrome in white and non-white patients. *Journal of Supportive Oncology*. 2007. 5(7): 337–43.

Son HS, Lee WY, Lee WS, Yun SH, Chun HK. Compliance and effective management of the hand-foot syndrome in colon cancer patients receiving capecitabine as adjuvant chemotherapy. *Yonsei Medical Journal*. 2009. 50(6): 796–802.

Susser WS, Whitaker-Worth DL, Grant-Kels JM. Mucocutaneous reactions to chemotherapy. *Journal of the American Academy of Dermatology*. 1999. 40(3): 367–98; quiz 99–400. Epub 10 March 1999.

Renal failure and hydronephrosis

Acute kidney injury

Acute Kidney Injury (AKI) is the acute loss of renal function. The grading of AKI is shown in Table 3.40. AKI is diagnosed through one of the following findings:
- Increased serum creatinine of 26 µmol/L within 48 hours OR
- Increased serum creatinine 1.5 x baseline value within three months OR
- Urine output below 0.5 ml/kg/hr for ≥6 hours

Causes
- Pre-renal: hypotension, sepsis.
- Renal: prolonged hypoperfusion, nephrotoxins (including NSAIDs, antibiotics and chemotherapeutic agents), glomerulonephritis, infiltrative disease, tumour lysis syndrome.
- Post-renal: obstruction or ureter or bladder outflow.
- Risk factors include: chronic kidney disease (eGRF <60), cardiac failure, liver disease, diabetes, nephrotoxins (IV contrast, NSAIDs, gentamicin, platinum chemotherapy).

Assessment and investigations
- Identify signs and any possible source of sepsis.
- Volume status: capillary refill time, pulse, JVP, skin turgor, pedal or pulmonary oedema, urine output.
- Examine for palpable bladder.
- Signs of vasculitis: rash, uveitis, joint swelling.

Table 3.40 CTCAE (V4.03) grading of acute kidney injury.

Grade	Criteria
1	Creatinine level increase of >0.3 mg/dL; creatinine 1.5–2.0 x above baseline.
2	Creatinine 2–3 x above baseline.
3	Creatinine >3 x baseline or >4.0 mg/dL; hospitalisation indicated.
4	Life-threatening consequences; dialysis indicated.
5	Death.

From the website of the National Cancer Institute (http://www.cancer.gov).

- Bloods: FBC, U&E, bicarbonate, LFT, calcium, phosphate.
- Urine dipstick.
- CXR, renal tract USS.

Management
- Optimise volume status and treat underlying cause, for example sepsis, obstruction
- Treat complications of AKI:
  - Hyperkalaemia.
  - Pulmonary oedema:
    - Sit patient upright and apply oxygen.
    - GTN spray may resolve symptoms.
    - Consider furosemide if passing urine.
    - GTN infusion – seek specialist advice and consider escalating care to HDU/ITU.
    - Renal replacement therapy (RRT) – careful patient selection.
  - Acidosis:
    - Consider treatment if below pH 7.2.
    - IV isotonic sodium bicarbonate 1.4% can be considered in stable patients. Senior discussion is needed as infusion may worsen intracellular acidosis and deliver an excess sodium load. Should not be used in patients with a low calcium.
  - Uraemia, consider RRT if pericarditis.
- Review medications:
  - Avoid nephrotoxic agents, for example NSAIDS, amphotericin B, aminoglycosides.
  - Adjust/stop renally excreted drugs: for example penicillins, LMWH, vancomycin, cephalosporins and morphine

Renal replacement therapy
Considered in patients with any of the following:
- Intractable hyperkalaemia
- Severe acidosis (pH <7.15)
- Intractable pulmonary oedema
- Uraemic complications: for example pericarditis, encephalopathy

Careful discussion is needed with the treating team and renal physicians/intensive care team about the appropriateness of RRT in oncological patients. If the insult to the kidneys is reversible or the prognosis is good then consideration should be undertaken and discussed early.

Chemotherapeutic agents and AKI
Renal toxicity is an important consideration when commencing chemotherapy. It can be a direct result of the chemotherapeutic agent, such as cisplatin, or secondary to other toxicities, such as diarrhoea, leading to dehydration and AKI with 5-FU or capecitabine.

The more commonly used renal toxic chemotherapy agents include:
- Alkylating agents: cisplatin, ifosfamide, nitrosoureas
- Antitumour antibiotics: mitomycin C
- Antimetabolites: high-dose methotrexate
- Biologic agents: interferon, interleukin-2

Consider performing an isotope renal scan (EDTA or DTPA) to accurately measure patients' GFR prior to commencing treatment in patients at high risk of AKI (e.g. patients with existing renal impairment). Renal function should be checked with each cycle of treatment and any possible cause considered, such as ongoing nausea and poor oral intake.

It is important to consider a dose reduction if the renal function has deteriorated as a direct or indirect consequence of chemotherapy. Curative and high-dose regimes should have all other causes considered and a senior discussion before any dose adjustment. The dose of carboplatin is calculated according to patients' GFR and therefore may be preferred to cisplatin in patients with renal impairment.

Hydronephrosis

Hydronephrosis is the distension of the ureter and collecting ducts of the kidney secondary to urinary outflow obstruction. It is an important cause of AKI in cancer patients.

Causes include:
- Non-malignant – urinary tract embolism, benign prostatic hypertrophy, post-surgical stenosis, retroperitoneal fibrosis, ureteric stone disease, TB, ovarian cysts.
- Malignant:
  - Invasion of ureter by primary, metastatic or nodal disease. Most common in patients with cervical, bladder, prostate, colorectal or gynaecological primaries.
  - Bladder outflow obstruction secondary to prostate cancer.

Signs and symptoms
- Flank pain and reduced urine output.
- Symptoms of underlying pathology – ureteric colic (urinary stones), bladder distension (bladder outflow obstruction).
- Signs and symptoms of sepsis are important – acute treatment is needed to relieve obstruction.

Investigations and management
- Investigations: FBC, U&E, LFT, coagulation screen, urine dipstick, USS renal tract, CT abdomen/pelvis.
- Systemic anti-cancer treatment may be appropriate, particularly in responsive cancers such as ovarian cancer.
- Treatment of obstruction depends on overall prognosis and severity of AKI:
  - Asymptomatic patients with normal renal function may be monitored in the first instance, especially those with only mild hydronephrosis.

- o Intervention is considered in those patients that have deterioration in renal function or symptoms (e.g. prolonged infection with a hydronephrotic kidney as a possible source).
- o The choice of intervention is dependent on the site of disease, performance status, and further cancer treatment options. Interventional options include:
  - Percutaneous nephrostomy
  - Anterograde ureteric stent (requires nephrostomy placement – temporarily or prior)
  - Retrograde ureteric stent
  - Anatomical stent (subcutaneous stent placement)

Other relevant sections of this book
- Chapter 3, sections on haematuria, proteinuria
- Chapter 9, section on nephrostomies and ureteric stents

References

Lewington A, Kanagasundarum S. UK Renal Association. *UK Renal Association Clinical Practice Guideline on Acute Kidney Injury*, fifth edition. 2011. Available from: http://www.renal.org (accessed 1 January 2014).
Logothetis CJ, Assikis V, Sarriera E. Diagnosis, treatment, and prevention of nephrotoxicity of cancer therapeutic agents. In: Kufe DW, Poolock RE, Weichselbaum RR, Bast RC Jr, Gansler TS, Holland JF, *et al. Cancer Medicine*, sixth edition. BC Decker: Hamilton. 2003.
NHS Choices. Hydronephosis. Available from: http://www.nhs.uk/Conditions/Hydronephrosis/Pages/Introduction.aspx (accessed 1 January 2014).

Sexual dysfunction

Sexual dysfunction
Definition: sexual dysfunction can describe a wide range of symptoms including erectile dysfunction, dyspareunia, changes in libido, delayed orgasm, vaginal dryness and treatment-induced menopause.

Chemotherapy, radiotherapy and hormonal therapies can all contribute to sexual dysfunction. Sexual dysfunction is reported in up to 100% in some groups of cancer survivors and if profound, has been shown to have a significant effect on quality of life. Patients can feel unprepared for the sexual changes after treatment and support can be difficult to access.

Symptoms and signs
Prostate cancer
- Up to 90% of patients who have had treatment for prostate cancer report erectile dysfunction. Other side effects of treatment include incontinence, painful orgasm, dry ejaculation or climacturia (loss of urine on climax).
- Surgery: newer surgical approaches to radical prostatectomy, including nerve-sparing and laparoscopic procedures, reduce the risk of post-operative

dysfunction but the majority of patients do not recover pre-operative levels of function.

- Radiotherapy:
  - Subsequent brachytherapy or external beam radiotherapy can exacerbate erectile dysfunction.
  - The combination of brachytherapy and radiotherapy carries the highest risk of erectile dysfunction.
- Androgen deprivation therapy (ADT):
  - Nearly 50% of all prostate cancer patients receive ADT during their treatment.
  - Sexual side effects include: penile shortening, erectile dysfunction, testicular atrophy, reduced libido, loss of body hair, weight gain, hot flushes and gynaecomastia.
  - Up to 30% of patients receiving ADT report significant fatigue, and sexual self-image can also be influenced by mood changes and depression.
  - Up to 70% of patients gain 10 lbs of central weight in the first year of ADT therapy but lose muscle mass and so can feel increasingly feminised when this is accompanied by loss of body hair and gynaecomastia.

Breast and gynaecological cancers

- Many patients with cervical, ovarian or breast cancer report sexual dysfunction post treatment.
- Symptoms include vaginal dryness, dyspareunia, lack of sensation, vaginal bleeding, decreased frequency of orgasm, reduced libido, urinary or bowel incontinence, fatigue and treatment-induced menopause.
- As with ADT, use of anti-oestrogens such as tamoxifen or aromatase inhibitors increases the risk of sexual dysfunction.

Other cancers

- Treatment for other types of cancer can also result in similar issues with sexual function.
- Colorectal cancer treatment can involve extensive pelvic surgery and radiation, with the additional challenge of resuming sexual activity with a stoma.
- Up to 60% of patients who have been treated for head and neck cancer report sexual dysfunction, possibly due to altered body image or loss of natural saliva.
- Bone marrow transplantation and subsequent immunosuppression can result in graft-versus-host disease. This can cause genital scarring and curvature of the penis or vaginal pain and stenosis.
- Patients also report concern about intimate contact in the setting of immunosuppression.

Emotional and social factors

- Emotions that can directly relate to treatment include mood changes, anxiety and depression.
- Body changes as a result of cancer or treatment can cause concerns about self-image, fear of embarrassment or fear of discomfort.
- Some patients report a fear of causing a cancer recurrence with intercourse.

- Other social concerns include the sexual needs of their partner, the partner's reaction to the body changes and coping with loss of fertility.
- Some cancer survivors fear that a partner's loss of interest in sex will result in marital separation.

Management
General management
- The ideal would be that all multidisciplinary teams include a sex therapist, but this is often not realistic.
- This can be a difficult issue to discuss, and patients from different cultural backgrounds may approach this topic differently, for example opinions regarding masturbation. Do not make pre-judgements regarding patients who are single, older or widowed.
- Examples of patient resources include Macmillan Cancer Support, the Sexual Advice Association or the College of Sexual and Relationship therapists.
- Referrals to appropriate medical specialists such as urology or gynaecology should be considered as required.

Physical symptoms
Erectile dysfunction
- No large prospective clinical trials have been performed and there are no current international recommendations. The grading of erectile dysfunction is shown in Table 3.41.
- Use of phosphodiesterase type 5 (PDE-5) inhibitors, for example sildenafil (Viagra®), alone or in combination with other treatments has been advocated.
- Other treatments include intercavernosal injections of alprostadil, paperverine and phentolamine; intraurethral alprostadil, vacuum erection devices or penile prostheses.
- Men prefer non-invasive treatments such as PDE-5 inhibitors.

Table 3.41 CTCAE (V4.03) grading of erectile dysfunction.

Grade	Criteria
1	Decrease in erectile function (frequency or rigidity of erections) but intervention not indicated.
2	Decrease in erectile function, erectile intervention indicated (e.g. medication or mechanical devices such as penile pump).
3	Decrease in erectile function but erectile intervention not helpful; placement of a permanent penile prosthesis indicated (not previously present).
4	—
5	—

From the website of the National Cancer Institute (http://www.cancer.gov).

- Alternatives to penile/vaginal intercourse, for example vibrators or oral sex could be explored.
- Even if interventions are successful, 50% of couples do not persist with the intervention after one year.

Vaginal dryness and stenosis

- The grading of vaginal dryness is shown in Table 3.42 and the grading of vaginal stricture in Table 3.43.
- Systemic hormone replacement therapy should be considered following radiotherapy to the pelvis, but increases the risk of recurrence in patients with hormone-sensitive breast cancer.
- Use of topical hormonal and non-hormonal preparations can improve symptoms of dryness and dyspareunia.
- Non-hormonal preparations include Replens® cream or water-based lubricants such as Senselle®.
- Women can be anxious about use of an oestrogen-containing topical preparation following treatment for breast cancer, but it is the most effective intervention.
- Some low-dose vaginal preparations with low oestrogen concentrations and limited systemic absorption such as vaginal promestriene may be helpful.

Table 3.42 CTCAE (V4.03) grading of vaginal dryness.

Grade	Criteria
1	Mild vaginal dryness not interfering with sexual function.
2	Moderate vaginal dryness interfering with sexual function or causing frequent discomfort.
3	Severe vaginal dryness resulting in dyspareunia or severe discomfort.
4	—
5	—

From the website of the National Cancer Institute (http://www.cancer.gov).

Table 3.43 CTCAE (V4.03) grading of vaginal stricture.

Grade	Criteria
1	Asymptomatic; mild vaginal shortening or narrowing.
2	Vaginal narrowing and/or shortening not interfering with physical examination.
3	Vaginal narrowing and/or shortening interfering with the use of tampons, sexual activity or physical examination.
4	—
5	—

From the website of the National Cancer Institute (http://www.cancer.gov).

- May benefit from rinsing vagina with a benzydamine douche.
- Other options include use of vaginal dilators or vibrators and self-touch can increase vaginal blood flow and prevent atrophy.

Hot flushes
- Oestrogen supplementation for prostate cancer patients on ADT has been suggested and in a small study, diethylstilbestrol improved hot flashes, fatigue, cognition and libido. There are, however, concerns about the thromboembolic and cardiovascular side effects and so this is yet to be prospectively validated.
- Female patients may benefit from acupuncture or pharmacological interventions such as venlafaxine, clonidine or gabapentin.

Other symptoms
- *Climacturia*: using a condom, emptying the bladder pre-intercourse or lying on the side or back during orgasm may limit climaturia.
- *Gynaecomastia*: irradiation of breast tissue or bicalutamide (150 mg daily) can limit gynaecomastia. Established gynaecomastia can be treated by a subcutaneous mastectomy or liposuction.

Other relevant sections of this book
Chapter 5, section on genitourinary side effects

References

Abbott-Anderson K, Kwekkeboom KL. Systematic review of sexual concerns reported by gynaecological cancer survivors. *Gynecologic Oncology*. 2012. 124(3): 477–89.

Baumgart J, Nilsson K, Evers AS, Kallak TK, Poromaa IS. Sexual dysfunction in women on adjuvant endocrine therapy after breast cancer. *Menopause*. 2013. 20(2): 162–8.

Bobez SL, Varela VS. Sexuality in adult cancer survivors: challenges and intervention. *Journal of Clinical Oncology*. 2012. 30: 3712–19.

Del Pup L. Management of vaginal dryness and dyspareunia in estrogen sensitive cancer patients. *Gynecolical Endocrinology*. 2012. 28(9): 740–5.

Higano CS. Sexuality and intimacy after definitive treatment and subsequent androgen deprivation therapy for prostate cancer. *Journal of Clinical Oncology*. 2012. 30(30): 3720–25.

Lammerink EA, de Bock GH, Schoder CP, Mourit MJ. The management of menopausal symptoms in breast cancer survivors: case-based approach. *Maturitas*. 2012. 73(3): 265–8.

Thrombocytopenia

Thrombocytopenia is defined as a reduction in the platelet count on laboratory testing. The grading of thrombocytopenia is shown in Table 3.44.

Aetiology
Reduced platelets may be secondary to reduced production, increased consumption or increased destruction. In patients treated for cancer, it is most commonly seen as a result of treatment such as chemotherapy. In haematological malignancies both

Table 3.44 CTCAE (V4.03) grading of thrombocytopenia.

Grade	Criteria
1	< LLN to 75 x10 ^{9}/L
2	< 75 x10 ^{9}/L to 50 x10 ^{9}/L
3	< 50 x10 ^{9}/L to 25 x10 ^{9}/L
4	< 25 x10 ^{9}/L
5	—

LLN = lower limit of normal.
From the website of the National Cancer Institute (http://www.cancer.gov).

the disease and the treatment may result in thrombocytopenia. In solid tumours, the disease is less likely to result in thrombocytopenia, but can be seen in those with a relatively heavy burden of disease within the bone marrow, secondary to prostate or breast cancer.

The causes of thrombocytopenia may be attributed to:
- Treatment:
  - Chemotherapy
  - Radiotherapy – large pelvic doses
  - Heparin-induced thrombocytopenia
  - Other, for example antibiotics (e.g. sulphonamides, rifampicin)
- DIC – secondary to cancer or its complications
- Cancer:
  - Most commonly leukaemia or lymphoma
  - Bone metastases, especially from prostate or breast cancer
  - Splenomegaly
  - Paraneoplastic syndrome associated with thrombocytopenia (rare)
- Other:
  - Prolonged bleeding on the background of malnutrition/treatment
  - Platelet dysfunction
  - Viral infection – parvovirus, rubella, mumps, varicella, hepatitis C, EBV, HIV
  - Long-term alcohol abuse
  - B12 or folic acid deficiency
  - Immune thrombocytopenia (ITP)
  - Thrombotic thrombocytopenic purpura – haemolytic uraemic syndrome (TTP-HUS)
  - Pseudothrombocytopenia – clumping of the platelets analysed from blood samples collected in EDTA bottles:
    - Leads to an artificially low platelet count.
    - Occurs in 0.1% of population.
    - Discussion with the haematology lab is advised who may then perform a blood film or smear test

Symptoms

Symptoms vary greatly, depending on the severity of bleeding and the site. Blood loss may be very apparent, as in PR bleeding, or less so, such as small bowel blood loss or blood loss from the urinary system. Patients may have nosebleeds, menorrhagia and easy bruising. Purpura may occur if platelet count < 50 x10⁹/L.

Severity is often categorised by the insult needed to cause bleeding:
- Major haemorrhage
- Bleeding after minor injury
- Spontaneous bruising
- Spontaneous bleeding – unusual if platelet count >20 x10⁹/L

Investigations
- FBC, clotting, LFT, U&E
- Radiological imaging may be useful and will be guided by symptoms: bone scan, CT of area with bleed
- Urinalysis

Management
Treatment is dependent on the cause and severity of the thrombocytopenia:
- Bleeding – treat as described in Chapter 2.
- Treat underlying cause if possible.
- Consider platelet transfusion: the values below are guidelines, individuals should be assessed for their own bleeding risk – this is often higher in patients with necrotic tumours:
  - Thrombocytopenia without haemorrhage – transfuse if platelets < 10 x10⁹/L
  - Thrombocytopenia with bleeding or pyrexia – transfuse platelets to maintain above 20 x10⁹/L
- Thrombopoetic agents have been used, but only in the research setting
- General measures:
  - If thrombocytopenia is secondary to treatment then the chemotherapy or radiotherapy should be reviewed with regards to its timing, dosage and the use of supportive medication.
  - Co-existing toxicities should be checked prior to the next treatment.
  - Concomitant medications should be reviewed, for example stop aspirin, NSAIDs.
  - Lifestyle factors – use of a soft toothbrush, avoidance of heavy contact sports, etc.

Heparin induced thrombocytopenia (HIT)

Immune-mediated HIT (with or without arterial thrombosis) can be a life-threatening complication. It is associated with up to 5% patients treated with unfractionated heparin and 0.5% of patients treated with LMWH.

HIT typically occurs within 5–10 days of starting heparin and should be considered if there is a 30% drop in the platelet count (note the low platelet count may still be within normal range).

There is a pre-test probability score available (the 4 Ts test, see *BJH* guidelines referenced below). If the pre-test score is not low, proceed with HIT management.

Management
- Stop all heparin treatment (including hep-lock etc.) prior to serological confirmation.
- Serological confirmation of diagnosis.
- Discuss with a haematologist.
- It may be inappropriate to stop anticoagulation in some patients; alternatives should be discussed with a haematologist and relevant treating teams (e.g. cardiology for post coronary artery stent placement).
- Prophylactic platelet transfusions should not be used, consider platelets in the presence of bleeding.

Other relevant sections of this book
Chapter 2, section on bleeding

References

Schiffer CA, Anderson KC, Bennett CL, Bernstein S, Elting LS, Goldsmith M, *et al.* Platelet transfusion for patients with cancer: clinical practice guidelines of the Amercian Society of Clinical Oncology. *Journal of Clinical Oncology.* 2001 19(5): 1519–538.

Watson H, Davidson S, Keeling D. Guidelines on the diagnosis and management of heparin-induced thrombocytopenia: second edition. *British Journal of Haematology.* 2012. 159(5): 528–540.

Thromboembolism

Venous thromboembolism (VTE)
- VTE includes deep vein thrombosis (DVT) and pulmonary embolus (PE). The grading of VTE is shown in Table 3.45.
- Patients with cancer have a seven-fold increased risk of VTE and 20% of patients experiencing a first episode of VTE have cancer.
- VTE may decrease quality of life and may also be associated with a reduction in overall survival.

Risk factors
- Patient factors:
  - Increasing age
  - Female sex
  - Black ethnicity
  - Comorbidities, for example hypertension, renal impairment, obesity, pulmonary disease, infection

Table 3.45 CTCAE (V4.03) grading of thromboembolic events.

Grade	Criteria
1	Venous thrombosis (e.g. superficial thrombosis).
2	Venous thrombosis (e.g. uncomplicated DVT), medical intervention indicated.
3	Thrombosis (e.g. uncomplicated PE (venous), non-embolic cardiac mural (arterial) thrombus), medical intervention indicated.
4	Life-threatening (e.g. PE, cerebrovascular event, arterial insufficiency); haemodynamic or neurologic instability; urgent intervention indicated.
5	Death.

From the website of the National Cancer Institute (http://www.cancer.gov).

- ○ Prior history of DVT
- ○ High platelet count pre-chemotherapy – highest risk if platelets >443 x10^9/L
- Disease factors:
  - ○ Stage of cancer – higher risk with metastatic disease
  - ○ Time since diagnosis – highest risk is in first three months
- Primary site of cancer: gastric and pancreatic cancer have the highest risk of VTE
- Treatment-related factors:
  - ○ Surgery
  - ○ Chemotherapy – 6.5 fold increased risk of VTE
  - ○ Hormonal or anti-angiogenic therapy
  - ○ Presence of central venous catheter (CVC)
  - ○ Use of erythropoeisis-stimulating agents

Specific anti-cancer agents
Hormonal therapy
Adjuvant hormonal therapy (especially tamoxifen) in breast cancer patients increases the risk of VTE by up to sevenfold.

Thalidomide
- Thalidomide in combination with dexamethasone or chemotherapy (e.g. anthracyclines, melphalan or doxorubicin) increases the risk of VTE by 26–28%.
- ASCO guidelines recommend prophylactic LMWH or adjusted-dose warfarin (aiming for INR 1.5) for any patient receiving thalidomide or lenalidomide in combination with dexamethasone or chemotherapy.

Bevacizumab
- There is an established increased risk of arterial thromboembolism. A pooled analysis of clinical trials with bevacizumab did not show a significant increase in risk of VTE, but larger meta-analyses have reported an increase in risk by a third.
- Due to the increase in bleeding associated with bevacizumab, the risk-benefit of VTE prophylaxis is still uncertain.

Symptoms and signs
- Swollen, painful, erythematous limb.
- CVC associated thrombosis may present with upper limb swelling, pain and erythema.
- PE may present with tachypnoea, tachycardia, pleuritic chest pain, haemoptysis and evidence of right heart strain (depending on thrombus location).
- Cerebral venous thrombosis is rare, but can present with headache, motor deficits, papilloedema, cranial nerve palsies, seizures or altered consciousness.
- VTE may be diagnosed incidentally on imaging, for example portal vein thrombosis or asymptomatic peripheral pulmonary emboli.

Investigations
- DVT or CVC associated thrombus – ultrasound
- PE – CTPA
- If a contrast enhanced CT is non-diagnostic, MR or CT venogram can be useful.

Management
Treatment of established VTE
- Anticoagulation is the recommended treatment, but has risks which need to be considered. These include:
  - Active bleeding (absolute contraindication)
  - Recent surgery, head trauma
  - Thrombocytopenia (avoid if platelet count <75 x10^9/L or platelet dysfunction)
  - Falls in elderly patients
  - Severe uncontrolled hypertension
  - Pericarditis or bacterial endocarditis
  - Epidural catheter
  - Coagulopathy
- There is limited data available concerning the safety of anticoagulation in patients with primary or metastatic brain disease.
- LMWH:
  - Recommended for at least the first 5–10 days of anticoagulation.
  - Duration: at least six months. Indefinite continuation of LMWH should be considered for patients on active treatment or with metastatic disease.
  - Side effects: clinically significant osteoporosis and heparin induced thrombocytopenia are uncommon.
- Major thrombosis, such as life-threatening PE or unresolving ileo-femoral thrombus should be treated with systemic thrombolysis.
- Some patients may require consideration of thrombectomy. Indications for this are the same as with patients without malignancy.

Treatment with warfarin
- The use of warfarin to treat VTE in cancer patients can be challenging and is not usually recommended. LMWH is preferred as it results in fewer recurrent VTE and a lower risk of bleeding over a six-month period.

- Disadvantages of warfarin:
  - Frequent monitoring is required to achieve the target INR (2.0–3.0 for VTE) and VTE can still occur when INR is in target range.
  - Increased risk of bleeding in cancer patients even at the target INR.
  - The onset of anticoagulation is slow and drug clearance is also slow (2–5 days).
  - Oncology patients frequently undergo procedures, for which anticoagulation needs to be temporarily discontinued.
  - Warfarin pharmacokinetics can be affected by interactions with anti-cancer therapy (e.g. 5-FU and capecitabine).
  - Nutritional status, dietary and herbal supplements and emesis can affect warfarin absorption and metabolism.

Treatment of CVC-associated thrombus
- Thrombotic complications of CVCs are more common than mechanical or infective complications and can occur in up to 66% of patients with a CVC.
- CVC-associated thrombi have been linked with significant morbidity and mortality.
- The risk of DVT with a CVC peaks 4–8 weeks after CVC insertion. Ipsilateral subclavian vein thrombus is the most common thrombotic event and is often asymptomatic.
- Trials investigating thromboprophylaxis for patients with CVCs have shown mixed results, possibly due to small sample size, and so this is not currently recommended.

Treatment of recurrent VTE
- The rate of recurrent VTE whilst on LMWH in clinical trials is 7–10%.
- In patients with recurrent VTE despite adequate anticoagulation, alternative anticoagulation can be used, for example switch to LMWH if previously treated with a Vitamin K antagonist.
- Haematology advice should be sought if there is complex coagulopathy.
- Vena cava (IVC) filters:
  - Studies in patients with malignancy are limited, particularly with removable IVC filters.
  - Two studies have suggested that IVC filter placement is associated with poorer survival in patients with malignancy. This may be due to an increase in distant metastatic disease and is under further evaluation.

Thromboprophylaxis
- Prophylactic anticoagulation significantly reduced VTE incidence in acutely unwell hospitalised patients and this has been extrapolated to include cancer patients. However, few studies have included a significant proportion of cancer patients.
- Currently, thromboprophylaxis is not recommended for ambulatory cancer patients except during treatment with thalidomide or lenalidomide in combination with other agents as previously described.

- VTE is a common complication of surgery and the risk of DVT is doubled to 80% in patients with malignancy. All patients undergoing more than a 30-minute procedure are at high risk of VTE.
  - Passive or active mechanical prophylaxis or pharmacological prophylaxis alone reduces DVT risk by 66% and PE risk by 31%. The combination of both methods is four times more effective than LMWH alone.
  - LMWH is as efficacious as unfractionated heparin at reducing VTE risk. There is some indication that fondiparinux may be more effective than LMWH in patients with malignancy.
  - Around 40% of post-operative thrombotic events occur following hospital discharge. It is recommended that pharmacological thromboprophylaxis continues for 7–10 days post surgery. For cancer patients with previous VTE, residual malignant disease and obesity, it should continue for up to four weeks.

Arterial thromboembolism (ATE)

Patients with malignancy are also at risk of arterial thrombotic events such as cerebrovascular events and MI, particularly as a result of anti-VEGF therapies (which also increase the risk of hypertension):

- Sunitinib and sorafenib: increase the risk of ATE threefold, independent of the type of cancer.
- Bevacizumab:
  - Significantly increases the risk of all grades of ATE by 44%.
  - A meta-analysis of trials using bevacizumab did not show a significant increase in risk of stroke, but there was an increase in the risk of high-grade cardiac ischaemia (relative risk 2.14).
  - The highest risk of ATE was seen in patients with NSCLC, renal or pancreatic cancer.

References

Barginear MF, Lesser M, Akerman ML, Strakhan M, Shapira I, Bradley T, *et al*. Need for inferior vena cava filters in cancer patients: a surrogate marker for poor outcome. *Clinical and Applied Thrombosis/Hemostasis*. 2009. 15(3): 263–9.

Choueiri TK, Schutz FAB, Je Y, Rosenberg JE, Bellmunt J. Risk of arterial thromboembolic events with sunitinib and sorafenib: a systematic review and meta-analysis of clinical trials. *Journal of Clinical Oncology*. 2010. 28(13): 2280–85.

Hanna DL, White RH, Wun T. Biomolecular markers of cancer-associated thromboembolism. *Critical Reviews in Oncology/Hematology*. 2013. 88(1): 19–29.

Khorana AA. Cancer and thrombosis: implications of published guidelines for clinical practice. *Annals of Oncology*. 2009. 20(10): 1619–30.

Lyman GH, Khorana AA, Falanga A, Clarke-Pearson D, Flowers C, Jahanzeb M, *et al*. American Society of Clinical Oncology guideline: recommendations for venous thromboembolism prophylaxis and treatment in patients with cancer. *Journal of Clinical Oncology*. 2007. 25(34): 5490–505.

Martinelli I. Cerebral vein thrombosis. *Thrombosis Research*. 2013. 131(Suppl. 1): S51–4.

Matsuo K, Carter CM, Ahn EH, Prather CP, Eno ML, Im DD, *et al*. Inferior vena cava filter place-ment and risk of haemotogenous distant metastasis in ovarian cancer. *American Journal of Clinical Oncology*. 2013. 36(4): 362–7.

Ranpura V, Hapani S, Chuang J, Wu S. Risk of cardiac ischemia and arterial thromboembolic events with the angiogenesis inhibitor bevacizumab in cancer patients: a meta-analysis of randomized controlled trials. *Acta Oncologica*. 2010. 49(3): 287–97.

Vaccinations and immunoglobulin

Vaccinations

There are two main types of vaccine:

- *Live attenuated vaccines*:
  - These should not be given to immunosuppressed patients as they have the potential to cause unchecked proliferation of the attenuated strains.
  - Include: MMR, measles, rubella, BCG, yellow fever, oral typhoid.
- *Inactivated vaccines*:
  - These are usually safe to administer to immunosuppressed patients unless they have any other contraindications to the vaccine.
  - Include: diphtheria, tetanus, pertussis, influenza, hepatitis A and B, cholera, meningitis, polio and IM typhoid.

Recommendations

- Both the annual influenza vaccination and the one-off pneumococcal vaccina-tion are recommended in the UK for patients at increased risk of infection. Treatment should not be delayed in order to give the vaccinations.
- In order to minimise the risk of transmitting infection:
  - Close contacts should be fully immunised according to the UK schedule.
  - Close contacts should also be offered vaccination against varicella and influenza.

Timing of vaccinations

- Immunosuppressed patients mount a variable response to vaccination and therefore vaccination should ideally be performed at least two weeks prior to starting immunosuppressive treatment. If this is not possible, then it may be appropriate for the patient to have immunisation during treatment and con-sider re-immunisation once treatment is completed.
- If given during chemotherapy, the best time to administer the vaccination is immediately prior to or immediately after each cycle. Vaccinating patients at the nadir of their leucocyte count does not seem to be harmful but may be less effective.
- After finishing any immunosuppressive treatment, it is recommended that patients wait for at least three months before having the pneumococcal vaccination. Vaccination with live vaccines can be considered in patients who are in remission and who have completed chemotherapy at least six months previously.

Bone marrow transplants

Patients who have received a bone marrow transplant are likely to lose any natural or immunisation-derived protective antibodies. A re-immunisation programme should be considered, but this is beyond the scope of this book.

Exposure to chickenpox

The risk of severe infection in immunocompromised patients exposed to varicella zoster can be reduced by the administration of varicella zoster immunoglobulin (VZIG). Patients should still be monitored because despite the use of VZIG, approximately 50% of susceptible patients will develop chickenpox (which can be fatal) and another 15% will have subclinical infection. The varicella vaccination is contraindicated in immunosuppressed patients.

Management of patients who have been exposed to varicella

1 Are they at increased risk of severe varicella? At risk patients include: patients undergoing chemotherapy or radiotherapy, patients who have previously received chemotherapy or radiotherapy (for at least six months following treatment), patients who have had a bone marrow transplant (for at least 12 months post transplant, longer if they had graft-versus-host disease) and patients who received high-dose steroids.
2 Does the index case have chickenpox or herpes zoster? VZIG should be considered for patients in whom the index case has chickenpox, disseminated zoster, exposed zoster lesions (e.g. ophthalmic zoster), or has zoster and is immunocompromised (as viral shedding may be greater). The risk of infection from immunocompetent people with non-exposed zoster lesions is remote.
3 Was the contact significant?
    (a) Contact in the same room (house, classroom, ward) for at least 15 minutes, face-to-face contact (e.g. during conversation). Airborne transmission at a distance has been reported in large, open wards.
    (b) VZIG is not given to 'contacts of contacts'.
    (c) Was it during the infectious period?
        (i) *Zoster*: VZIG is usually restricted to patients exposed between the day vesicles appear until the lesions have crusted.
        (ii) *Chickenpox*: VZIG is usually restricted to patients exposed between 48 hours before onset of the rash until the lesions have crusted.
4 What is the patient's varicella zoster antibody status?
    (a) Whenever possible, patients should be tested regardless of their past history of chickenpox.
    (b) *Positive*: VZIG not indicated.
    (c) *Negative*: give VZIG if it can be given within ten days of exposure (ideally within seven days).
    (d) *Unknown*: if it is possible to test the patient and give VZIG within seven days of exposure then test the patient; if this is not possible then give VZIG.

5 Consider prophylaxis with acyclovir:
   (a) Dose: 40 mg/kg per day in four divided doses.
   (b) Can be given in addition to VZIG or when VZIG is not indicated.

References

Cancer Research UK. Travelling abroad. 2011. Available from: http://cancerhelp.cancerre-searchuk.org/coping-with-cancer/coping-practically/travel/travelling-abroad#vaccine (accessed 1 January 2014).

Melcher L. Recommendations for influenza and pneumococcal vaccinations in people receiving chemotherapy. *Clinical Oncology* (R Coll Radiol). 2005. 17(1): 12–15.

Public Health England. Immunisation against infectious disease. 2013. Available from: https://www.gov.uk/government/collections/immunisation-against-infectious-disease-the-green-book (accessed 1 January 2014).

Visual symptoms

Eye disorders

Visual symptoms in cancer patients can be secondary to disorders of various parts of the eye as well as extra-orbital lesions. The grading of common eye disorders in clinical practice is shown in Table 3.46. Symptoms can be due to the disease or anti-cancer treatment:

- Intracranial and meningeal disease can cause cranial nerve palsies and visual impairment.
- Disease can affect the sympathetic nervous system, including Pancoast tumours and cause ptosis.

Ocular toxicity
Ocular toxicity secondary to chemotherapy

Cytotoxic chemotherapy can cause reversible and irreversible ocular toxicity. Some of the more common ocular toxicities associated with chemotherapy are detailed in Table 3.47.

Ocular toxicity secondary to targeted agents

Newer targeted therapies can also cause ocular toxicity, and ophthalmology input has been critical to early phase trials of some agents, for example MEK inhibitors and gefitinib. The ocular toxicities of targeted therapies are summarised below:

- ALK-MET inhibitors (e.g. crizotinib): trails of light, particularly when changing from light to dark.
- AKT inhibitors (e.g. perifosine): ulcerative keratitis.
- Anti-angiogenic agents (e.g. bevacizumab, sunitinib, sorafenib, pazopanib, regorafenib, aflibercept): hypertensive retinopathy (secondary to systemic

Table 3.46 CTCAE (V4.03) grading of eye disorders.

Grade	Dry eye	Keratitis	Retinopathy
1	Asymptomatic; clinical or diagnostic observations only; mild symptoms relieved by lubricants.	—	Asymptomatic; clinical or diagnostic observations only.
2	Symptomatic; multiple agents indicated; limiting instrumental ADL.	Symptomatic; medical intervention indicated (e.g. topical agents); limiting instrumental ADL.	Symptomatic with moderate decrease in visual acuity (20/40 or better); limiting instrumental ADL.
3	Decrease in visual acuity (< 20/40); limiting self-care ADL.	Decline in vision (worse than 20/40 but better than 20/200); limiting self-care ADL.	Symptomatic with marked decrease in visual acuity (worse than 20/40); disabling; limiting self-care ADL.
4	—	Perforation or blindness (20/200 or worse) in the affected eye.	Blindness (20/200 or worse) in the affected eye.

From the website of the National Cancer Institute (http://www.cancer.gov).

Table 3.47 Ocular complications occurring with ≥ 20% probability on administration of chemotherapy.

Site	Symptom	Agent
Retina	Macular pigment changes (reversible)	Cisplatin
Cornea	Keratitis	Cytosine arabinoside
Lacrimal drainage	Epiphora (watery eyes)	5-FU
Conjunctiva	Keratoconjuncitivitis sicca	Cyclophosphamide, busulfan
	Conjunctivitis	5-FU
Orbit	Periorbital oedema	5-FU, methotrexate
	Eye pain	5-FU
Cranial nerves 3–6	Cranial nerve palsies	Vincristine, vinblastine, vindesine, vinorelbine
	Ptosis	Vincristine, vinblastine, vindesine, vinorelbine
Vision	Blurred vision	Busulfan, 5-FU
	Photophobia	5-FU

Adapted from Schmid KE, Kornek GV, Scheithauer W, Binder S. Update on ocular complications of systemic cancer cemotherapy. *Survey of Ophthalmology*. 2006. 51(1): 19–40. (STM opt-out, Reproduced with permission of Elsevier).

hypertension), retinal artery/vein occlusion, optic neuropathy, posterior reversible leukoencephalopathy syndrome (PRLS). Sunitinib can also cause eyelid oedema and conjunctivitis.

- BCR-ABL and C-KIT inhibitors (e.g. imatinib, dasatinib, nilotinib): peri-orbital oedema, epiphora, optic neuritis.
- EGFR inhibitors (e.g. cetuximab, panitumumab, erlotinib, gefitinib): trichomegaly, eyelid irritation, entropion/ectropion, dry eye, blepharitis, conjunctivitis, conjunctival hyperaemia, corneal erosions, episcleritis, keratitis, photophobia.
- Heat shock protein-90 inhibitors: blurred vision, flashes in vision, night blindness.
- Ipilimumab: blurred vision and eye pain is common. Less common side effects include blepharitis, conjunctivitis, episcleritis, scleritis, uveitis and temporal arteritis.
- MEK inhibitors: blurred vision, increased lacrimation, central serous retinopathy, eyelid oedema, retinal detachment, retinal vein occlusion and subconjunctival haemorrhage.
- Tamoxifen: optic neuropathy or central visual field loss secondary to macular oedema can rarely occur.

Ocular toxicity secondary to radiotherapy
The lens of the eye has a low tolerance to treatment with radiation. If the radiotherapy field includes the lens there is a significant risk of developing cataracts in the long term.

Supportive medications and ocular toxicity
Dexamethasone is frequently used as an anti-emetic during chemotherapy and as an adjunct to radiotherapy. It is associated with the development of cataracts, raised intraocular pressure and glaucoma.

Management
General management
- If infective blepharitis or conjunctivitis is suspected, swab the affected eye for micro-organisms.
- Counsel the patient to avoid using contact lenses and to bathe the eyelid in warm water twice daily.
- A course of antibiotics (e.g. chloramphenicol eye drops) or anti-virals may be appropriate.
- If symptoms do not improve or there are marked symptoms, ophthalmology review is advised.
- Peri-orbital oedema due to imatinib does not usually require treatment. Diuretics may be indicated in extreme cases.

Management of ocular toxicity due to cytotoxic chemotherapy
- Refer symptomatic patients to ophthalmology.
- Ocular toxicity can be treated if detected at the early stages. Mild to moderate ocular toxicity may be reversible on withdrawal of the anti-cancer agent.
- Significant toxicity may mandate dose reduction or withdrawal of treatment to preserve vision.
- Baseline ophthalmology review has been suggested for patients starting treatment with 5-FU, docetaxel, methotrexate and cytosine arabinose due to the likely need for tear substitutes and the possibility of canalicular or nasolacrimal duct obstruction, but this is not currently routine practice.

Cytosine arabinoside
- Glucocorticoid eye drops or 2-deoxycytidine eye drops prior to starting treatment with cytosine arabinose can help prevent or improve photophobia and conjunctivitis.
- Saline eye washes and betamethasone eye drops can also reduce ocular side-effects.

5-FU
- Mild ocular toxicities are common (see Table 3.47).
- A break of 1–2 weeks off chemotherapy usually resolves the symptoms.
- Topical corticosteroids may also be useful.
- Some patients can develop stenosis of the lacrimal canaliculus, which results in severe epiphora. In patients with marked symptoms, ophthalmologic review is recommended. Surgical intervention may be indicated.
- Methylcellulose or dexamethasone eyedrops can improve ocular symptoms.

Management of ocular toxicity due to newer targeted agents
- These drugs are usually given within a clinical trial. As the full ocular toxicity profile of newer agents is as yet unknown, baseline ophthalmologic review, including visual acuity, fundoscopy and tonemetry (measurement of intraoptic pressure) is often recommended as part of clinical trial protocols.
- Visual field testing and retinal photographs are recommended for agents likely to cause retinal pathology.
- For agents that may cause anterior chamber symptoms, slit lamp examination should be performed.
- Monitoring during treatment should be at regular intervals and there should be a reassessment at least 4–8 weeks post starting treatment.
- If a patient develops ocular symptoms, the agent should be withheld until ophthalmologic review.

References

Electronic Medicines Compendium. Summaries of Product Characteristics 2012 (updated 15 December 2012). Available from: http://www.medicines.org.uk/EMC/default.aspx (accessed 1 January 2014).

Peterson JD, Bedrossian EH Jr. Bisphosphonate-associated orbital inflammation-a case report and review. *Orbit.* 2012. 31(2): 119–23.

Renouf DJ, Velazquez-Martin JP, Simpson R, Siu LL, Bedard PL. Ocular toxicity of targeted therapies. *Journal of Clinical Oncology.* 2012. 30(26): 3277–86.

Schmid KE, Kornek GV, Scheithauer W, Binder S. Update on ocular complications of systemic cancer chemotherapy. *Survey of Ophthalmology.* 2006. 51(1): 19–40.

CHAPTER 4

Introduction to radiotherapy

Emma Dugdale, Alexandra Gilbert and Robin Prestwich

St James's Institute of Oncology, UK

Introduction to radiotherapy

Radiotherapy is the use of radiation in the management of cancer. Radiotherapy is a locoregional treatment with curative potential in the absence of distant metastatic disease. It forms part of the management of 40% of patients cured of their disease, but is also widely used to palliate symptoms. This chapter aims to provide an introduction to radiotherapy. The side-effects of radiotherapy are discussed in the next chapter.

Indications for radiotherapy
- *Radical/curative*: delivered as the sole treatment modality, for example prostate cancer. In locally advanced disease, radiotherapy may be combined with chemotherapy to improve efficacy.
- *Neo-adjuvant*: to improve the chances of curative surgery, for example pre-operatively for rectal cancer.
- *Adjuvant*: to reduce the risk of local recurrence following surgery, for example post-operatively for breast cancer.
- *Palliative*: palliation of symptoms and sometimes improved survival, when cure is not possible.

Radiotherapy dose and fractionation
- The absorbed dose of radiation within tissue is expressed in the unit gray (Gy).
- Commonly delivered as a series of smaller doses called fractions rather than as a single dose.

Clinical Problems in Oncology: A Practical Guide to Management, First Edition.
Edited by Sing Yu Moorcraft, Daniel L.Y. Lee and David Cunningham.
© 2014 John Wiley & Sons, Ltd. Published 2014 by John Wiley & Sons, Ltd.

- The number of fractions and the dose given in each fraction (Gy) depends on the treatment intent:
  - Radical/curative treatments require large doses of radiotherapy overall. The total dose is divided into multiple small fractions (often giving 2 Gy at a time daily Monday to Friday) to reduce the severity of acute and late toxicity, for example 70 Gy in 35 fractions over seven weeks for head and neck cancer.
  - Palliative radiotherapy is delivered in a smaller number of fractions, giving more than 2 Gy per fraction but to a lower total dose, for example 8 Gy in 1 fraction or 30 Gy in 10 fractions.
- The dose and fractionation used for each tumour type and indication may vary from one treatment centre to another. Some examples of typical treatment regimes will be given in the following chapter.

Efficacy of radiotherapy
- Factors affecting tumour kill and toxicity:
  - Total dose, total volume treated, dose per fraction, overall treatment time
  - Comorbidities (e.g. diabetes, inflammatory bowel disease)
  - Smoking – reduces efficacy and increases toxicity
  - Radiogenomics
  - Additional treatment modalities (chemotherapy, surgery, biological therapies)
- Gaps in radiotherapy treatment can reduce efficacy as tumour cells can proliferate during treatment. This is particularly important in fast growing squamous cell carcinomas, such as cervical, anal and head and neck cancers. Acute side effects are intensively managed to ensure that treatment can continue as prescribed.
- Chemoradiotherapy:
  - Chemotherapy given during radiotherapy treatment is called concurrent chemotherapy or chemoradiotherapy.
  - Concurrent chemotherapy is thought to act as a radiosensitiser, increasing the sensitivity of the cells to radiation.
  - It leads to improved efficacy of the radiotherapy treatment, but also increases radiation-related side effects (in addition to the expected side effects of the chemotherapy).

Methods of delivery of radiotherapy

There are a number of different ways radiotherapy can delivered – external beam radiotherapy, brachytherapy and radioisotopes. The radiotherapy treatment process is shown in Figure 4.1.

External beam radiotherapy
- This is the most common form of radiotherapy used in the UK and is delivered by a linear accelerator (see Figure 4.2). It can be given in two forms:
  - *Photons (high energy X-rays)*:
    - Photons penetrate deep into body tissue where they produce secondary electrons that cause DNA damage to both cancer cells and normal cells.
    - The majority of radiotherapy treatments use photons.

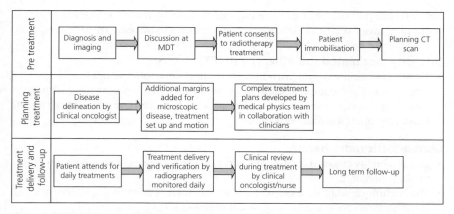

Figure 4.1 Flow diagram of radiotherapy treatment process.

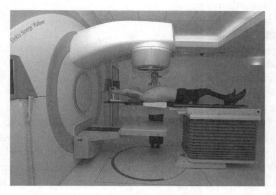

Figure 4.2 Linear accelerator. Image courtesy of Medical Illustrations, St James' Institute of Oncology. To see a colour version of this figure, see Plate 4.2.

- ○ *Electrons*:
  - ▪ Electrons damage DNA directly and deliver their dose superficially just below the skin surface.
  - ▪ Typically, electrons are used to treat skin lesions.
- Normal cells can often repair the DNA damage and therefore survive. Conversely, cancer cells commonly have defective DNA repair pathways and are unable to repair radiotherapy induced DNA damage. Cancer cells subsequently undergo cell death at the time of cell division (mitotic cell death) or apoptotic cell death.
- There are strict radiation protection laws governing the delivery of radiotherapy for protection of patients, staff and the wider public.

Newer techniques using external beam radiotherapy

New techniques have been developed and brought into clinical use over the past decade. Currently, they are not routinely available in every radiotherapy centre.

These techniques can be used to reduce the dose to surrounding normal tissues in order to reduce toxicity, or perhaps to escalate doses to increase treatment efficacy.

Intensity modulated radiotherapy (IMRT)

- This uses multiple beams with non-uniform dose across the field.
- Allows for more complex shaping of the beam with more sparing of normal tissues and steep dose gradients. The process is more time consuming during treatment planning and verification.

Stereo-tactic radiotherapy

- This is a highly targeted treatment, for which the patient may be fully immobilised to allow precision.
- The technique may be used to treat intracranial lesions (e.g. cyberknife) and certain extracranial lesions (e.g. small peripheral lung tumours).
- Treatment is often given in fewer fractions with a higher dose per fraction than conventional radiotherapy.

Proton therapy

Uses protons to damage DNA. This is not discussed in this book as it is not currently in clinical use in the UK. Patients can be referred to Europe or USA if appropriate after specialist review.

Brachytherapy

Brachytherapy is a form of radiation treatment where radiation sources are placed within or close to the tumour. It allows the delivery of a localised high radiation dose to a small tumour volume, thereby increasing the chance of tumour control whilst minimizing the dose to surrounding normal tissue. The commonest cancers treated with brachytherapy are prostate cancer, gynaecological cancers, oesophageal cancer and head and neck cancers. It may be used alone or in combination with external beam radiotherapy.

Delivery of brachytherapy

- The radiation is provided by radioactive decay of radionuclides such as Iridium-192 and Iodine-125 which are implanted within the body.
- The two main types of brachytherapy are:
  - *Intracavity*: radioactive material is placed inside a body cavity, for example uterus.
  - *Interstitial*: radioactive material is put into the target tissue, for example prostate.
- The implants can be temporary or permanent.
- There are different dose rates (high, low and pulsed), which relate to how quickly a dose is given and therefore how long it will take to deliver the required total dose.
- How brachytherapy is given to any one patient will depend on the local expertise and equipment available, which is variable across the UK. Detailed discussions of the techniques used are outside the scope of this book.

- Side effects will be localised to the anatomical treatment site. For example, radioactive seeds placed inside the prostate to treat prostate cancer may cause intense urinary symptoms in the weeks after placement.

Radiation protection
- Radiation protection is of particular importance in brachytherapy.
- Brachytherapy implant insertion is carried out in a dedicated theatre.
- Whilst the radioactive source is *in situ* the patient will be radioactive. High dose rate patients will complete treatment, and therefore only be radioactive, whilst in theatre (temporary implant).
- Following brachytherapy implant insertion low dose rate patients (permanent seed brachytherapy) may be treated on the ward in a lead-lined room to which access will be controlled until the radioactive levels emitted are low (usually 1–2 days). If in doubt ask a senior member of nursing or medical staff.
- Before discharge a patient will be advised about their ongoing radiation risk to others.

Radioisotopes
- A radioisotope is an unstable form of a chemical element, which emits radiation when it decays and is another method of radiation delivery.
- The most commonly used form is radioactive iodine, I-131, which is used in the management of the most common forms of thyroid cancer.
- Following total thyroidectomy a patient is given a capsule of I-131. The iodine is preferentially taken up by and concentrated in any remaining thyroid tissue (normal or malignant) where it emits radiation and ablates the cells. As there are few other tissues in the body that take up iodine this is a way to selectively deliver radiation.
- Excess I-131 is excreted in sweat, urine and faeces. The patient is kept in a lead-lined room until the level of radiation they are emitting is low enough not to provide a risk to others, usually around four days.
- Side effects of treatment are minimal, but include mild nausea, possible mild neck pain and swelling, swollen salivary glands, a dry mouth and taste change. These all resolve after a few days.
- Radiation protection is extremely important and local protocols should be followed. If in doubt ask a senior member of nursing or medical staff.

Palliative radiotherapy
- Radiotherapy can be very useful in palliating symptoms caused by cancer, which may be from the primary disease, nodal disease or metastases. The aim should be to keep side effects to a minimum whilst improving symptoms. In some cases the dose may be high enough to improve overall survival.
- Response to treatment is not immediate (particularly for pain, which may take a few weeks to respond). Therefore other management, for example analgesia, should be optimised. Treatment of bone metastases causes a pain flare in the

days after receiving radiotherapy in approximately 15% of patients. This responds to a temporary increase in analgesia.

- Important factors when deciding on the length of treatment include: extent of disease, comorbidity and performance status.
- Table 4.1 provides examples of indications and treatment regimes. Spinal cord compression is discussed in Chapter 2.

Paediatric radiotherapy

Radiotherapy is used in the management of paediatric cancers and is highly specialised. The long-term side effects are of particular importance. Further discussion is outside the remit of this book.

Table 4.1 Examples of palliative treatment regimes and treatment indications.

Diagnosis	Site treated	Symptom to palliate	Example of dose and fractionation
Lung cancer	Primary disease Nodal masses	Cough, pain, haemoptysis and dyspnoea	10 Gy in 1 fraction 16 Gy in 2 fractions 20 Gy in 5 fractions 36 Gy in 12 fractions
Oesophageal cancer	Primary disease Nodal masses	Pain, bleeding and dysphagia	20 Gy in 5 fractions 30 Gy in 10 fractions
Pancreatic cancer	Primary disease Nodal masses	Pain	8 Gy in 1 fraction 20 Gy in 5 fractions
Rectal cancer	Primary disease Nodal masses	Pain, bleeding, discharge	8 Gy in 1 fraction 20 Gy in 5 fractions 30 Gy in 10 fractions
Bladder cancer	Primary disease Nodal masses	Pain, bleeding	8 Gy in 1 fraction 20 Gy in 5 fractions 30 Gy in 10 fractions 21 Gy in 3 fractions
Endometrial/ cervical cancer	Primary disease Nodal masses	Pain, bleeding	8 Gy in 1 fraction 20 Gy in 5 fractions 30 Gy in 10 fractions
Prostate cancer	Primary disease Nodal masses	Pain, bleeding	8 Gy in 1 fraction 20 Gy in 5 fractions 30 Gy in 10 fractions

Continued

Table 4.1 Continued

Any	Whole brain Gamma knife considered if small number of metastases	Controversy remains about the effectiveness of radiotherapy for brain metastases in reducing symptoms or improving survival.	20 Gy in 5 fractions 30 Gy in 10 fractions
Any	Bone	Pain, 60–70% response rate	8 Gy in 1 fraction 20 Gy in 5 fractions 30 Gy in 10 fractions
Any	Skin and soft tissue deposits	Pain, bleeding, ulceration	8 Gy in 1 fraction 20 Gy in 5 fractions
Head and neck cancer	Primary disease Nodal masses	Pain, bleeding, ulceration	8 Gy in 1 fraction 20 Gy in 5 fractions

References

Ahmad SS, Duke S, Jena R, Williams MV, Burnet NG. Advances in radiotherapy. *British Medical Journal.* 2012. 345: e7765.

Hanna L, Crosby T, Macbeth F (eds). *Practical Clinical Oncology,* first edition. Cambridge University Press: Cambridge. 2008.

Hoskin P (ed.). *Radiotherapy in Practice. External Beam Therapy,* second edition. OUP: Oxford. 2012.

CHAPTER 5

Radiotherapy side effects and their management

Alexandra Gilbert, Emma Dugdale and Robin Prestwich
St James' Institute of Oncology, UK

Overview of radiotherapy toxicity

Radiotherapy itself is painless during delivery. Radiotherapy is a localised treatment and therefore other than treatment-related fatigue, side effects are related to the anatomical area of the body that is receiving treatment. For example treatment to the thorax will not cause lower GI symptoms such as diarrhoea.

There are a number of clinician reported acute and late toxicity grading systems in clinical use, including the Common Terminology Criteria for Adverse Events (CTCAE version 4).

There are three types of toxicity:
1 *Acute toxicity*: for example mucositis
  (a) Develops during treatment, usually after the first 5–10 fractions and peaks at 2–4 weeks post completion.

Clinical Problems in Oncology: A Practical Guide to Management, First Edition.
Edited by Sing Yu Moorcraft, Daniel L.Y. Lee and David Cunningham.
© 2014 John Wiley & Sons, Ltd. Published 2014 by John Wiley & Sons, Ltd.

(b) Increases during treatment and is maximal in the first few weeks following the end of treatment.

(c) Generally reversible but must be managed appropriately to ensure patient compliance with full course of treatment.

2 *Delayed toxicity*: for example radiation pneumonitis. develops at least six weeks after completion of radiotherapy and must be recognised as such to ensure it is appropriately managed.

3 *Late toxicity*: for example skin atrophy, lung fibrosis:

(a) Develops at least three months after radiotherapy and sometimes manifests years later.

(b) Often irreversible and may worsen over time. It can be difficult to treat, requiring multidisciplinary management.

Risk of second malignancies

- Radiotherapy itself is carcinogenic and there is a risk of a second malignancy developing as result of treatment.
- The risk increases over the decades after treatment and depends on the treated volume and dose.
- It has been difficult to quantify the risk because there are many contributing factors, but for women receiving radiotherapy for breast cancer there is an excess absolute risk of a second malignancy of 2–4 cases per 10,000 person years. The risk is significantly greater for younger patients treated for a good prognosis cancer (e.g. Hodgkin's lymphoma).

Causes of toxicity

- The acute toxicity of radiotherapy is due to damage of normal tissue. The ability of normal cells to repair the damage also explains why the acute toxicity recovers once treatment has finished.
- Long-term toxicity occurs as some of the damage cannot be repaired by normal cells, partly due to the development of fibrosis and blood vessel damage within the irradiated tissue.

The effect of radiotherapy schedules on toxicity

- Radiotherapy schedules delivered with curative intent usually involve high total doses, leading to significant acute and late toxicities. Acute toxicities must be appropriately managed during treatment to ensure patients are able to complete a full course of treatment with no delays.
- While there may be some toxicity associated with palliative treatments, side effects are generally less severe and shorter lived in keeping with the aim of improving quality of life.

Overview of radical radiotherapy treatment and side effect management by anatomical treatment site

Brain

- When radically treating a patient with glioblastoma multiforme (GBM), radiotherapy is only given to the area of the brain where the cancer is situated. For other indications, such as palliative radiotherapy for cerebral metastases, prophylactic cranial irradiation (PCI) and cerebral lymphoma, it is given to the whole brain.
- Patients will usually wear a mask covering their face and neck during each radiotherapy fraction to ensure reproducible set-up each day.
- Most patients will be on steroids (usually dexamethasone) to help with symptoms. The dose should be established and modified as required.
- The side effects of brain radiotherapy are shown in Table 5.1.

Indications and example radical regimes

- *Radical/adjuvant*: GBM: 60 Gy in 30 fractions. Often given with oral temozolamide.
- *Prophylactic cranial irradiation (PCI)*: given to patients with small cell lung cancer (SCLC) after chemotherapy to prevent the development of brain metastases.

Table 5.1 Side effects and management of radiotherapy to the brain.

Side effects	Early	Late	Notes
Alopecia	***	*	Dependent on area in radiotherapy field. Patchy re-growth possible.
Cognitive decline	N/A	**	Dose dependent. Non-reversible.
Fatigue	***	*	Common during and in the first few weeks post treatment.
Headache	**	N/A	Usually responds to starting/increasing steroids.
Hearing loss	*	N/A	Dependent on area in radiotherapy field.
Loss of taste	*	N/A	Dependent on area in radiotherapy field.
Nausea and vomiting	**	N/A	Consider steroids in addition to anti-emetics.
Pituitary dysfunction	N/A	***	May require referral to an endocrinologist.
Scalp erythema	**	N/A	*See skin toxicities section.*
Somonolence syndrome	***	N/A	Occurs 4–6 weeks after radiotherapy has finished. Self-limiting, no specific treatment.

Table key for all side effects: * = rare, ** = uncommon, *** = frequent, N/A = not applicable (frequency of side effects for each site adapted from Ahmad SS, Duke S, Jena R, Williams MV, Burnet NG. Advances in radiotherapy. *British Medical Journal*. 2012. 345: e7765).

25 Gy in 10 fractions for limited stage disease; 20 Gy in 5 fractions for extensive stage disease.
- *Other/rarer indications*: meningioma, pituitary adenoma, cerebral lymphoma.

Head and neck
- Head and neck cancers include cancers of the oral cavity, larynx, pharynx, nasopharynx, lip, nasal cavity and paranasal sinuses. Over 90% of head and neck cancers are squamous cell carcinomas (HNSCC).
- Surgery and radiotherapy are the treatment modalities used with curative intent in head and neck cancer. The majority of patients present with locally advanced disease and require a combined approach to treatment.
- Radiotherapy can be used as an alternative to surgery for organ preservation.
- If fit, patients may receive chemo-radiotherapy.
- The majority of centres have adopted the use of image modulated radiotherapy (IMRT) in the treatment of HNSCC, with the aim of reducing side effects.
- In all radical and palliative treatments patients will wear a mask for radiotherapy treatment to ensure reproducible set-up from day to day (see Figure 5.1).
- All patients will be advised to stop smoking and not drink alcohol.

Indications and example radical regimes
- *Radical*: 70 Gy in 35 fractions over 49 days. Concurrent cisplatin or carboplatin may be given.
- *Induction chemotherapy*: role is uncertain, but potential options include docetaxel, cisplatin and 5-fluorouracil (TPF).
- *Adjuvant radiotherapy*: 60–66 Gy in 30–33 fractions.

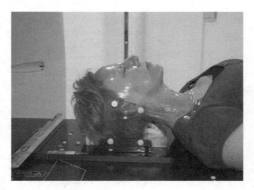

Figure 5.1 Example of a perspex mask used in head and neck radiotherapy. Image courtesy of Medical Illustrations, St James' Institute of Oncology. To see a colour version of this figure, see Plate 5.1.

Head and neck radiotherapy side effects

- Managing a patient's toxicity as they go through radiotherapy for a head and neck cancer requires a multidisciplinary team approach, including doctors, nurses, radiographers, dieticians and speech and language therapists. Side effects of radiotherapy to the head and neck are shown in Table 5.2.
- The main side effects are mucositis (see Table 5.3 for grading) and skin toxicity (see the skin toxicity section of this chapter for more details).
- Patients require regular review (at least weekly) during treatment to ensure toxicity is managed appropriately to ensure patient comfort and compliance with treatment.
- Decisions to allow breaks in treatment should only be taken by the treating clinical oncologist.
- Recovery after treatment is a long process that requires ongoing input from the multidisciplinary team.

Management of early head and neck toxicity

- *Mouth care*:
  - Mucositis of the upper airway tract is the main toxicity in head and neck radiotherapy. It makes eating, talking and even opening the mouth difficult. It cannot be prevented and must be appropriately managed.
  - Regular rinsing of the mouth with normal saline removes debris and secretions.
  - There are a number of preparations available that form a protective layer over the inflamed mucosa, for example Gelclair® and MuGard®, that can be tried.
  - Analgesia should be prescribed according to the WHO analgesic ladder. Opiates are very often required and consider using the trans-dermal route. Gargled aspirin can sometime be helpful.
  - Thick oral secretions develop. The colour can range from clear to yellowy-green and may contain streaks of blood. Nebulised normal saline can be helpful in loosening these secretions so they are easier to expectorate.
  - Have a low threshold for suspecting oral thrush and treat using high dose fluconazole (e.g. 100 mg once a day for 1–2 weeks).
- *Nutrition*:
  - Nutrition and hydration are vital. Dietetic input can be very valuable. Stability of weight is important to ensure both treatment set up accuracy as well as ensuring that the increased nutritional requirement of the body through treatment and recovery are met.
  - Despite optimal analgesia severe mucositis can prevent a patient from swallowing sufficient fluid and nutrition including nutritional supplements.
  - Enteral feeding should be considered if the patient is unable to maintain an adequate calorific intake and certainly if a patient loses > 10% of the starting body weight. If extensive mucositis is expected from the treatment, a prophylactic gastrostomy may be placed prior to treatment, otherwise an NG tube will need to be passed.

Table 5.2 Side effects of head and neck radiotherapy.

Side effects	Early	Late	Notes
Alopecia	**	*	Dependent on area in radiotherapy field.
Aspiration risk	**	**	*See management of early head and neck toxicity section.*
Cataracts	N/A	*	Dependent on area in radiotherapy field.
Dental problems	N/A	*	All patients are seen by a dentist prior to start of radiotherapy treatment to extract any diseased teeth, with the aim of preventing osteonecrosis. Dry mouth post radiotherapy increases the risk of dental decay.
Dry mouth (xerostomia)	**	***	*See management of late head and neck toxicity section.*
Dysgeusia (altered taste/smell)	***	***	Taste generally improves in the months post radiotherapy.
Dysphagia	***	**	May require enteral feeding and analgesia. May develop oesophageal stricture in long term.
Fatigue	***	*	Common during and in the first few weeks post treatment.
Hoarseness	**	**	Speech generally improves within a few months and with SALT support.
Hearing loss	*	*	Related to cisplatin use and dependent on area in radiotherapy field.
Lymphoedema (under the chin)	N/A	*	
Mucositis (oral)	***	N/A	*See management of early head and neck toxicity section.*
Odynophagia	***	N/A	*See upper GI side effects section.*
Osteonecrosis of the jaw	N/A	**	Teeth extractions and high doses of radiotherapy to the mandible increase risk.
Pituitary dysfunction	N/A	*	Dependent on area in radiotherapy field.
Skin reaction (acute)	***	N/A	*See skin toxicities section.*
Skin reaction (chronic)	N/A	**	*See skin toxicities section.*
Trismus (jaw stiffness)	N/A	*	Risk depends of position of radiotherapy. If this is a risk patients will be given jaw opening exercises.
Throat secretions	***	N/A	*See management of early head and neck toxicity section.*
Thyroid gland dysfunction	N/A	*	Dependent on area in radiotherapy field.

Table key for all side effects: * = rare, ** = uncommon, *** = frequent, N/A = not applicable (frequency of side effects for each site Ahmad SS, Duke S, Jena R, Williams MV, Burnet NG. Advances in radiotherapy. *British Medical Journal*. 2012. 345: e7765).

Table 5.3 CTCAE (V4.03) grading of mucositis.

Grade	Criteria
1	Asymptomatic or mild symptoms; intervention not indicated.
2	Moderate pain; not interfering with oral intake; modified diet indicated.
3	Severe pain; interfering with oral intake.
4	Life-threatening consequences; urgent intervention indicated.
5	Death.

From the website of the National Cancer Institute (http://www.cancer.gov).

- *Difficulties / unsafe swallowing*:
  - Mucositis also causes difficulty swallowing due to oedema and inflammation of the oropharynx and its musculature. There is reduction in movement and loss of co-ordination, which can make the swallow unsafe as the epiglottis and larynx become involved. Speech and language therapy input is therefore vital.
  - It may be appropriate to place the patient NBM as treatment progresses and therefore enteral feeding is required.
- *Aspiration pneumonia*:
  - An unsafe swallow increases the risk of aspiration pneumonia, which can be further complicated by neutropenia if they are receiving concurrent chemotherapy.
  - Symptoms such as cough after swallowing, a wet gurgly voice or clinical evidence of a chest infection may indicate a high risk of aspiration and the patient's swallow should be formally assessed.
  - Thick oral secretions alone are not a reason to treat for a chest infection (they are a normal response and can often look 'dirty'). If there is any doubt aspiration pneumonia should be excluded.
  - The patient will require admission, to be NBM and be treated with intravenous antibiotics and fluids as per local protocol. A normal CXR does not exclude the diagnosis in the early stages.

Management of late head and neck toxicity
- *Dry mouth (xerostomia)*:
  - The salivary glands are radiosensitive and if irradiated the patient will suffer from long-term xerostomia.
  - This makes eating and speaking difficult and has significant implications for oral hygiene.
  - Newer radiotherapy techniques (IMRT) have been shown to be effective in sparing the parotid glands and therefore reduce the incidence and severity of xerostomia.
  - Artificial saliva can be tried and the patient advised to take small sips of fluid regularly throughout the day and to see a dentist on a regular basis.

- *Decreased oral movement*:
  - Fibrosis of the musculature of the oropharynx and larynx can cause a long-term reduction in oral movement, which hinders the recovery of the swallow.
  - Oral exercises during treatment can help reduce this problem. Long-term speech and language therapy input may be required.
  - Enteral feeding may be stopped only once a safe and functional swallow has returned.
- *Laryngeal cartilage necrosis*: this is rare but can lead to an unsafe swallow. In such case a laryngectomy may be required even if the cancer has been cured.

Other relevant sections of this book
Chapter 3, sections on dental disorders, mucositis

Breast
- Radiotherapy to the breast following a wide local excision, or to the chest wall following mastectomy, is the most common indication for radiotherapy in the UK. It is proven to reduce the risk of local recurrence of breast cancer and improve overall survival.
- The supra-clavicular fossa may be treated for some node positive patients. The axilla is increasing being treated now. Practice has recently changed.
- *Adjuvant radiotherapy*: the commonest fractionations used in the UK are 40 Gy in 15 fractions and 50 Gy in 25 fractions.
- *Acute toxicities include*:
  - A localised skin reaction, most pronounced in the infra-mammary fold and can sometime be severe (moist desquamation). Application of cream twice a day and dressings are generally sufficient to manage the skin reaction.
  - Discomfort, swelling and shooting pains in the breast can occur, and should be managed expectantly.
  - Fatigue is often experienced.
- *Late toxicities include*:
  - A permanent change in the shape and feel of the breast, although the cosmetic result is better with the use of current treatment techniques.
  - A small amount of lung is included in the treatment field with resulting lung fibrosis, but this is clinically not significant for most women.
  - Rib fractures are uncommon.
  - Treatment for a left-sided cancer does involve a dose of radiation to the heart and may lead to a small long-term increased risk of cardiac disease.

Thorax
- This section discusses radical radiotherapy to the thorax for lung cancer and oesophageal cancer
- When treating a lung cancer, respiratory toxicity (see Table 5.4 for grading) should be expected, but gastrointestinal (GI) symptoms may also occur if the disease is central, that is, lying in close proximity to the oesophagus.

Table 5.4 CTCAE (V4.03) grading of respiratory toxicity.

Grade	Cough	Pneumonitis	Pulmonary fibrosis
1	Mild symptoms; non-prescription intervention indicated.	Asymptomatic; clinical or diagnostic observations only; intervention not indicated.	Mild hypoxemia; radiologic pulmonary fibrosis < 25% of lung volume.
2	Moderate symptoms, medical intervention indicated; limiting instrumental ADL.	Symptomatic; medical intervention indicated; limiting instrumental ADL.	Moderate hypoxemia; evidence of pulmonary hypertension; radiographic pulmonary fibrosis 25–50%.
3	Severe symptoms; limiting self-care ADL.	Severe symptoms; limiting self-care ADL; oxygen indicated.	Severe hypoxemia; evidence of right-sided heart failure; radiographic pulmonary fibrosis > 50–75%.
4	—	Life-threatening respiratory compromise; urgent intervention indicated (e.g. tracheotomy or intubation).	Life-threatening consequences (e.g. haemodynamic/pulmonary complications); intubation with ventilatory support indicated; radiographic pulmonary fibrosis > 75% with severe honeycombing.
5	—	Death.	Death.

From the website of the National Cancer Institute (http://www.cancer.gov).

- When treating oesophageal cancer, GI toxicity will occur and patients may also experience respiratory symptoms, as although the beam of radiation is focused on the site of disease it has to pass through lung tissue to get there.
- The volume of normal lung tissue treated should always be kept to a minimum and there are recommended dose constraints, as this is a recognised risk factor for the development of pneumonitis.
- For patients who are at risk of oesophagitis/dysphagia, their weight should be monitored as they may require nutritional support for significant weight loss e.g. 10–15%.
- See Table 5.5 for an overview of side effects of radiotherapy to the thorax.

Indications and example radical regimes
- NSCLC:
  - *Radical*: 60–66 Gy in 30–33 fractions with concurrent cisplatin and etoposide or carboplatin and taxol; or 55 Gy in 20 fractions without chemotherapy. Stereotactic ablative radiotherapy is available in certain units, giving a large dose (50–60 Gy) over 3–8 fractions.
  - *Adjuvant*: 40 Gy in 15 fractions.
- SCLC:
  - *Radical*: 40 Gy in 15 fractions with or without cisplatin/carboplatin and etoposide (followed by consideration of prophylactic cranial irradiation (see section on brain for details).

Table 5.5 Side effects of radiotherapy to the thorax.

Side effects	Early	Late	Notes
Anorexia	**	N/A	Encourage eating regular small amounts to maintain nutrition. Manage any nausea. Steroids can be used but only as a short-term measure.
Chest pain/discomfort	**	N/A	Usually relieved by simple analgesia.
Cough	**	*	*See management of early respiratory toxicity section.*
Dysphagia	***	*	Dependent on area in radiotherapy field. *See upper GI side effects section.*
Dyspnoea	*	*	Need to consider infection, pleural effusion, lobar collapse and disease progression. Optimise COPD management.
Fatigue	**	*	Common during and in the first few weeks post treatment.
Haemoptysis	*	*	During treatment if small amounts produced then no treatment is required. If larger volume then consider stopping any anti-coagulants and anti-platelet medication and starting tranexamic acid. *Also see management of late respiratory toxicity section.*
Lung fibrosis	N/A	**	*See management of late respiratory toxicity section.*
Myocardial ischaemia	N/A	*	Cardiology referral appropriate.
Nausea and vomiting	*	N/A	Dependent on area in radiotherapy field.
Oesophageal stricture	N/A	**	Dependent on area in radiotherapy field. *See upper GI side effects section.*
Odynophagia	***	N/A	Dependent on area in radiotherapy field. *See upper GI side effects section.*
Pneumonitis	**	N/A	*See management of early respiratory toxicity section.*
Rib fracture	N/A	*	Symptomatic management.
Skin reaction	**	*	*See skin toxicities section.*
Tracheo-oesophageal fistula	N/A	*	Can occur with radiotherapy for a proximal oesophageal cancer. A covered stent can be used to close fistula.

Table key for all side effects: * = rare, ** = uncommon, *** = frequent, N/A = not applicable (frequency of side effects for each site adapted from Ahmad SS, Duke S, Jena R, Williams MV, Burnet NG. Advances in radiotherapy. *British Medical Journal.* 2012. 345: e7765).

- Oesophageal cancer:
  - *Radical*: 50 Gy in 25 fractions with cisplatin and 5-FU or capecitabine. Or 50–55 Gy in 16–20 fractions without chemotherapy.
  - *Other/rarer indications*: lymphoma, mesothelioma, thymoma, sarcoma.

Management of early respiratory toxicity
- *Cough*:
  - Often dry and irritant.
  - Consider infection and send sputum for culture.
  - Simple linctus and codeine linctus can be useful, but caution if cough is productive. Can use opiates such as Oramorph®.
  - Nebulised normal saline can be useful for both productive and irritant coughs.
  - Carbocisteine can be used to reduce the viscosity of sputum.
- *Pneumonitis*:
  - This typically develops 6–12 weeks after radiotherapy has finished.
  - Presents with acute cough, dyspnoea and chest tightness or fever.
  - CXR typically shows haziness in area that received radiotherapy.
  - Patient requires admission and urgent CT scan to diagnose.
  - Treated with oxygen, high dose steroids (typically prednisolone 60 mg OD for 10–14 days and then tapered over several weeks) and antibiotics if any suggestion of infection.
  - Although the process starts in the irradiated area it can become a systemic process and affect the contra-lateral lung, which carries a more severe prognosis. Respiratory support may be required.

Management of late respiratory toxicity
- *Fibrosis*:
  - Although radiologically there will be an area of lung fibrosis it may not be clinically apparent.
  - Pre-existing fibrosis will make symptoms more likely and therefore is a relative contraindication to radiotherapy.
  - Radiotherapy induced fibrosis is an irreversible change and requires medical management, often by a respiratory physician. Long-term oxygen may be required in severe cases.
- *Haemoptysis*: this can occur secondary to the development of telangiectasia within the respiratory tree. A malignant cause, such as local recurrence, should be excluded. The area of telangiectasia can be treated by Yag-laser (requires referral to the respiratory team).

Upper gastrointestinal side effects
Toxicity relating to the upper GI tract can occur when treating disease within the thorax or upper abdomen.

Table 5.6 CTCAE (V4.03) grading of dysphagia.

Grade	Criteria
1	Symptomatic, able to eat regular diet.
2	Symptomatic and altered eating/swallowing.
3	Severely altered eating/swallowing; tube feeding or TPN or hospitalisation indicated.
4	Life-threatening consequences, urgent intervention indicated.
5	Death.

From the website of the National Cancer Institute (http://www.cancer.gov).

Management of early upper gastrointestinal toxicity
- *Dysphagia and odynophagia*:
- Occurs secondary to disease or localised mucositis of the oesophagus.
- Grade severity of dysphagia using the CTCAE grading system (see Table 5.6) or Mellow-Pinkas score (0 = normal diet, 1 = can eat some but not all solids, 2 = soft foods only, 3 = liquid diet, 4 = unable to swallow anything).
- Assess nutritional status and electrolyte balance.
- Modify diet texture (e.g. soft, liquidised) and nutritional supplements if appropriate.
- May require NG feeding during treatment.
- Analgesia prescribed as per WHO analgesia ladder and antacid and oxetacaine oral suspension as a local anaesthetic used prior to mealtimes.

Management of late upper gastrointestinal toxicity
- *Oesophageal strictures*:
  - Can develop months to years after treatment.
  - Exclude a malignant cause, such as local recurrence, via endoscopy.
  - Benign strictures should be dilated. Malignant causes may be stented or treated with further radiotherapy or chemotherapy if appropriate.
- *Gastric and/or GI perforation*:
  - Patients receiving radical radiotherapy to the pancreas are at risk of perforation and should therefore be commenced on a PPI before radiotherapy starts. This should be continued for at least six months.
  - A perforation or a bleed should be managed according to the clinical situation and disease status at the time it occurs.

Other relevant sections of this book
Chapter 3, section on dysphagia

Abdomen
It is uncommon to give radiotherapy to the abdominal area, the most common site being the pancreas. Radiotherapy is not used to treat stomach or renal cancer except in exceptional circumstances.

Table 5.7 Side effects of radiotherapy to the abdomen.

Side effects	Early	Late	Notes
Abdominal/back pain	*	N/A	May respond to simple analgesia.
Anorexia	**	N/A	Encourage eating regular small amounts to maintain nutrition. Manage any nausea. Steroids can be used but only as a short-term measure.
Diabetes	N/A	*	Requires medical management.
Diarrhoea	**	*	*See lower GI side effects section.*
Fatigue	**	*	Common during and in the first few weeks post treatment.
Gastric perforation	N/A	*	*See upper GI side effects section.*
GI bleeding	N/A	*	*See upper GI side effects section.*
Malabsorption	***	***	All patients should be on pancreatic enzyme replacement (Creon®) and the dose modified as appropriate.
Nausea and vomiting	*	N/A	Dependent on area in radiotherapy field.
Skin reaction	*	N/A	Expected to be minimal. *See skin toxicities section.*

Table key for all side effects: * = rare, ** = uncommon, *** = frequent, N/A = not applicable (frequency of side effects for each site adapted from Ahmad SS, Duke S, Jena R, Williams MV, Burnet NG. Advances in radiotherapy. *British Medical Journal*. 2012. 345: e7765).

Indications and typical radical regimes

- Radical treatment of pancreatic cancer: 50.4 Gy in 28 fractions given concurrently with either capecitabine or gemcitabine.
- Other/rarer indications: cholangiocarcinoma, HCC, lymphoma, sarcoma, germ cell.

Abdominal radiotherapy side effects

Radiotherapy to the abdomen mainly results in upper and lower GI side effects (see sections above and below and Table 5.7).

Pelvis

- There are six disease sites treated with radiotherapy in the pelvis – anal, bladder, cervical, endometrial, prostate and rectal cancer.
- Radiotherapy is often used in combination with surgery and chemotherapy to increase efficacy, which increases the risk of acute and late side effects.
- GI side effects predominate, with 80% developing early GI side effects and 50% long-term GI side effects (see Table 5.8) often with an associated reduction in their quality of life.
- Pelvic radiotherapy may be given externally (EBRT) or as brachytherapy or as a combination of both.

Table 5.8 Side effects of pelvic radiotherapy.

Side effects	Early	Late	Notes
Alopecia	***	*	Dependent on area in radiotherapy field.
Anaemia	*	N/A	Pancytopenia associated with bone marrow irradiation (and associated chemotherapy).
Bone toxicity	N/A	**	Chronic insufficiency fractures, osteoporosis.
Bowel symptoms	***	***	Urgency, incontinence, bleeding, constipation, diarrhoea, malabsorption, obstruction, fistula, bloating, perforation, nausea and vomiting, dyspepsia. *See lower GI side effects section.*
Electrolyte abnormalities	**	*	Secondary to diarrhoea and chemotherapy – hypokalaemia and hypomagnesaemia. *See Chapter 8*
Fatigue	***	*	Common during and in the first few weeks post treatment.
Haematological toxicity	*	N/A	Acute bone marrow suppression (lymphopenia most common). Consider thrombocytopenia as a complication causing rectal bleeding.
Lymphoedema	N/A	**	Often more severe following surgical lymph node removal.
Sexual dysfunction (male and female)	N/A	***	Reduced libido, changes to orgasm, early menopause, infertility, erectile dysfunction, dry ejaculation or reduced semen production. *See management of late male and female sexual dysfunction sections.*
Skin reaction (acute – dermatitis radiation)	***	N/A	Skin in treated area becomes red from second week.
Skin reaction (chronic)	N/A	**	Skin may become hyperpigmented, fibrosed and have telengectasia present.
Urinary symptoms	***	*	Cystitis (non-infective), frequency, urgency, incontinence, retention, fistula, obstruction, pain. Bladder spasm and perforation.
Uterine symptoms	N/A	*	Haemorrhage, obstruction and fistula.
Vaginal symptoms	N/A	***	Dryness, stricture, stenosis, increased risk of thrush, dyspareunia, irritation secondary to semen. *See management of late female sexual dysfunction section.*

Table key for all side effects: * = rare, ** = uncommon, *** = frequent, (frequency of side effects for each site adapted from Ahmad SS, Duke S, Jena R, Williams MV, Burnet NG. Advances in radiotherapy. *British Medical Journal.* 2012. 345: e7765).

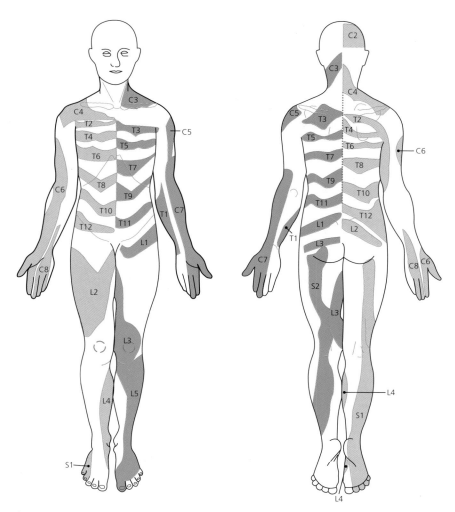

Plate 2.1 Dermatomal distributions. There is individual variation in the distribution of dermatomes. This figure illustrates the likely distribution of dermatomes, but there is overlap between dermatomes areas of increased individual variability. Blank areas illustrate areas of greatest variability and overlap. Source: Lee MWL. *et al Clinical Anatomy*. 2008. 21(5): 363–73. Reproduced with permission of John Wiley and Sons.

Clinical Problems in Oncology: A Practical Guide to Management, First Edition.
Edited by Sing Yu Moorcraft, Daniel L.Y. Lee and David Cunningham.
© 2014 John Wiley & Sons, Ltd. Published 2014 by John Wiley & Sons, Ltd.

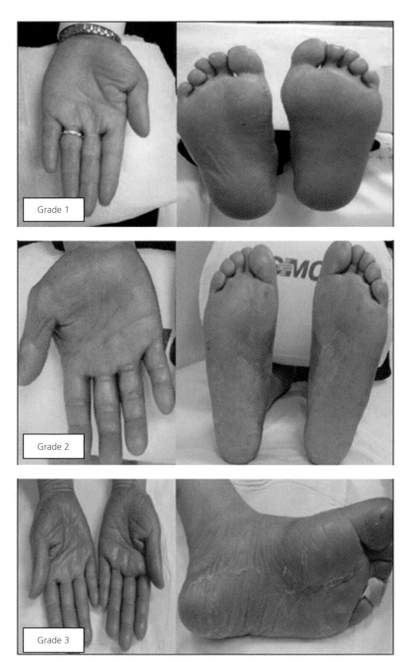

Plate 3.2 Hand foot syndrome secondary to capecitabine. Reproduced from Son HS, Lee WY, Lee WS, Yun SH, Chun HK. Compliance and effective management of the hand-foot syndrome in colon cancer patients receiving capecitabine as adjuvant chemotherapy. *Yonsei Medical Journal.* 2009. 50(6): 796–802 (open access article).

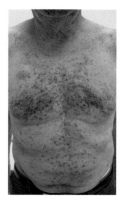

Plate 3.3 Panitumumab-related rash. Reproduced from Fabbrocini G, Cameli N, Romano MC, Mariano M, Panariello L, Bianca D, et al. Chemotherapy and skin reactions. *Journal of Experimental & Clinical Cancer Research.* 2012. 31: 50 (open access article).

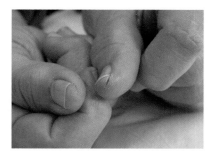

Plate 3.4 Fissures of the fingertips in a patient treated with taxanes. Reproduced from Fabbrocini G, Cameli N, Romano MC, Mariano M, Panariello L, Bianca D, et al. Chemotherapy and skin reactions. *Journal of Experimental & Clinical Cancer Research.* 2012. 31: 50. BioMed Central (open access article).

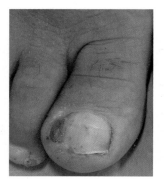

Plate 3.5 Paronychia in a patient treated with lapatinib. Reproduced from Fabbrocini G, Cameli N, Romano MC, Mariano M, Panariello L, Bianca D, et al. Chemotherapy and skin reactions. *Journal of Experimental & Clinical Cancer Research.* 2012. 31: 50. BioMed Central (open access article).

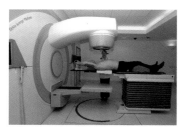

Plate 4.2 Linear accelerator. Image courtesy of Medical Illustrations, St James' Institute of Oncology.

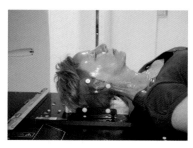

Plate 5.1 Example of a perspex mask used in head and neck radiotherapy. Image courtesy of Medical Illustrations, St James' Institute of Oncology.

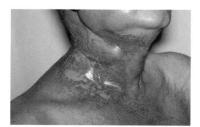

Plate 5.2 Example of acute radiotherapy skin reaction: CTCAE grade 3 confluent moist desquamation. Image courtesy of Medical Illustrations, St James' Institute of Oncology.

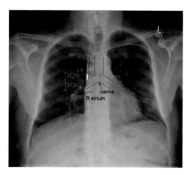

Plate 9.2 Ensuring the ideal position for the catheter tip for central venous access devices. The CXR shows a left-sided PICC line with its tip (white square) lying in the long axis of the superior vena cava (SVC) just above the carina. The boundaries of the safe zone are shown by the red dotted lines, lying 2 cm above and 2 cm below the carina respectively.

- It is important for cervical cancer patients to have their haemoglobin level maintained > 10 g/dL during radiotherapy treatment as anaemia has been found to reduce efficacy.

Indications and typical radical regimes
- Anal cancer:
  - *Radical:* T1–4 and node positive/negative: 50.4 Gy in 28 fractions with mitomycin and 5-FU.
- Bladder cancer:
  - *Radical:* 55 Gy in 20 fractions or 52.5 Gy in 20 fractions if given neoadjuvantly or with gemcitabine.
- Cervical cancer:
  - *Radical:* Stage Ib2–IV – 48 Gy in 24 fractions with weekly cisplatin, followed immediately by intracavity brachytherapy (21 Gy in 3 fractions).
  - *Adjuvant:* 45 Gy in 25 fractions +/– cisplatin.
- Endometrial cancer:
  - *Adjuvant:* 45 Gy in 25 fractions +/– cisplatin.
- Prostate cancer:
  - *Radical:* 76 Gy in 37 fractions.
  - *Adjuvant:* 52.5 Gy in 20 fractions.
- Rectal cancer:
  - *neoadjuvant:*
  - T1–3 (Circumferential Resection Margin (CRM) clear): short course radiotherapy with 25 Gy in 5 fractions. Surgery within 7–14 days.
  - T4 or involved CRM: 45 Gy in 25 fractions with either capecitabine or 5-FU. Surgery after six-week delay.

Lower gastrointestinal side effects
- The volume and dose given to the small bowel, rectum and anal sphincters (when not the tumour site) should be minimised as this is a known predictor of long-term side effects. Dose constraints for these organs exist.
- Late lower GI side effects may be related to small bowel irradiation, causing intestinal hurry, rectal and anal sphincter irradiation causing fibrosis and reduced storage capacity, or may be related to alternative diagnoses, such as bile acid malabsorption or small bowel bacterial overgrowth.
- Assess grade of toxicity (see Table 5.9 and Chapter 3, section on diarrhoea), consider comorbidities known to increase risk of toxicity (such as inflammatory bowel disease, previous abdominal surgery) and the impact on quality of life and electrolyte balance.

Management of early lower gastrointestinal toxicity
- *Diarrhoea:*
  - Grade 1: continue radiotherapy and chemotherapy treatment. Monitor symptoms
  - Grade 2: admit if adverse features – nausea and vomiting, neutropenic. Send stool cultures, including for *C. difficle*. Consider stopping radiotherapy and

Table 5.9 CTCAE (V4.03) grading of lower GI side effects.

Grade: early and late	Incontinence	Bleeding	Diarrhoea
1	Occasional use of pads.	Mild/no intervention needed.	Increase < 4 per day over baseline.
2	Daily pads required.	Moderate. Medical intervention needed.	Increase of 4–6 times per day over baseline.
3	Severe symptoms – operative intervention.	Transfusion. Operative intervention.	Increase of > 7 stools per day/ incontinence/hospitalisation.
4		Life threatening.	Life threatening.

From the website of the National Cancer Institute (http://www.cancer.gov).

chemotherapy treatment until symptoms settle (discuss with senior colleagues). Start loperamide.
- Grade 3: admit patient. As per Grade 2 but also start IV fluids. If neutropenic start IV antibiotics (consider GCSF).
- Grade 4: as above. Also consider starting octreotide and codeine. Consider urgent cross-sectional imaging if it will help further assessment/management.
- *Incontinence*: patients with severe incontinence prior to commencing treatment with pelvic radiotherapy may be recommended to have a defunctioning colostomy.
- *Tenesmus*:
  - The sensation can be improved with analgesia.
  - Patients may feel more confident wearing an incontinence pad.
  - To reduce flatulence reduce carbonated drinks and advise eating slowly.

Management of late lower gastrointestinal toxicity
- Long term GI symptoms post pelvic radiotherapy may be referred to as 'radiation proctitis'. Persistent symptoms resistant to simple treatment measures require referral for specialist gastrointestinal advice.
- *Diarrhoea and urgency*:
  - Consider diet modifications (increase or decrease fibre intake, excess lactose or fat).
  - Consider anti-diarrhoeal medications – loperamide or codeine.
  - Recommend anal sphincter and pelvic floor exercises to improve the capacity of the bowel.
- *Incontinence*: affects one in five post pelvic radiotherapy. Consider diet modifications, antidiarrhoeal medications and pelvic floor exercises.
- *Rectal bleeding*:
  - Secondary to telangiectasia. If bleeding is > grade 2 and impacting on quality of life stop/reduce anticoagulants.
  - Consider use of sucralfate enemas.
  - Discuss definitive ablative treatment for telangiectasia – hyperbaric oxygen therapy, argon plasma coagulation, formalin therapy.

- *Mucus discharge*:
  - ○ Ensure fibre intake is not excessive.
  - ○ Provide pelvic floor exercises.
  - ○ Consider a stool bulking agent and/or anti-diarrhoeal medication.
- *Excess rectal flatulence*:
  - ○ Consider dietary modifications: increase or decrease fibre intake and ensure adequate fluid intake.
  - ○ Consider alternative causes: colonic faecal loading, small intestinal bacterial overgrowth, organic causes, for example inflammatory bowel disease, neoplasia.

Genitourinary side effects

- During and after radiotherapy treatment for pelvic cancer, patients may have symptoms of urinary and sexual dysfunction. Side effects are often multifactorial, relating to the type of radiotherapy schedule and also to the effects of any surgery and/or hormone therapy.
- Urinary symptoms are related to inflammation and fibrosis of the bladder wall as well as damage to the pelvic floor muscles. Patients may also develop a urethral stricture following radiotherapy.
- Sexual difficulties are often unreported. Side effects related to fibrotic changes following radiotherapy, such as vaginal dryness and atrophic vaginitis, are compounded by radiation induced ovarian failure, resulting in decreased vaginal lubrication and vaginal thinning.
- In anal cancer patients there is an additional risk of hypogonadism due to irradiation of the testes.
- Assessment should include the grade of toxicity (see Table 5.10) and consideration of comorbidities known to increase risk of toxicity (such as diabetes, arterial disease, tumour bulk).

Management of early urinary toxicity

- *Non-infective cystitis*:
  - ○ Affects approximately 1 in 20 patients during and shortly after pelvic radiotherapy.
  - ○ Recommend avoiding caffeine and alcohol, which may irritate bladder.
  - ○ Advise patients to drink at least 2 L of fluid a day. Occasionally patients may require catheterisation.
- *Urinary retention*: catheterisation and consider starting an alpha blocker (e.g. tamsulosin).
- *Incontinence*: may find difficulties with incontinence for first few months following treatment. In the short term recommend use of incontinence pads.

Management of late urinary symptoms

- *Infective cystitis*: more common post radiotherapy. Treat as for infective cystitis.
- *Urinary frequency/urgency/irritation*:
  - ○ Bladder irritation usually settles after a few weeks/months. Avoid caffeine, fizzy drinks and alcohol.
  - ○ Avoid constipation. Stop or reduce smoking.

Table 5.10 CTCAE (V4.03) grading of genitourinary side effects.

Grade: early and late	Cystitis (non-infective)	Vaginal dryness	Erectile dysfunction
1	Microscopic haematuria, minimal increase in frequency, urgency, dysuria or nocturia.	Mild, not interfering with sexual function.	Decrease in erectile function (frequency/rigidity of erections) but erectile aids not indicated.
2	Moderate haematuria, moderate increase in frequency, dysuria, urgency or nocturia; bladder irrigation or catheter indicated.	Moderate, interfering with sexual function or causing discomfort.	Decrease in erectile function (frequency/rigidity of erections), erectile aids indicated.
3	Gross haematuria; transfusion or hospitalization indicated.	Severe dryness resulting in dyspareunia or severe discomfort.	Decrease in erectile function (frequency/rigidity of erections), but erectile aids not helpful; penile prosthesis indicated.
4	Life threatening consequences.		

From the website of the National Cancer Institute (http://www.cancer.gov).

- ○ If symptoms persist investigate with urine dip/MC&S; check renal function; consider urological ultrasound/KUB X-ray.
- ○ May need referral for consideration of cystoscopy.
- *Incontinence*:
  - ○ May need referral to physiotherapist or continence adviser to guide pelvic floor exercises.
  - ○ Avoid strain to pelvic floor, for example constipation, heavy lifting and high BMI. Consider use of anti-spasmodic medication (e.g. oxybutynin).
  - ○ Incontinence pads.
  - ○ Will need referral to urology if simple measures are not effective.
- *Nocturia*: secondary to overactive bladder. Consider anti-spasmodic medications and referral for bladder training.
- *Haematuria*:
  - ○ If symptomatic anaemia then consider tranexamic acid and may need referral for bladder washouts.
  - ○ In resistant cases patients may need cystoscopy and cauterisation.

Management of late female sexual dysfunction

- *Vaginal stenosis and pain during intercourse*:
  - ○ Using a dilator regularly post treatment will improve symptoms. Aim to start use two weeks post treatment (as acute side effects allow) using 3–4 times per week. Use may need to be life-long.
  - ○ Pelvic floor exercises at the same time may improve effectiveness.

- *Vaginal dryness*:
  - Water-based lubricating gel or vaginal moisturisers can improve dryness.
  - Consider starting hormone replacement therapy (HRT) or vaginal oestrogen creams if HRT contraindicated.
  - May have benefit from rinsing vagina with a benzydamine douche.
  - Increased risk of thrush – water-based lubricants and dilators reduce risk of occurrence.
- *Bleeding*: secondary to telangiectasia. Monitor symptoms. If irregular or severe will need investigation.
- *Vaginal irritation secondary to semen*: occurs in first few months post radiotherapy. Use extra lubricant gels (consider silicone-based lubricants).
- *Changes in orgasm*: thought to be secondary to changes in blood flow and nerve damage following radiotherapy. May need referral to sexual counsellor.
- *Infertility and early menopause*:
  - Post radiotherapy to the pelvis all women will be infertile due to effects on the ovaries and uterus. Careful counselling before and after treatment is important.
  - It will take approximately three months post radiotherapy for the ovaries to stop producing eggs.
  - In a young patient it is important to advise them not to get pregnant and to use contraception during this time.
  - Consider HRT if not contraindicated.
  - Consider risk of osteoporosis with early menopause.

Management of late male sexual dysfunction
- The main side effects following pelvic radiotherapy are erectile dysfunction and change to ejaculation (see Chapter 3 section on sexual dysfunction).
- Testes are very sensitive to radiotherapy and patients are likely to become infertile post treatment. Consider sperm banking and referral to a counsellor.
- Recommend that all patients continue to use contraception for at least six months to two years post treatment due to possible risks of teratogenicity.
- Reduced libido may be related to low testosterone levels, which can be replaced if low.

Other relevant sections of this book
Chapter 3, sections on diarrhoea, fertility and pregnancy, sexual dysfunction

Skin toxicities

- Caused by damage to the basal cell layer of skin.
- Symptoms typically start 10–14 days after the first fraction of radiotherapy and severity peaks 7–10 days after radiotherapy has finished.
- Usually healed 4–6 weeks after radiotherapy has finished.
- The severity of the skin reaction is dependent on a number of factors; a higher total dose, electron therapy, the use of bolus and the concomitant use of chemotherapy radiosensitisers such as 5-FU, mitomycin C, and cisplatin, all of which will increase severity.

- Severe skin reactions more commonly occur at treatment sites where the depth of the tumour from the surface of the skin is small and therefore the dose received by the skin is higher, for example head and neck, anus, penis and vulva.
- Other factors known to worsen the skin reaction are poor nutrition, smoking and the use of metal-containing dressings and creams on the skin in the treatment field.

Assessment of skin reactions

- Assess the amount of skin area affected and the grade of skin reaction (see Table 5.11 and Figure 5.2).
- Look for any signs of infection. It is normal for a greenish/yellow exudate to be present within areas of moist desquamation; this is a normal tissue response and should not be cleaned off (unless there are excessive amounts) as it assists with the healing process and provides pain relief by bathing the exposed nerve endings within the area of moist desquamation.
- Assess the amount of pain the patient is in and associated symptoms such as oral mucositis in head and neck patients.

Table 5.11 CTCAE (V4.03) grading of radiation dermatitis.

Grade	Criteria
1	Faint erythema or dry desquamation.
2	Moderate to brisk erythema; patchy moist desquamation, mostly confined to skin folds and creases; moderate oedema.
3	Moist desquamation in areas other than skin folds and creases; bleeding induced by minor trauma or abrasion.
4	Life-threatening consequences; skin necrosis or ulceration of full thickness dermis; spontaneous bleeding from involved site; skin graft indicated.
5	Death.

From the website of the National Cancer Institute (http://www.cancer.gov).

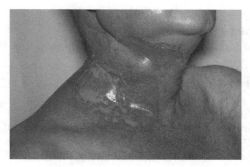

Figure 5.2 Example of acute radiotherapy skin reaction: CTCAE grade 3 confluent moist desquamation. Image courtesy of Medical Illustrations, St James' Institute of Oncology. To see a colour version of this figure, see Plate 5.2.

Management of early skin toxicity

- Patients may continue to use soap and water to clean themselves during treatment, but are advised to aim to maintain skin integrity and avoid any products that cause skin irritation.
- See Table 5.12 for guidance on the management of skin toxicity.
- Infection is uncommonly associated with the acute skin reaction, but if suspected appropriate swabs should be taken and if clinically possible results awaited before starting antibiotics.
- For patients receiving radiotherapy to the perineal area (anal, penile, vulva cancers) dressing application can be difficult. Patients may require catheterisation but this must be discussed with the treating clinical oncologist first. Constipation must be avoided.

Management of late skin toxicity

- The extent and grade of late skin toxicity is dependent on numerous factors, including total dose, dose per fraction and size of treatment field.
- The changes are often progressive and irreversible. There is no specific treatment.
- Sun exposure to the treatment site should be kept to a minimum and high factor sun cream used to prevent secondary skin cancer developing.
- Corrective plastic surgery would not be considered except for very extreme cases of functional loss. Camouflage make-up is available.

Table 5.12 Guidance on the management of early skin toxicity. Adapted from The Princess Royal Radiotherapy Review Team. Managing Radiotherapy Induced Skin Reactions – A Toolkit for Healthcare Professionals.

CTCAE grade	Management
0	For all patients. Apply aqueous cream or a sodium lauryl sulphate (SLS) free emollient cream, twice daily to skin within the treatment field. This is to promote hydrated skin and maintain skin integrity.
1	Increase application of cream as needed. A 1% hydrocortisone cream may also be prescribed for symptomatic relief. Commence analgesia as guided by WHO analgesic ladder.
2	Continue to apply cream on unbroken skin and increase application of cream as needed. Stop cream and hydrocortisone on moist/broken skin. Apply an appropriate dressing to moist desquamation areas (hydrocellular foam or silicone based dressings). Analgesia as guided by WHO analgesic ladder – opiate analgesia may be needed. Advise loose fitting clothing.
3	Stop using cream on all moist/broken skin. Continue with CTCAE 2 interventions.
4	Seek specialist advice ASAP.

From the website of the National Cancer Institute (http://www.cancer.gov).

Total body irradiation

Total body irradiation (TBI) is used, along with high dose chemotherapy, prior to bone marrow transplant for the cure and long-term remission of haematological malignancies such as acute lymphatic and acute myeloid leukaemia, lymphoma and myeloma.

- All patients will be in-patients on the bone marrow transplant unit at the time of treatment.
- The whole body is treated, with the aim of eliminating residual malignant disease and to ablate residual bone marrow to allow engraftment of peripheral stem cells or bone marrow.
- There are a number of different regimes from 2 Gy in a single fraction to 14.4 Gy in 8 fractions. When a patient is having more than 1 fraction they will receive 2 fractions a day. A lower total dose is used as the whole body is being treated.
- *Early side effects include*: a generalised skin reaction, nausea and vomiting, mucositis (oropharyngeal/oesophageal), temporary global hair loss, pneumonitis, diarrhoea, fatigue, parotid swelling, hepatic veno-occlusive disease and somnolence syndrome.
- *Late effects include*: cataracts, cardiac and lung side effects, renal damage, ovarian failure, infertility in men and women, hypothyroidism, neuropsychiatric effects and an increased risk of second malignancy.
- Patients are advised not to smoke and to protect the skin from burning.

References

Ahmad SS, Duke S, Jena R, Williams MV, Burnet NG. Advances in radiotherapy. *British Medical Journal*. 2012. 345: e7765.

Andreyev HJ, Davidson SE, Gillespie C, Allum WH, Swarbrick E. Practice guidance on the management of acute and chronic gastrointestinal problems arising as a result of treatment for cancer. *Gut*. 2012. 61(2): 179–92.

The Princess Royal Radiotherapy Review Team. Managing Radiotherapy Induced Skin Reactions: A Toolkit for Healthcare Professionals. St James's Institute of Oncology, Leeds. Available from: http://www.yorkshire-cancer-net.org.uk/html/publications/guidelines_rt.php (accessed 14 March 2014).

CHAPTER 6

Endocrine therapy, immunotherapy and targeted therapies

Samantha Turnbull

St James' Institute of Oncology, UK

> **CHAPTER MENU**
>

Endocrine therapy

Breast cancer

Some breast cancers have high levels of expression of oestrogen and/or progesterone receptors. As the growth of hormone-receptor positive breast tumours can be dependent on oestrogen activity, endocrine treatments for breast cancer generally rely on its suppression, which can be done in a variety of ways.

Selective oestrogen receptor modulators (SERMs)

- Tamoxifen is a SERM that is used for the treatment of oestrogen receptor (ER) positive breast cancer.
- Tamoxifen binds to the oestrogen receptor of different tissues and exerts either agonistic or antagonistic effects, depending on the expression of either β-oestrogen or α-oestrogen receptors. It has an antagonistic effect on oestrogen receptors in mammary tissue, but an agonistic effect on the endometrium and therefore increases the risk of endometrial cancer.
- *Other side effects include*: increased risk of VTE, myalgia and hot flushes. Vaginal bleeding/discharge is also common and care should be taken to investigate this as appropriate, given the risk of endometrial malignancy.

Clinical Problems in Oncology: A Practical Guide to Management, First Edition.
Edited by Sing Yu Moorcraft, Daniel L.Y. Lee and David Cunningham.
© 2014 John Wiley & Sons, Ltd. Published 2014 by John Wiley & Sons, Ltd.

Oestrogen receptor antagonists

Fulvestrant is a pure oestrogen antagonist, with no agonistic properties like the SERMs. It is given IM and the most frequent adverse events associated with its use are hot flushes, nausea, myalgia and arthralgia, increased risk of VTE and vaginal bleeding.

Aromatase inhibitors

- These are used in post-menopausal women with ER-positive breast cancer.
- They bind to and inhibit aromatase (the enzyme responsible for oestrogen synthesis). This is thought to have increased activity within breast tumours.
- They can be classified into first, second and third generation, as well as steroidal inhibitors (e.g. exemestane) and non-steroidal inhibitors (e.g. anastrozole and letrozole).
- *Side effects include*: hot flushes, headache, fatigue, arthralgia/myalgia, nausea, vomiting and diarrhoea. As they do not have an agonist effect on bone they can be associated with loss of bone density and osteoporotic fractures. However, the risk of secondary endometrial cancers is lower when compared to tamoxifen.

Prostate cancer

Androgen blockade is one of the mainstays of treatment of prostate cancer. Surgical castration (bilateral orchidectomy) is one mechanism of controlling the growth of tumours of the prostate, but there are also a number of medical therapies used.

Gonadotrophin releasing hormone (GnRH) agonists

- Also known as lutenising-hormone-releasing hormone (LHRH) agonists, these cause so-called 'medical castration' via androgen suppression.
- These drugs (e.g. goserelin and leuprolide) mimic the naturally occurring hormone (GnRH) that is released from the hypothalamus, which stimulates the anterior pituitary to produce LH and FSH that stimulate the testes to produce androgens.
- *Tumour flare*:
  o When initially given, a GnRH agonist can cause overstimulation of the pituitary, causing a brief rise in androgen production. This is called 'tumour flare' and can lead to potentially harmful exacerbation of clinical symptoms, such as precipitation of spinal cord compression in patients with bone metastases.
  o This phenomenon can be counteracted by giving concurrent anti-androgen therapy (e.g. bicalutamide) for a short period of time.
  o After this initial flare the production of androgens slows as the pituitary becomes desensitised to GnRH stimulation and androgen levels fall significantly.
- *Side effects include*: decreased libido, low mood, hot flushes and erectile dysfunction.

Gonadotrophin releasing hormone (GnRH) antagonists

- The GnRH antagonist degarelix blocks the effect of GnRH on the pituitary directly.
- Unlike the GnRH agonists, there is no tumour/clinical flare syndrome associated with its use.
- *Side effects include*: gynaecomastia, erectile dysfunction, hot flushes and raised liver enzymes.

Anti-androgens

- Bicalutamide and nilutamide are examples of non-steroidal anti-androgens. They act by blocking androgen receptors, and thus the binding of testosterone.
- *Side effects include*: GI disturbance, gynaecomastia (especially if single agent therapy), hot flushes and hepatotoxicity.

Inhibitors of steroidogenesis

- Over time, androgen production, PSA and tumour growth can start to increase despite androgen blockade/inhibition. This is termed castration-resistant prostate cancer (CRPC).
- Abiraterone inhibits an enzyme (CYP17) involved in androgen synthesis in the testes and prostate (and therefore the tumour itself). This enzyme can be overexpressed in prostate cancer cells.
- *Side effects include*: fatigue, nausea, elevated hepatic transaminases and hypertension.
- Blockage of the CYP17 enzyme conversely leads to increased mineralocorticoid levels. This causes hypokalaemia, hypertension and peripheral oedema. This secondary hyperaldosteronism is prevented through the concomitant use of prednisolone, which should be continued throughout the duration of abiraterone treatment.

Other relevant sections of this book

Chapter 3, sections on bone metastases and osteoporosis, sexual dysfunction

References

Conn PM, Crowley WF, Jr. Gonadotropin-releasing hormone and its analogues. *New England Journal of Medicine*. 1991. 324(2): 93–103.

de Bono JS, Logothetis CJ, Molina A, Fizazi K, North S, Chu L, *et al*. Abiraterone and increased survival in metastatic prostate cancer. *New England Journal of Medicine*. 2011. 364(21): 1995–2005.

McLeod DG. Tolerability of nonsteroidal antiandrogens in the treatment of advanced prostate cancer. *Oncologist*. 1997. 2(1): 18–27.

Riggs BL, Hartmann LC. Selective estrogen-receptor modulators – mechanisms of action and application to clinical practice. *New England Journal of Medicine*. 2003. 348(7): 618–29.

Robertson JF. Fulvestrant (Faslodex) – how to make a good drug better. *Oncologist*. 2007. 12(7): 774–84.

Shore ND. Experience with degarelix in the treatment of prostate cancer. *Therapeutic Advances in Urology.* 2013. 5(1): 11–24.

Smith IE, Dowsett M. Aromatase inhibitors in breast cancer. *New England Journal of Medicine.* 2003. 348(24): 2431–42.

Immunotherapy

Introduction
There are currently a number of strategies for utilising the immune response in cancer therapy, including monoclonal antibodies and cancer vaccines. In recent years there have been a number of significant developments in this area.

Ipilumumab and CTLA-4
- Ipilimumab is a fully human monoclonal antibody against cytotoxic T-lymphocyte antigen 4 (CTLA-4) and is used in the treatment of patients with melanoma.
- Ipilimumab activates T-cell proliferation, resulting in an immune-mediated anti-tumour effect against proteins present on the melanoma cell surface.
- Caution should be exercised when assessing response to treatment. In the first few months, tumour size can increase (pseudoprogression) prior to subsequent tumour shrinkage. This may be due to an inflammatory reaction to the treatment.
- *Side effects*
  Toxicities are generally immune related, particularly:
  ○ Colitis (diarrhoea, bloody stools, nausea and vomiting)
  ○ Rash
  ○ Hepatitis with elevated transaminases and/or bilirubin
  ○ Hypophysitis (pituitary gland dysfunction)
- *Management of side effects*:
  ○ Topical steroids and anti-pruritics can be used for rash.
  ○ Oral or IV corticosteroids may be required in cases of colitis and hepatitis. Ipilimumab may need to be discontinued.
  ○ In severe cases other immunosuppressive therapies (e.g. infliximab or mycophenolate) may be indicated.
  ○ In cases of hypophysitis, including adrenal insufficiency, steroid therapy should be initiated first, followed by endocrine therapy as required.

Interleukin-2 (IL-2)
- IL-2 is a cytokine that stimulates further cytokine production as well as T-cell function, which is how it is thought to exert its anti-cancer activity. It is used in the treatment of RCC.
- *Side effects include*:
  ○ Diarrhoea, fever, nausea, rash and myelosuppression.

○ 'Capillary-leak syndrome' is also a recognised side-effect, with fluid shifts leading to hypotension, oedema, pleural effusions, ascites and adult respiratory distress syndrome (ARDS). The hypotension that results from this can lead to end-organ damage including renal failure.

Interferon-α (IFN-α)

- The interferons are also a group of cytokines used in the treatment of a number of solid tumours, including melanoma, RCC and some leukaemias.
- They are thought to have a number of anti-tumour actions, including enhancement of natural killer cell and macrophage activity. They also have anti-proliferative and anti-angiogenic effects.
- *Side effects*: these can be numerous and include flu-like symptoms, myalgia/arthralgia, fatigue, fever, neutropenia, hepatotoxicity, mood disturbance and depression.

Intravesical immunotherapy

- Bacille Calmette-Guérin (BCG) is used intravesicularly for the treatment and prophylaxis of superficial bladder cancer after transurethral resection of bladder tumour (TURBT).
- Although the exact mechanism of action is poorly understood, BCG can initiate an immune response in the bladder mucosa and infiltration of the bladder wall with cytokines, including TNF-α, interleukins and interferon, as well as T-cells and macrophages. It is this inflammatory immune response which is thought to have anti-tumour activity.

Cancer vaccines

- Some vaccines can help prevent the development of different types of malignancy, for example vaccines against viral hepatitis (associated with HCC) and human papilloma virus (associated with cervical cancer).
- There are a number of therapeutic cancer vaccines that are currently being developed or in clinical trials. Sipuleucel-T, for example, is a vaccine used in metastatic prostate cancer.

Future treatments

There are a number of other immunotherapies that have shown promise in clinical trials. For example:

- Binding of the programmed death (PD) protein to its ligand (PD-L1) causes T-cell inhibition and allows tumour cells to evade the normal host immune response.
- In Phase I trials, anti-PD-L1 antibodies have resulted in responses in patients with a variety of solid tumours including NSCLC, RCC and melanoma.
- *Side effects include*: infusion reactions, diarrhoea, fever, hepatitis, rash and hypothyroidism.

Other relevant sections of this book

Chapter 3, section on diarrhoea

References

Brahmer JR, Tykodi SS, Chow LQ, Hwu WJ, Topalian SL, Hwu P, *et al*. Safety and activity of anti-PD-L1 antibody in patients with advanced cancer. *New England Journal of Medicine*. 2012. 366(26): 2455–65.

Kahler KC, Hauschild A. Treatment and side effect management of CTLA-4 antibody therapy in metastatic melanoma. *Journal der Deutschen Dermatologischen Gesellschaft* (Journal of the German Society of Dermatology). 2011. 9(4): 277–86.

Kantoff PW, Higano CS, Shore ND, Berger ER, Small EJ, Penson DF, *et al*. Sipuleucel-T immunotherapy for castration-resistant prostate cancer. *New England Journal of Medicine*. 2010. 363(5): 411–22.

Kirchner GI, Franzke A, Buer J, Beil W, Probst-Kepper M, Wittke F, *et al*. Pharmacokinetics of recombinant human interleukin-2 in advanced renal cell carcinoma patients following subcutaneous application. *British Journal of Clinical Pharmacology*. 1998. 46(1): 5–10.

Sabel MS, Sondak VK. Pros and cons of adjuvant interferon in the treatment of melanoma. *Oncologist*. 2003. 8(5): 451–8.

Shintani Y, Sawada Y, Inagaki T, Kohjimoto Y, Uekado Y, Shinka T. Intravesical instillation therapy with bacillus Calmette-Guerin for superficial bladder cancer: study of the mechanism of bacillus Calmette-Guerin immunotherapy. *International Journal of Urology*. 2007. 14(2): 140–6.

Weber J. Review: anti-CTLA-4 antibody ipilimumab: case studies of clinical response and immune-related adverse events. *Oncologist*. 2007. 12(7): 864–72.

Zigler M, Shir A, Levitzki A. Targeted cancer immunotherapy. *Current Opinion in Pharmacology*. 2013. 13(4): 504–10.

Targeted therapies

Some newer anti-cancer therapies focus on selecting targets involved in cellular signalling pathways which may be mutated, up-regulated or over-expressed in malignant cells. Targeted treatments may have single or multiple sites of action, but work in a different way to chemotherapy agents and are therefore associated with different toxicities.

Types of targeted therapies
Tyrosine kinase inhibitors (TKIs)

- Tyrosine kinases are enzymes that can transfer a phosphate group from ATP to the tyrosine amino acid of cell surface receptors (receptor tyrosine kinases). This leads to activation of intracellular signalling pathways.
- TKIs are small molecules that block the binding of ATP to the receptor at their intracellular binding site.
- TKIs can bind to and block a number of different targets and therefore can be more imprecise than monoclonal antibodies.

Monoclonal antibodies

- Monoclonal antibodies can act to inhibit the proliferation, replication and survival of cancer cells either directly (by blocking cellular receptors responsible for activation of intracellular signalling pathways), or indirectly via antibody dependent cytotoxicity.
- The suffix 'mab' in the name indicates that the drug in question is an antibody.

Examples of targeted therapies

Targeted treatments are constantly evolving and expanding, with newer therapies currently being developed and undergoing clinical trials. The following is not an exhaustive list, but gives examples of the more commonly used therapies and their targets.

CD20

- CD20 is expressed on the surface of B cells. Rituximab is a monoclonal antibody against the CD20 antigen and is used in the treatment of lymphomas and CLL.
- *Common side effects include*: infusion reactions, fever, chills, arthralgia and neutropenia (which can persist after treatment is complete).
- *Other serious side effects include*: progressive multifocal encephalopathy and potential reactivation of hepatitis B. Patients should be screened for hepatitis prior to commencing treatment.

Anaplastic lymphoma kinase (ALK)

- The abnormal EML4-ALK fusion gene can be found in a very small number of patients with NSCLC.
- Crizotinib is an oral inhibitor of the ALK and MET tyrosine kinases, and has been shown to have a dramatic effect on disease in patients with this mutation.
- *Side effects include*: neutropenia, nausea, vomiting, diarrhoea, peripheral neuropathy, elevated LFTs, oedema and visual disturbance.

BRAF

- Vemurafenib is an oral inhibitor of mutated BRAF and is used in the treatment of melanoma.
- *Side effects include*: rash, arthralgia, fatigue, nausea, diarrhoea, QT interval prolongation and photosensitivity. Patients also have a higher risk of developing squamous cell carcinomas of the skin.

C-KIT and BCR-ABL

- Imatinib:
  - Imatinib is an oral TKI widely used in the treatment of CML as it inhibits the BCR-ABL fusion gene product, leading to complete haematological response in a high number of patients.
  - Imatinib also inhibits platelet derived growth factor receptor (PDGFR) and c-KIT and is used in the treatment of GI stromal tumours (GIST), with the

most dramatic responses seen in patients with specific mutations in exon-11 of KIT.
  ○ *Side effects include*: GI disturbance, raised liver enzymes, fluid retention, arthralgia/myalgia and myelosuppression.
• Dasatinib is another small molecule TKI with similar targets of action, and can be used in patients who have refractory CML.

Epidermal growth factor receptor (EGFR)
• Cetuximab and panitumumab:
  ○ Monoclonal antibodies which bind to the extracellular domain of EGFR.
  ○ They are used in patients with colorectal and head and neck malignancies who are KRAS wild-type (i.e. do not have a KRAS mutation).
  ○ *Side effects include*: acneiform rash, diarrhoea, electrolyte disturbance (e.g. hypomagnesaemia) and rarely interstitial pneumonitis. The rash may have to be managed with topical steroids or antibiotics, but oral steroids may be warranted in severe cases.
• Gefitinib and erlotinib:
  ○ These are TKIs which inhibit the binding of ATP to EGFR.
  ○ *Side effects include*: acneiform rash, dry skin, nausea, vomiting, diarrhoea, fatigue, increased transaminases and, rarely, interstitial lung disease or pneumonitis.

Human epidermal growth factor (HER-2)
• Trastuzumab:
  ○ Trastuzumab is a humanised monoclonal antibody which binds to the extra-cellular domain of the HER-2 receptor.
  ○ *Side effects include*: infusion reactions (rash, hypotension, rigors, dyspnoea) and cardiac dysfunction (especially when combined with other cardiotoxic agents such as anthracyclines).
  ○ Patients should have regular assessment of cardiac function (echocardiogram/MUGA scan) prior to initiation of therapy, and trastuzumab should be discontinued if left ventricular function falls significantly. ACE-inhibitors are sometimes required.
  ○ Does not cross the blood–brain barrier, so patients can relapse with brain metastases.
• Lapatinib:
  ○ Lapatinib is a TKI used in breast cancer which targets the intracellular portion of the HER-1 and HER-2 receptors and can cross the blood brain barrier.
  ○ *Side effects include*: diarrhoea, nausea, heart failure, hepatotoxicity, nail changes and acneiform rash.

Mammalian target of rapamycin (mTOR)
• Everolimus is an oral inhibitor of mTOR that is similar to tacrolimus, which is used in patients who have received solid organ transplants. It is used in the treatment of RCC and neuroendocrine tumours.

- *Side effects include*: nausea, diarrhoea, hyperlipidaemia, rash and thrombocytopenia. Mucositis can be a particular problem. There is also a risk of raised ALP and hyperglycaemia, which in some cases will require hypoglycaemic therapy.

Vascular endothelial growth factor (VEGF)

- Expression of VEGF allows cancers to grow and metastasise. As tumours grow within their local environment, cells can become hypoxic, which stimulates vasculogenesis via the up-regulation of proteins such as VEGF. This is known as the 'angiogenic switch' and stimulates formation of new blood vessels.
- VEGF binds to the VEGF-receptor (VEGFR 1, 2 or 3) on the cell surface.
- Sorafenib:
  - This is a TKI which targets VEGFR 1, 2 and 3 and PDGFR as well as inhibiting intracellular Raf-kinases and is used in RCC and HCC.
  - *Side effects include*: diarrhoea, nausea, hand-foot syndrome, myelosuppression and fatigue. Both bleeding and thrombosis can be seen, as well as elevated serum lipase levels. Hypertension is also well recognised in all inhibitors of VEGF and may require pharmacological intervention.
- Sunitinib:
  - This is a TKI of multiple targets including VEGFR 1, 2 and 3, PDGFR and KIT (stem cell factor receptor) amongst others.
  - Used in RCC and GIST.
  - Side effects are similar to those seen with sorafenib. Thrombocytopenia and neutropenia are common, along with GI disturbance, fatigue and hand-foot syndrome.
- Bevacizumab:
  - This is a humanised antibody which binds to VEGF and is used in many different tumour types, including colorectal, lung and gynaecological cancer.
  - *Side effects include*: hypertension, proteinuria, bleeding, VTE, arterial thrombosis, delayed wound healing and GI perforation.
  - Should be avoided in patients who have colonic stents *in situ* and withheld for at least four weeks pre- and post surgical procedures.
  - Blood pressure should be monitored and anti-hypertensive treatment or discontinuation of bevacizumab may be required.
  - Urinalysis should be performed prior to each administration; 24-hour urine collection is indicated if >3+ proteinuria on dipstick. Severe or non-resolving proteinuria may lead to discontinuation of therapy.
- Aflibercept:
  - Aflibercept is a 'VEGF trap' compromised of the extracellular portions of the VEGF receptor, bound to immunoglobulin. This creates a fusion protein which has a high affinity for VEGF and 'traps' it, preventing its own binding to the cellular VEGF receptors.
  - *Side effects include*: hypertension, bleeding and thrombosis, as well as GI perforation.

Other relevant sections of this book

- Chapter 3, sections on chest pain and other cardiac complications, hypertension, rash, renal failure and hydronephrosis
- Chapter 10, section on personalised medicine and molecular testing

References

Chapman PB, Hauschild A, Robert C, Haanen JB, Ascierto P, Larkin J, *et al*. Improved survival with vemurafenib in melanoma with BRAF V600E mutation. *New England Journal of Medicine*. 2011. 364(26): 2507–16.

Davis TA, Grillo-Lopez AJ, White CA, McLaughlin P, Czuczman MS, Link BK, *et al*. Rituximab anti-CD20 monoclonal antibody therapy in non-Hodgkin's lymphoma: safety and efficacy of re-treatment. *Journal of Clinical Oncology*. 2000. 18(17): 3135–43.

Gerber HP, Ferrara N. Pharmacology and pharmacodynamics of bevacizumab as monotherapy or in combination with cytotoxic therapy in preclinical studies. *Cancer Research*. 2005. 65(3): 671–80.

Hudis CA. Trastuzumab – mechanism of action and use in clinical practice. *New England Journal of Medicine*. 2007. 357(1): 39–51.

Jonker DJ, O'Callaghan CJ, Karapetis CS, Zalcberg JR, Tu D, Au HJ, *et al*. Cetuximab for the treatment of colorectal cancer. *New England Journal of Medicine*. 2007. 357(20): 2040–8.

Klumpen HJ, Beijnen JH, Gurney H, Schellens JH. Inhibitors of mTOR. *Oncologist*. 2010. 15(12): 1262–9.

Kwak EL, Bang YJ, Camidge DR, Shaw AT, Solomon B, Maki RG, *et al*. Anaplastic lymphoma kinase inhibition in non-small-cell lung cancer. *New England Journal of Medicine*. 2010. 363(18): 1693–703.

Llovet JM, Ricci S, Mazzaferro V, Hilgard P, Gane E, Blanc JF, *et al*. Sorafenib in advanced hepatocellular carcinoma. *New England Journal of Medicine*. 2008. 359(4): 378–90.

Motzer RJ, Hutson TE, Tomczak P, Michaelson MD, Bukowski RM, Rixe O, *et al*. Sunitinib versus interferon alfa in metastatic renal-cell carcinoma. *New England Journal of Medicine*. 2007. 356(2): 115–24.

Moy B, Goss PE. Lapatinib-associated toxicity and practical management recommendations. *Oncologist*. 2007. 12(7): 756–65.

Ono M, Kuwano M. Molecular mechanisms of epidermal growth factor receptor (EGFR) activation and response to gefitinib and other EGFR-targeting drugs. *Clinical Cancer Research*. 2006. 12(24): 7242–51.

Van Cutsem E, Tabernero J, Lakomy R, Prenen H, Prausova J, Macarulla T, *et al*. Addition of aflibercept to fluorouracil, leucovorin, and irinotecan improves survival in a phase III randomized trial in patients with metastatic colorectal cancer previously treated with an oxaliplatin-based regimen. *Journal of Clinical Oncology*. 2012. 30(28): 3499–506.

CHAPTER 7

Electrolyte abnormalities

Sing Yu Moorcraft

The Royal Marsden NHS Foundation Trust, UK

Hypocalcaemia

The normal range of total calcium is usually 2.12–2.65 mmol/L (8–10 mg/dl). Hypocalcaemia is defined as a low concentration of calcium in the blood. The grade of hypocalcaemia is shown in Table 7.1.

Pseudohypocalcaemia

This is when variation in protein concentrations (particularly albumin) leads to fluctuations in total calcium level, but ionised calcium levels remain relatively stable. For example, patients with chronic illnesses such as cancer can have a low total plasma calcium but normal ionised calcium. Therefore calcium levels should be corrected for albumin as follows: corrected calcium (mmol/L) = measured calcium (mmol/L) + 0.02 * (40 – patient's albumin (g/L)).

Symptoms/signs

- *Symptoms/signs*: Chvostek's sign (tapping over the facial nerve causes facial twitching), Trousseau's sign (carpopedal spasm when brachial artery occluded), tetany, depression, perioral paraesthesiae, confusion, papilloedema.
- *ECG changes*: increased QT interval, T wave inversion, heart block.

Causes

- Tumour lysis syndrome
- Chronic renal failure

Clinical Problems in Oncology: A Practical Guide to Management, First Edition.
Edited by Sing Yu Moorcraft, Daniel L.Y. Lee and David Cunningham.
© 2014 John Wiley & Sons, Ltd. Published 2014 by John Wiley & Sons, Ltd.

Table 7.1 CTCAE (V4.03) grading of hypocalcaemia.

Grade	Criteria
1	Corrected serum calcium of < LLN – 8.0 mg/dL; < LLN – 2.0 mmol/L; ionised calcium < LLN – 1.0 mmol/L.
2	Corrected serum calcium of <8.0–7.0 mg/dL; < 2.0–1.75 mmol/L; ionised calcium < 1.0–0.9 mmol/L; symptomatic.
3	Corrected serum calcium of <7.0–6.0 mg/dL; < 1.75–1.5 mmol/L; ionised calcium < 0.9–0.8 mmol/L; hospitalisation indicated.
4	Corrected serum calcium of <6.0 mg/dL; < 1.5 mmol/L; ionised calcium <0.8 mmol/L; life-threatening consequences.
5	Death.

LLN = lower limit of normal.
From the website of the National Cancer Institute (http://www.cancer.gov).

- *Surgery*:
  - Thyroid or parathyroid surgery
  - Radical neck surgery
- *Endocrine*:
  - Hypoparathyroidism
  - Pseudohypoparathyroidism
- *Drugs*:
  - Bisphosphonates, denosumab
  - Phosphate therapy
  - Cisplatin
  - Foscarnet
  - Calcium channel blocker overdose
- *Gastrointestinal*:
  - Pancreatitis
  - Vitamin D malabsorption/deficiency
  - Re-feeding syndrome
- *Infections*:
  - Sepsis
  - Toxic shock syndrome
- Osteomalacia, bone metastases
- Hypomagnesaemia
- *Other*: acute hyperventilation, overhydration, rhabdomyolysis, low exposure to UV light, massive blood transfusion.

Management
- Correct abnormalities in potassium and magnesium
- Mild – moderate (calcium 1.88–2.11 mmol): oral calcium replacement:
  - For example: 1 tablet BD of Calcichew® or Adcal® (plus vitamin D if vitamin D deficient).

- ○ Give after meals to maximise absorption. May decrease the bioavailability of tetracyclines, fluoroquinolones, iron and atenolol.
- Moderate to severe (calcium < 1.88 mmol/L): IV calcium replacement:
  - ○ 10 ml of 10% calcium gluconate (2.2 mmol Ca^{2+}) IV over 20 minutes (max 2 ml/min). The effect is short-lasting and so this can be repeated as required or dilute 100 ml of 10% calcium gluconate in 1 L of 0.9% saline or 5% glucose, start at a rate of 50 ml/hour and adjust according to response.
  - ○ ECG monitoring should be performed (particularly in patients with heart disease or a high risk of arrhythmias).
  - ○ Risks of IV calcium: arrhythmias, hypotension, hypercalcaemia. Use cautiously in patients on digoxin as they are more sensitive to fluctuations in serum calcium and calcium can potentiate digoxin toxicity.
  - ○ Measure calcium regularly until within the normal range.
- *Further investigations*:
  - ○ Consider checking PTH levels in patients who are resistant to therapy (PTH is reduced or normal in hypoparathyroidism and hypomagnesaemia, but high in other causes of hypocalcaemia).
  - ○ Serum 25-hydroxyvitamin D levels can be useful in confirming vitamin D deficiency.

Other relevant sections of this book

- Chapter 2, sections on hypercalcaemia, tumour lysis syndrome
- Chapter 7, sections on hyperkalaemia and hypokalaemia, hypermagnesaemia and hypomagnesaemia

References

Cooper MS, Gittoes NJ. Diagnosis and management of hypocalcaemia. *British Medical Journal*. 2008. 336(7656): 1298–302.

Ecc Committee S, Task Forces of the American Heart A. 2005 American Heart Association guidelines for cardiopulmonary resuscitation and emergency cardiovascular care. *Circulation*. 2005. 112(24 Suppl.): IV1–203.

Joint Formulary Committee. *British National Formulary* (online). London: BMJ Group and Pharmaceutical Press. Available from: http://www.medicinescomplete.com (accessed 1 January 2014).

Nolan J, Soar J, Lockey A, Pitcher D, Gabbott D, *et al. Advanced Life Support*, fifth edition. Resuscitation Council (UK): London. 2008.

Hyperkalaemia and hypokalaemia

Hyperkalaemia

The normal range of potassium is usually 3.5–5.0 mmol/L. Hyperkalaemia is defined as an elevated concentration of potassium in the blood. The grade of hyperkalaemia is shown in Table 7.2.

Table 7.2 CTCAE (V4.03) grading of hyperkalaemia.

Grade	Criteria
1	> ULN – 5.5 mmol/L.
2	> 5.5–6.0 mmol/L.
3	> 6.0–7.0 mmol/L; hospitalisation indicated.
4	> 7.0 mmol/L; life-threatening consequences.
5	Death.

ULN = upper limit of normal.
From the website of the National Cancer Institute (http://www.cancer.gov).

Symptoms/signs

- *Symptoms/signs*: arrhythmias, sudden death, weakness, paraesthesiae, depressed tendon reflexes.
- *ECG changes*: flattened or absent P wave, wide QRS complex, tall-tented T wave, VF/VT, first degree heart block, ST segment depression, bradycardia.

Causes

- Artefact, for example due to haemolysis, delay in sample analysis, high WCC or platelet count.
- Oliguric renal failure.
- Tumour lysis syndrome.
- *Drugs*: excess potassium therapy, potassium-sparing diuretics, ACE inhibitors, digoxin.
- *Other*: Addison's disease, metabolic acidosis, burns, massive blood transfusion, haemolysis, rhabdomyolysis.

Management

- General management:
  - Perform an ECG
  - Stop all potassium containing drugs
  - Assess severity of hyperkalaemia:
    - *Mild*: 5.5–6 mmol/L
    - *Moderate*: 6.1–6.4 mmol/L
    - *Severe*: ≥ 6.5 or ECG changes or symptomatic
  - Low potassium diet (see hypokalaemia section for more details on potassium containing foods)
  - If the patient is hypovolaemic, give fluids to enhance urinary potassium excretion
- If potassium > 6.5 mmol/L or ECG changes:
  - Give 10 ml of 10% calcium gluconate (2.2 mmol Ca^{2+}) IV over two minutes repeated as necessary for cardioprotection (does not reduce the potassium

level). If the patient is on digoxin, rapid administration of calcium gluconate can cause myocardial digoxin toxicity. Therefore in these patients calcium gluconate should be given slowly over 20 minutes in 100 ml of 5% glucose.

o Insulin and glucose: for example 10 units of short-acting insulin (e.g. Actrapid®) and 250 ml of 10% glucose over 30–60 minutes (or 50 ml of 50% glucose IV over 5–15 minutes, preferably via a central line). Onset of action in 15–30 minutes, maximum effect at 30–60 minutes. Glucose should be checked 30 minutes after administration of insulin and then hourly for six hours as delayed hypoglycaemia can occur.

o Give 2.5–10 mg nebulised salbutamol (adjunct use only). Onset of action in 15–30 minutes. Use with caution in patients with tachycardia or ischaemic heart disease.

o Calcium resonium: there is little evidence for efficacy and it often causes constipation, leading to increased reabsorption of potassium.

o Consider dialysis.

o Consider IV sodium bicarbonate if patient is acidotic (pH 7.1–7.3), for example due to diabetic ketoacidosis.

o Check potassium at least twice daily until <6 mmol/L.

Hypokalaemia

Hypokalaemia is defined as a low concentration of potassium in the blood. The grade of hypokalaemia is shown in Table 7.3.

Symptoms/signs

• *Signs/symptoms*: arrhythmias, cramps, tetany, muscle weakness, hypotonia, fatigue.
• *ECG changes*: prolonged PR interval, ST depression, flattened T waves, prominent U wave (after T wave).

Causes

• *Gastrointestinal*: vomiting, diarrhoea, pyloric stenosis, intestinal fistulae.
• *Endocrine*: Cushing's syndrome, Conn's syndrome.

Table 7.3 CTCAE (V4.03) grading of hypokalaemia.

Grade	Criteria
1	< LLN – 3.0 mmol/L.
2	< LLN – 3.0 mmol/L; symptomatic; intervention indicated.
3	< 3.0–2.5 mmol/L; hospitalisation indicated.
4	< 2.5 mmol/L; life-threatening consequences.
5	Death.

LLN = lower limit of normal.
From the website of the National Cancer Institute (http://www.cancer.gov).

- *Drugs*: cisplatin, diuretics, laxatives, steroids, adrenaline, high dose penicillin, amphotericin B, insulin.
- Renal tubular failure.
- *Other*: magnesium depletion, alkalosis, poor dietary intake, purgative abuse.

Management
- General management:
  - ○ Check magnesium level and replace if low.
  - ○ *High potassium diet*: dried figs, molasses, dried fruits (dates, prunes), nuts, avocados, bran cereals, wheat germ, lima beans, spinach, tomatoes, broccoli, beets, carrots, cauliflower, potatoes, bananas, kiwis, oranges, mangoes, ground beef, steak, veal, lamb, chocolate.
  - ○ Measure serum potassium regularly until within the normal range.
- Mild (potassium 3.1–3.5 mmol/L, asymptomatic): give oral potassium, for example Sando-K® two tablets OD/BD. Side effects include nausea, vomiting, abdominal pain, diarrhoea and GI ulceration.
- Moderate (potassium 2.6–3.0 mmol/L): oral potassium, for example Sando-K® two tablets BD/TDS.
- Severe (potassium <2.5 mmol/L, dangerous symptoms), IV potassium:
  - ○ IV potassium should be given at a maximum rate of 20 mmol/hour.
  - ○ Concentrations of greater than 40 mmol/L should ideally be given in a critical care setting via a central line (or a large peripheral vein in emergency situations).
  - ○ Examples of IV potassium replacement:
    - ▪ 40 mmol of potassium in 1000 ml of 0.9% sodium chloride over at least four hours via a peripheral or a central line.
    - ▪ 40 mmol of potassium in 100 ml of 0.9% sodium chloride over at least 2–4 hours via a central line in an HDU/ITU setting.
  - ○ ECG monitoring is required if patient is at high risk of arrhythmias, rate of infusion 20 mmol/hour or potassium concentration >80 mmol/L.
  - ○ Rapid infusion can cause arrhythmias, heart block, hyperkalaemia, phlebitis, pain at the injection site and cardiac arrest.
- Unstable arrhythmias where cardiac arrest is imminent or has occurred: consider a more rapid infusion, for example 2 mmol/min for 10 minutes, followed by 10 mmol over 5–10 minutes with continuous cardiac monitoring.

References

Clinical Resource Efficiency Support Team (CREST). Guidelines for the treatment of hyperkalaemia in adults 2005. Available from: www.dhsspsni.gov.uk/publications/2005/hyperkalaemia-booklet.pdf (accessed 1 January 2014).

Cohn JN, Kowey PR, Whelton PK, Prisant LM. New guidelines for potassium replacement in clinical practice: a contemporary review by the National Council on Potassium in Clinical Practice. *Archives of Internal Medicine*. 2000. 160(16): 2429–36.

Ecc Committee S, Task Forces of the American Heart A. 2005 American Heart Association guidelines for cardiopulmonary resuscitation and emergency cardiovascular care. *Circulation.* 2005. 112(24 Suppl.): IV1–203.

Nolan J, Soar J, Lockey A, Pitcher D, Gabbott D, *et al. Advanced Life Support, fifth edition.* Resuscitation Council (UK): London. 2008.

Hypermagnesaemia and hypomagnesaemia

Hypermagnesaemia

The normal range of magnesium is usually 0.75–1.05 mmol/L. Hypermagnesaemia is defined as an elevated concentration of magnesium in the blood. The grade of hypermagnesaemia is shown in Table 7.4.

Symptoms/signs

- *Symptoms/signs*: drowsiness, confusion, decreased conscious level/coma, nausea, vomiting, muscular weakness, diminished/absent reflexes, hypoventilation, hypotension, bradycardia and arrhythmias.
- Associated with hypocalcaemia.
- *ECG changes*: prolonged PR interval, prolonged QT interval, peaked T waves and AV block.

Causes

- Renal failure
- Tumour lysis syndrome
- Drugs: excessive antacids or laxatives
- Iatrogenic (e.g. due to administration of IV magnesium, magnesium enema)
- Adrenal insufficiency

Management

- Hypermagnesaemia rarely requires treatment.
- Stop any oral or IV magnesium supplementation (commonly used in patients on cisplatin).

Table 7.4 CTCAE (V4.03) grading of hypermagnesaemia.

Grade	Criteria
1	> ULN – 3.0 mg/dL; > ULN – 1.23 mmol/L.
2	—
3	> 3.0–8.0 mg/dL; > 1.23–3.30 mmol/L.
4	> 8.0 mg/dL; > 3.30 mmol/L; life-threatening consequences.
5	Death.

ULN = upper limit of normal.
From the website of the National Cancer Institute (http://www.cancer.gov).

- If a patient is symptomatic or has severe hypermagnesaemia, consider:
  - 5–10 ml of 10% calcium chloride IV. This removes magnesium from serum and will often correct potentially fatal arrhythmias.
  - Cardiorespiratory support (if necessary and appropriate).
  - Dialysis.
  - Saline diuresis: if the patient has normal renal function and adequate cardiovascular function then 0.9% saline with 1 mg/kg of furosemide IV can increase urinary magnesium excretion. However, this can also lead to calcium excretion and hypocalcaemia will result in worsening symptoms and signs from hypermagnesaemia.
- Patients with renal failure should not receive magnesium-containing medication.

Hypomagnesaemia

Hypomagnesaemia is defined as a low concentration of magnesium in the blood. Hypomagnesaemia is much more common than hypermagnesaemia. The grading of hypomagnesaemia is shown in Table 7.5.

Symptoms/signs
- May be non-specific and be attributed to the patient's cancer or chemotherapy.
- Chronic hypomagnesaemia can occur after three weeks of chemotherapy (e.g. with cisplatin) and persist for months or years.
- *Symptoms/signs*: tetany, muscle weakness, paraesthesiae, seizures, tremor, ataxia, nystagmus, Chvostek's sign (tapping over the facial nerve causes facial twitching), Trousseau's sign (carpopedal spasm when brachial artery occluded), mental state changes (e.g. disorientation, irritability, psychoses), lethargy and arrhythmias.
- Associated with hypocalcaemia and hypokalaemia.
- *ECG changes*: prolonged PR interval, prolonged QT interval, ST segment depression, T wave inversion, flattened P waves, increased QRS duration, torsade de pointes.

Table 7.5 TCAE (V4.03) grading of hypomagnesaemia.

Grade	Criteria
1	< LLN – 1.2 mg/dL; < LLN – 0.5 mmol/L.
2	< 1.2–0.9 mg/dL; < 0.5–0.4 mmol/L.
3	< 0.9–0.7 mg/dL; < 0.4–0.3 mmol/L.
4	< 0.7 mg/dL; < 0.3 mmol/L; life threatening consequences.
5	Death.

LLN = lower limit of normal.
From the website of the National Cancer Institute (http://www.cancer.gov).

Causes

- *Gastrointestinal*: diarrhoea, vomiting, pancreatitis, gastrointestinal fistulae, surgical resection, malabsorption, starvation, TPN, refeeding syndrome.
- *Endocrine*: uncontrolled diabetes, ketoacidosis, SIADH, hyperthyroidism, hyper-parathyroidism, hyperaldosteronism.
- *Renal*: tubular defects, polyuria.
- *Drugs*:
  - Anti-cancer therapies: cisplatin, carboplatin (less than cisplatin), tacrolimus, cyclosporin, EGFR inhibitors (e.g. cetuximab, panitumumab), interleukin-2, pegylated liposomal doxorubicin, dasatinib, nilotinib.
  - Diuretics.
  - Proton pump inhibitors.
  - Aminoglycoside antibiotics.
  - Pentamidine, amphotericin B.
  - Bisphosphonates.
- *Other*: alcohol, blood transfusions

Management

- Correct calcium and potassium abnormalities.
- Foods that are high in magnesium: green leafy vegetables, seeds, nuts, peas, beans and cocoa.
- Mild – moderate (magnesium 0.4–7 mmol/L): magnesium replacement should be considered if the patient is symptomatic or following a risk/benefit decision.
- Severe (magnesium ≤0.4 mmol/L): magnesium replacement should be prescribed.
- Magnesium replacement:
  - Oral magnesium, for example magnesium glycerophosphate 1–2 tablets (4 mmol Mg^{2+}/tablet) TDS or up to three tablets every six hours (unlicensed). This can cause diarrhoea.
  - IV magnesium, for example 20 mmol (5 g) of magnesium sulphate in 1 L of 0.9% sodium chloride or 5% glucose over 3–5 hours. Local practice may vary and a longer infusion period may be more suitable for non-emergency situations.
  - Risks of IV magnesium:
    - Patients with renal failure are at risk of hypermagnesaemia. Magnesium should therefore be used with great caution, the dose reduced by 50–75% and magnesium levels closely monitored.
    - Rapid administration can cause cardiac arrest.
    - Can cause hypocalcaemia, hypotension and hypermagnesaemia.
- *Emergencies*:
  - *Torsade de points*: 8 mmol (2 g) of 50% magnesium sulphate IV over 15 minutes.
  - *Seizure*: 8 mmol (2 g) magnesium sulphate IV over 10 minutes.
  - Patients should have cardiac monitoring.
- Magnesium takes 36–48 hours to distribute to body tissues therefore recheck magnesium after 48 hours. Successful treatment usually takes 2–3 days.

References

Ecc Committee S, Task Forces of the American Heart A. 2005 American Heart Association guidelines for cardiopulmonary resuscitation and emergency cardiovascular care. *Circulation*. 2005. 112(24 Suppl.): IV1–203.

Nolan J, Soar J, Lockey A, Pitcher D, Gabbott D, *et al. Advanced Life Support*, fifth edition. Resuscitation Council (UK): London. 2008.

Saif MW. Management of hypomagnesemia in cancer patients receiving chemotherapy. *Journal of Supportive Oncology*. 2008. 6(5): 243–8.

UK Medicines Information Pharmacists. How is acute hypomagnesaemia treated in adults? 2010. Available from: http://www.evidence.nhs.uk/search?q=acute+hypomagnaesemia (accessed 1 January 2014).

Hypernatraemia and hyponatraemia

Hypernatraemia

The normal range for sodium is usually 135–145 mmol/L. Hypernatraemia is defined as an elevated level of sodium in the blood. The grading of hypernatraemia is shown in Table 7.6.

Symptoms/signs

- The severity of symptoms depends on the rate and severity of change in sodium concentration.
- *Symptoms/signs*: signs of dehydration, confusion, irritability, nausea, thirst, postural hypotension, oliguria, coma and seizures.

Causes

- IV fluids (e.g. excessive 0.9% sodium chloride).
- Fluid loss without water replacement, for example vomiting, diarrhoea.
- Osmotic diuresis (e.g. diabetic ketoacidosis, TPN).
- Medication: for example lithium, tetracyclines, amphotericin B.
- Other causes: diabetes insipidus (pituitary or nephrogenic), hyperaldosteronism (associated with hypertension and hypokalaemia).

Table 7.6 CTCAE (V4.03) grading of hypernatraemia.

Grade	Criteria
1	> ULN – 150 mmol/L.
2	> 150–155 mmol/L.
3	> 155–160 mmol/L; hospitalisation indicated.
4	> 160 mmol/L; life-threatening consequences.
5	Death.

ULN = upper limit of normal.
From the website of the National Cancer Institute (http://www.cancer.gov).

Management

- *Investigations*:
  - ○ Measure simultaneous plasma and urine osmolality and sodium.
  - ○ If urine osmolality is lower than that of plasma this indicates diabetes insipidus.
  - ○ If urine osmolality is high this suggests an osmotic diuresis or excessive extrarenal water loss.
- Treat the underlying cause if possible.
- Severe hypernatraemia (> 170 mmol/L) in hypovolaemic patients: 0.9% sodium chloride should be used initially to avoid rapid drops in serum sodium concentration, which could lead to cerebral oedema.
- Mild or moderate hypernatraemia: water orally if possible, or 5% dextrose slowly IV (e.g. approximately 4 L in 24 hours). Can also use 0.9% sodium chloride (especially if hypovolaemic) as this results in less marked fluid shifts.
- Monitor urine output and plasma sodium regularly.

Hyponatraemia

Hyponatraemia is a common problem in oncology patients, particularly in patients with SCLC. Hyponatraemia is defined as a low concentration of sodium in the blood and the grading of hyponatraemia is shown in Table 7.7.

Symptoms/signs

- Symptoms are rare unless there is an acute fall in sodium concentration or the sodium concentration is < 120 mmol/L.
- *Symptoms/signs*: confusion, irritability, headache, hypertension, oedema, nausea, vomiting, muscle weakness, cardiac failure and seizures.

Causes

- Overhydration with IV fluids (e.g. 5% dextrose)
- *Medication*:
  - ○ Diuretics
  - ○ Anti-cancer drugs: cisplatin, carboplatin, cyclophosphamide, ifosfamide, vinblastine, vincristine, methotrexate, interferon

Table 7.7 CTCAE (V4.03) grading of hyponatraemia.

Grade	Criteria
1	< LLN – 130 mmol/L.
2	—
3	< 130 – 120 mmol/L.
4	< 120 mmol/L; life-threatening consequences.
5	Death.

LLN = lower limit of normal.
From the website of the National Cancer Institute (http://www.cancer.gov).

- Opioids, NSAIDs
- Antidepressants: SSRIs, tricyclics, monoamine oxidase inhibitors, venlafaxine
- Anti-epileptics: sodium valproate, carbamazepine, lamotrigine
- Antipsychotics: haloperidol, risperidone
- PPIs: omeprazole, lansoprazole, pantoprazole
- Renal failure, nephrotic syndrome, interstitial renal disease
- Addison's disease, hypothyroidism
- Syndrome of inappropriate anti-diuretic hormone secretion (SIADH)
- Cirrhosis, CCF
- Diarrhoea, vomiting, small bowel obstruction, pancreatitis
- Pseudohyponatraemia, for example due to high lipids, protein or glucose

Syndrome of inappropriate antidiuretic hormone secretion (SIADH)

- Syndrome of inappropriate antidiuretic hormone secretion (SIADH) is a common cause of hyponatraemia in cancer patients, occurring in approximately 11–15% of patients with SCLC and approximately 3% of patients with head and neck cancers. SIADH can also occur in patients with other malignancies, for example lymphoma, prostate, thymus, pancreatic and brain tumours.
- Non-malignant causes of SIADH:
  - Pulmonary lesions: pneumonia, TB, lung abscess
  - CNS causes: meningitis, subdural haematoma, cerebral abscess, head injury
  - Metabolic: alcohol withdrawal, porphyria
  - Drugs (see above)
- *Investigations*: low plasma osmolality and high urine osmolality (in euvolaemic patients).
- *Treatment* – see below.

Management

- Assess the most likely cause and fluid status:
  - If dehydrated:
    - If urinary sodium >20 mmol/L: consider Addison's disease, renal failure, diuretics.
    - If urinary sodium <20 mmol/L: consider diarrhoea, vomiting, fistula, small bowel obstruction.
  - If not dehydrated:
    - If oedematous: consider nephrotic syndrome, cirrhosis, renal or cardiac failure.
    - If not oedematous and urine osmolality >500 mmol/kg: consider SIADH
  - If not oedematous and urine osmolality <500 mmol/kg: consider water overload, hypothyroidism, glucocorticoid insufficiency.
- Review patients' medication and, if possible, treat the cause of hyponatraemia.

- It is important to correct hyponatraemia gradually as rapid changes in sodium concentration can cause central pontine myelinolysis or coma.
- Asymptomatic patients with chronic hyponatraemia – fluid restriction (if patient is not dehydrated) or slow rehydration with 0.9% sodium chloride. If no improvement with a fluid restriction of 1 L/day, reduce to 500 ml/day.
- Symptomatic patients – slow correction with 0.9% sodium chloride. The rate of correction should be <10–12 mmol/L over 24 hours and <18 mmol/L over 48 hours. If hypovolaemic, try a fluid challenge of 0.5–1 L over 2–4 hours and recheck sodium. Patients with chronic hyponatraemia should have their sodium corrected at an even slower rate (< 10 mmol/L).
- For severely symptomatic patients who are euvolaemic/hypervolaemic (e.g. patients with SIADH), consider hypertonic (3%) saline via a continuous infusion or bolus. Seek specialist advice and monitor sodium at least every 1–2 hours. Correction beyond 10–12 mmol/L in the first 24 hours should be avoided.
- In patients with SIADH, consider demeclocycline 600–1200 mg daily if fluid restriction is ineffective.

References

Castillo J, Vincent M, Justice E. Diagnosis and management of hyponatraemia in cancer patients. *Oncologist*. 2012. 17(6): 756–65.

Ecc Committee S, Task Forces of the American Heart A. 2005 American Heart Association guidelines for cardiopulmonary resuscitation and emergency cardiovascular care. *Circulation*. 2005. 112(24 Suppl.): I V1–203.

Wakil A, Ng JM, Atkin SL. Investigating hyponatraemia. *British Medical Journal*. 2011. 342 d1118.

Hyperphosphataemia and hypophosphataemia

Hyperphosphataemia

The normal range for phosphate is usually 0.8–1.45 mmol/L. Hyperphosphataemia is defined as an elevated concentration of phosphate in the blood. There is no CTCAE grading for hyperphosphataemia.

Symptoms/signs

- Most patients are asymptomatic.
- Most symptoms are non-specific and are due to the underlying cause or associated hypocalcaemia, for example fatigue, anorexia, nausea, tetany, perioral numbness/tingling.
- Other symptoms include muscle weakness, rash, bone or joint pain.

Causes
- Tumour lysis syndrome
- Acute or chronic kidney disease
- Rhabdomyolysis
- Lactic acidosis
- *Endocrine*: hypoparathyroidism, acromegaly
- *Drugs*: phosphate-containing laxatives, for example Fleet Phospho-soda® (patients with renal impairment are at increased risk)
- Pseudohyperphosphataemia, for example due to haemolysis, hyperbilirubinaemia, hyperlipidaemia, hyperglobulinaemia (e.g. due to multiple myeloma)

Management
- Acute hyperphosphataemia:
  - In patients with normal renal function, acute hyperphosphataemia usually resolves within 6–12 hours.
  - Can be associated with symptomatic hypocalcaemia and be life-threatening.
  - IV fluids (0.9% sodium chloride) can increase phosphate excretion, but may worsen hypocalcaemia.
  - Consider haemodialysis, particularly if symptomatic hypocalcaemia and impaired renal function.
- Chronic hyperphosphataemia:
  - Refer to a dietician for advice on a low phosphate diet, for example minimise intake of dairy products, dark colas, fish, chocolate, bran, organ meats (e.g. liver).
  - Consider a phosphate binder in patients with renal failure, for example calcium acetate (e.g. Renacet®, PhosLo®, Phosex®). If calcium acetate is not tolerated, consider calcium carbonate (Calcichew®). Discuss with the renal team.

Hypophosphataemia
Hypophosphataemia is defined as a low concentration of phosphate in the blood. The grade of hypophosphataemia is shown in Table 7.8.

Table 7.8 CTCAE (V4.03) grading of hypophosphataemia.

Grade	Criteria
1	< LLN – 2.5 mg/dL; < LLN – 0.8 mmol/L.
2	< 2.5–2.0 mg/dL; < 0.8–0.6 mmol/L.
3	< 2.0–1.0 mg/dL; < 0.6–0.3 mmol/L.
4	< 1.0 mg/dL; < 0.3 mmol/L; life-threatening consequences.
5	Death.

LLN = lower limit of normal.
From the website of the National Cancer Institute (http://www.cancer.gov).

Symptoms/signs
- Most patients are asymptomatic.
- *Symptoms/signs*: arrhythmias, heart failure, respiratory muscle dysfunction (e.g. respiratory failure, difficulty weaning), muscle weakness, seizures, encephalopathy, altered mental status, confusion, polyneuropathy, central pontine myelinolysis, rhabdomyolysis, insulin resistance, haemolysis, leucocyte dysfunction.

Causes
- *Gastrointestinal*: diarrhoea, vomiting, malnutrition, nasogastric suction, vitamin D deficiency, TPN, refeeding syndrome
- *Drugs*:
  - Bisphosphonates
  - Acyclovir, foscarnet
  - Diuretics
  - Antacids
  - Salbutamol, theophylline
  - Phosphate binding agents
  - Glucocorticoids, oestrogens, insulin, catecholamines
  - Anti-cancer drugs: imatinib
- *Endocrine*: diabetic ketoacidosis, hyperparathyroidism.
- *Infections*: severe infections (especially Gram negative bacteraemia, *Legionella* infections).
- *Post-operative*: particularly after major hepatic surgery.
- *Secondary to malignancy*: for example acute leukaemia.
- *Other*: trauma, alcohol, metabolic acidosis, respiratory alkalosis, hungry bone syndrome, pseudohypophosphataemia.

Management
- Patients with hypocalcaemia should have this corrected prior to phosphate administration to prevent further hypocalcaemia.
- Assess severity of hypophosphataemia:
  - *Mild*: 0.65–0.8 mmol/L
  - *Moderate*: 0.32–0.65 mmol/L
  - *Severe*: < 0.32 mmol/L
- Asymptomatic patients with mild-moderate hypophosphatemia:
  - Give oral phosphate, for example two tablets BD/TDS of Phosphate-Sandoz® (contains 16.1 mmol of phosphate, 20.4 mmol of sodium and 3.1 mmol of potassium). These are effervescent tablets that must be dissolved in water and can cause nausea and/or diarrhoea. Oral magnesium, calcium or aluminium containing products can bind to Phosphate-Sandoz® and prevent its absorption if given at the same time of day.

- ○ If a patient is unlikely to absorb oral phosphate, IV phosphate can be used. There are a variety of suggested regimes. These include 0.2–0.5 mmol/kg/day of IV phosphate up to a maximum of 50 mmol, for example:
  - 40–60 kg: 10 mmol (100 ml) of Phosphate Polyfusor®
  - 61–80 kg: 15 mmol (150 ml) of Phosphate Polyfusor®
  - 81–120 kg: 20 mmol (200 ml) of Phosphate Polyfusor®
- Severe hypophosphataemia or symptomatic patients: administer IV phosphate. There are a variety of suggested regimes. These include 0.2–0.5 mmol/kg/day of IV phosphate up to a maximum of 50 mmol, for example:
  - ○ 40–60 kg: 25 mmol (250 ml) of Phosphate Polyfusor®
  - ○ 61–80 kg: 35 mmol (350 ml) of Phosphate Polyfusor®
  - ○ 81–120 kg: 50 mmol (500 ml) of Phosphate Polyfusor®
- IV phosphate:
  - ○ Each 500 ml of Phosphate Polyfusor® contains 50 mmol of phosphate, 9.5 mmol of potassium and 81 mmol of sodium.
  - ○ Phosphate Polyfusor® is usually given over 12–24 hours (but can be given over 6–12 hours).
  - ○ Initial dose should be halved in patients with renal impairment.
  - ○ Risks of IV phosphate: hyperphosphataemia, hypomagnesaemia, hypocalcaemia, hypotension and precipitation with calcium. Use with caution in patients with peripheral or pulmonary oedema or cardiac disease.

References

Geerse DA, Bindels AJ, Kuiper MA, Roos AN, Spronk PE, Schultz MJ. Treatment of hypophosphatemia in the intensive care unit: a review. *Critical Care*. 2010. 14(4): R147.

Liamis G, Milionis HJ, Elisaf M. Medication-induced hypophosphatemia: a review. *Quarterly Journal of Medicine*. 2010. 103(7): 449–59.

National Institute for Health and Care Excellence (NICE). Hyperphosphataemia in chronic kidney disease (CG157):.Available from: http://guidance.nice.org.uk/CG157/NICEGuidance/pdf/English (accessed 1 January 2014).

UK Medicines Information Pharmacists. How is acute hypophosphataemia treated in adults? Available from: http://www.evidence.nhs.uk/search?q=phosphate+polyfusor (accessed 1 January 2014).

CHAPTER 8

Palliative care and pain management

Karen Neoh

St Gemma's Academic Unit of Palliative Care, UK

Pain management

Overview of pain management

Pain is defined as an unpleasant sensory and emotional experience associated with actual or potential tissue damage, or described in terms of such damage. The majority of patients with cancer experience pain; therefore clinicians must understand the impact pain can have on patients and manage symptoms quickly and effectively.

Assessment

- Thorough clinical assessment including: site, character, radiation, exacerbating or relieving factors, timing and severity (see Table 8.1 for further details).
- On average cancer patients experience two distinct pains, so documentation of individual pains must be made.
- Full medication history, including topical, inhaled, as required and over-the-counter or complementary therapies. Establish which medications patients feel have been effective for their symptoms and any side effects experienced, as this affects adherence.
- Establish which medications patients have also tried that were ineffective and why.

Clinical Problems in Oncology: A Practical Guide to Management, First Edition.
Edited by Sing Yu Moorcraft, Daniel L.Y. Lee and David Cunningham.
© 2014 John Wiley & Sons, Ltd. Published 2014 by John Wiley & Sons, Ltd.

Table 8.1 'SOCRATES': a common mnemonic acronym for assessing pain.

S	Site	Where is the pain, or the maximal site of the pain?
O	Onset	When did the pain start, was it sudden or gradual? Is the pain progressive or regressive?
C	Character	What is the pain like? An ache? Stabbing? Sharp?
R	Radiation	Does the pain radiate anywhere?
A	Associations	Any other signs or symptoms associated with the pain such as dyspnoea or nausea.
T	Time course	Does the pain follow any pattern?
E	Exacerbating/relieving factors	Does anything change the pain?
S	Severity	How bad is the pain? 1–10 with 10 representing the most severe pain.

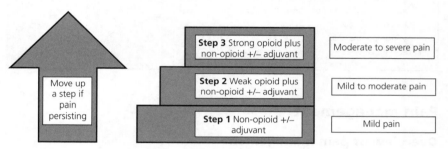

Figure 8.1 Based on the World Health Organisation (WHO). Adapted with permission, from the World Health Organisation, *WHO's Pain Ladder for Adults 2013*. Available from: http://www.who.int/cancer/palliative/painladder/en/ (accessed 1 January 2014).

Choice of analgesic

- The World Health Organisation (WHO) analgesic ladder (see Figure 8.1) provides the basis for initiating and titrating analgesia. It considers the severity of pain and previous analgesia. Start at the step appropriate for the patient's level of pain.
  - Simple analgesics include paracetamol and NSAIDs.
  - Weak opioids refer to codeine and tramadol. Strong opioids include morphine, oxycodone, fentanyl and buprenorphine. Strong opioids are indicated if pain is moderate to severe in intensity or if pain has not responded to weaker analgesia.
  - Adjuvant medications are drugs which were not originally marketed for pain but have been found to be effective in certain situations, for example antidepressants and anticonvulsants for neuropathic pain and bisphosphonates for bone pain.
- **Paracetamol** should be prescribed in all patients unless there is a contraindication. It has a synergistic effect with opioids. The dose may need to be reduced with liver impairment or in patients weighing less than 50 kg.

- **NSAIDs** are indicated for pain with an inflammatory component or bone pain, but have serious side effects, including gastric ulceration or bleeding and renal impairment:
  - Patients on steroids already have a higher risk of GI problems. Concomitant aspirin and SSRIs also greatly increase the risk of bleeding.
  - Palliative care patients may have pre-existing renal impairment which can be exacerbated, so renal function should be monitored and NSAIDs used with caution.
  - Consider starting a PPI concurrently.
  - Ibuprofen: 400 mg every 8 hours (max 2.4 g in 24 hours, but 1.2 g in 24 hours is usually sufficient for maintenance) is the safest NSAID in terms of GI and cardiovascular toxicity. Consider the risks and benefits on an individual basis.
  - Newer COX-2 selective NSAIDs can be given once daily, so reduce tablet burden, but have increased cardiovascular risks; therefore risk of stroke or MI should be balanced against potential benefit, even with short-term use.
  - The important message when prescribing an NSAID is to evaluate patients individually and consider their risk of GI, renal and cardiovascular complications.
- **Weak opioids**: codeine 30–60 mg QDS is an effective step 2 analgesic and should be co-prescribed with paracetamol. A combination preparation is available (co-codamol 30/500 mg) which reduces tablet burden. Codeine is metabolised to morphine via CYP2D6; however, it is not metabolised (and therefore ineffective) in up to 10% of people, and can be constipating and cause nausea which can limit the useful dose. See the opioid prescribing section for more details.
- **Strong opioids**: see the opioid prescribing section for more details.
- **Adjuvants**: these include antidepressants, anti-epileptics and bisphosphonates. Examples include gabapentin, amitriptyline and pregabalin for neuropathic pain:
  - These can cause drowsiness so need to be titrated and monitored closely. They should be started by a senior doctor or by those with specialist knowledge, such as the palliative care and pain team.
  - Gabapentin is started at a dose of 300 mg nocte and titrated upwards (increase by 300 mg a day) to a maximum of 600 mg TDS.
  - Pregabalin is started at 75 mg nocte and titrated upwards to a maximum of 300 mg BD.
  - Amitriptyline is started at 10 mg nocte and titrated gradually every 5–7 days up to 75 mg. Higher doses (up to 150 mg/day) may be used following specialist advice, but are associated with side effects that outweigh their analgesic benefit. Patients should be advised that sleepiness can persist to the next morning and may impair their ability to drive.

Renal and liver failure

- *Liver failure*: morphine is relatively safe in liver failure, but metabolites may accumulate, paracetamol should be reviewed and patients may need a dose reduction.

- *Renal failure*:
  - Morphine can accumulate quickly in those with renal failure as it is renally excreted.
  - Oxycodone has less toxic metabolites and patients with a mild level of impairment may be started on or switched to oxycodone.
  - Alfentanil does not rely on renal excretion and therefore is useful in patients in renal failure. As it has a very short half-life it should be given as a continuous infusion:
    - To convert oral morphine doses to alfentanil the 24-hour dose should be divided by 30.
    - The breakthrough analgesia in those with severe renal impairment who have an alfentanil infusion should be oxycodone (as alfentanil is very short acting).
    - Alfentanil does not accumulate and is not removed by dialysis.
  - Buprenorphine and fentanyl can also be used.
- In renal impairment and end-stage renal failure, regardless of the opioid used, extra caution is always required whether or not the patient is on dialysis. This is particularly necessary in patients with rapidly deteriorating renal function or when acutely unwell.
- NSAIDs are generally avoided in renal failure. However, if a patient's pain is due to bony metastases and other inflammatory processes, which may respond to NSAIDs, cautious use with monitoring of renal function can be trialled if alternative analgesia is ineffective.

Bone pain
Bone pain can be managed with radiotherapy, bisphosphonates and NSAIDs (see section on NSAIDs above). Following treatment with bisphosphonates or radiotherapy pain may improve dramatically, sometimes allowing a reduction in the doses of regular analgesia.

Radiotherapy
- In patients with good enough performance status, pain from bone metastases often responds well to radiotherapy.
- Factors that need to be considered include prognosis and previous radiotherapy. If a patient has had previous radiotherapy the maximum dose must be calculated and cannot be exceeded.
- Following radiotherapy there may be an exacerbation of pain before an improvement, for which steroids may be helpful.
- It takes 1–2 weeks before any improvement is seen. Patients therefore need to have a minimum prognosis of several weeks to benefit from radiotherapy.

Bisphosphonates
- Bisphosphonates may be effective in malignant bone pain and can be used in patients with a shorter prognosis. An effect is generally seen within two weeks.

- Bisphosphonates are given intravenously and can be given as an outpatient day case procedure; if patients are not well enough to attend outpatients they are unlikely to benefit from it.
  - Common (> 10%) side effects include transient pyrexia and flu-like symptoms, fatigue, headache, hypocalcaemia and bone pain. Less common side effects include sleep disturbances, arrhythmias, deterioration in renal function and osteonecrosis of the jaw. Bronchospasm and anaphylaxis occurs very rarely.
  - Milder side effects can be treated with paracetamol or NSAIDs.
  - Renal function must be checked prior to administration and patients may require a period of IV hydration prior to bisphosphonate infusion.
  - To reduce the risk of osteonecrosis of the jaw patients should have any pending dental work carried out prior to starting a bisphosphonate and if they have poor oral hygiene they should also have a dental review.
  - Example bisphosphonate prescriptions:
    - Pamidronate 90 mg IV in 500 ml 0.9% saline over 2–4 hours.
    - Zoledronic acid 4 mg IV in 100 ml 0.9% saline or 5% dextrose over 15 minutes (dose reductions required if creatinine clearance less than 60 ml/minute).
    - Infusion rate and amount of prehydration should take into account pre-existing renal disease to avoid fluid overload.

Opioid prescribing in palliative care

In 2012 the National Institute for Health and Care Excellence (NICE) published '*Safe and effective prescribing of strong opioids in palliative care of adults*' based on systematic reviews of the best available evidence. The recommendations are summarised below:

- **Patient advice**: side effects and common queries associated with opioid medications when commencing treatment need to be highlighted to avoid unnecessary anxiety or worries such as addiction and tolerance. Patients should be told that analgesia will be reviewed and that all medication changes will be discussed with their GP so they can seek their help if required. In addition to verbal advice, written guidance can help to reinforce information. NICE recommend that the following should be included:
  - When and why strong opioids are used to treat pain
  - How effective they are likely to be
  - Taking strong opioids for background and breakthrough pain, addressing:
    - How, when and how often to take strong opioids
    - How long pain relief should last
  - Side effects and signs of toxicity:
    - Safe storage
    - Follow-up and further prescribing
    - Information on who to contact out of hours, particularly during initiation of treatment
- Advise patients that it is important to take pain medication regularly to prevent the pain from coming on, rather than waiting until the pain is unbearable. If

patients are struggling with oral intake, a change to liquid form, injection, syringe driver or patches is possible.

General principles of opioid prescribing

- There is no maximum dose of opioid, but if patients are requiring very high doses re-assess the pain and consider reversible causes or whether the pain is non-responsive to opioids.
- Do not prescribe more than one opioid at a time.
- Ensure an immediate release opioid for episodes of breakthrough pain is prescribed and patients know that they can take these medications in addition to any regular modified release preparations to control pain (see the initiating strong opioids section for details on how to calculate breakthrough doses).

Management of side effects

- *Constipation*: inform patients that constipation affects nearly everyone receiving strong opioids and prescribe regular laxative treatment for all patients. Laxatives (e.g. Movicol® 1–2 sachets once or twice a day or docusate 100–200 mg BD) need to be taken regularly before considering switching to a different strong opioid.
- *Nausea*: advise patients that nausea may occur when starting strong opioid treatment or when the dose is increased, but that it is likely to be transient. Prescribe anti-emetics, for example cyclizine PO 50 mg TDS. If nausea persists, optimise anti-emetic treatment before considering switching to a different opioid (examples of oral anti-emetics include metoclopramide 10 mg up to TDS and levomepromazine 6 mg up to QDS). Metoclopramide should be avoided in those with Parkinsonism and levomepromazine can be sedating and so should be given at night.
- *Drowsiness*: advise patients that mild drowsiness or impaired concentration may occur when they start strong opioid treatment or when the dose changes, but that these are often transient. Warn patients that impaired concentration may affect their ability to do manual tasks such as driving.

Initiating opioid analgesia

Pain is managed in a stepwise manner using the WHO analgesic ladder. Patients may be started on a weak opioid such as codeine, which can be started PRN and then prescribed regularly.

- Codeine is commonly found in combination with paracetamol and the lowest dose is co-codamol 8/500 mg, (two tablets QDS maximum). As this contains paracetamol it must be explicitly stated to patients not to take additional paracetamol. This can then be increased to co-codamol 30/500 mg (two tablets QDS maximum).
- Codeine also comes without paracetamol and can be prescribed as codeine 30–60 mg QDS maximum.
- If this is ineffective then a strong opioid should be considered. The NICE recommendation is to commence morphine.

Initiating strong opioids

- Offer regular, oral sustained-release or oral immediate-release morphine (depending on patient preference), with rescue doses of oral immediate-release morphine for breakthrough pain.
- For example, typical daily starting doses for opioid naive patients:
  - 20–30 mg oral sustained-release morphine given as 10–15 mg twice daily with 5 mg oral immediate-release morphine for breakthrough pain.
  - 5–10 mg oral immediate release morphine at four-hourly intervals, with access to PRN doses for breakthrough pain.
  - Lower doses may be required for patients with renal impairment (see above), opioid-sensitive, frail or elderly patients.
- Oramorph® comes in two concentrations: 10 mg/5 ml or the stronger concentration of 100 mg/5 ml. The strength needs to be stipulated on a prescription.

Maintenance phase

- Continue oral sustained-release morphine and offer oral immediate-release morphine for the first-line breakthrough medication.
- The recommended dose of immediate release morphine for breakthrough pain is the equivalent of one-sixth of the total 24-hour morphine dose:
  - For example, if a patient is taking 30 mg twice a day of MST then the total dose is 60 mg, 60/6 = 10 mg. Breakthrough dose 10 mg of Oramorph® PRN.
  - Remember to change the breakthrough dose if the long-acting dose is modified.
  - A maximum dose for 'as required' medications must be indicated. This may be a total dose in 24 hours or how regularly the patient can have the breakthrough dose, such as two or four hourly.
- Incident pain is a type of breakthrough pain that is related to a specific event and can be classified into three subtypes:
  - *Volitional* – precipitated by a voluntary act (e.g. walking).
  - *Non-volitional* – precipitated by an involuntary activity (e.g. coughing).
  - *Procedural* – related to a therapeutic intervention (e.g. dressing changes).
- If oral morphine is being used pre-emptively to treat incident pain, this should be taken 30–60 minutes before the precipitating event.
- Immediate-release fentanyl preparations (e.g. lozenges, tablets or nasal sprays) have a rapid onset of action (about 10–15 minutes) and therefore may be useful for breakthrough pain, especially short-lived incident pain. However, these preparations should not be used if the patient is taking < 60 mg morphine/day and should usually only be prescribed by a palliative care specialist.
- If oral opioids are not suitable (patients with swallowing problems or if oral absorption is impaired) consider transdermal patches and subcutaneous opioids (see below for conversions).
- Seek specialist advice if pain is difficult to control or side effects persist. Consider reduced doses or alternative opioids if the patient has moderate to severe hepatic or renal impairment. Adjust the dose to balance pain control and side effects, with frequent review.

Writing opioid prescriptions

Examples of in-patient prescriptions are shown in Figure 8.2. These are examples only and drug charts will vary locally.

Below is an example of how to prescribe controlled drugs on a discharge letter. Please refer to your local prescribing guidelines as there will be local variances. Some trusts will prefer the brand name and/or the generic name of a medication to be used. There is a section in the *BNF* which stipulates the legal requirements for prescribing controlled drugs. If your trust uses electronic (typed) discharge letters the controlled drugs will still need to be handwritten.

The principles are:

- Drug name and strength/concentration
- Form (tablets/capsules/patch/injection/liquid)
- Dose
- Total quantity in words and figures
- For injectable medications the ampoule size must be stipulated

For example:

Morphine sulphate modified release capsules (Zomorph®) 10 mg twice a day. Please supply 28 (twenty eight) capsules.

Morphine sulphate injection 10 mg in 1 ml ampoule. 2.5 mg subcutaneously as required. Maximum 2 hourly. Please supply 5 (five) ampoules.

Oxycodone (OxyNorm) oral solution 5 mg in 5 ml. 5 mg as required. Maximum 4 hourly. Please supply 250 ml (two hundred and fifty millilitres).

Regular medication

Drug			Dose	Time
Morphine sulphate MR tablets (MST)			15 mg	08.00
Route	Special directions		Frequency	
PO	Do not crush or chew		BD	
Start date	Signature		Pharm	20.00
1/3/13	A Doctor			

As required medication

Drug		Dose
Morphine sulphate (Oramorph) liquid 10 mg in 5 ml		5 mg
Route	Special directions/indications	Frequency
PO	If 3 consecutive doses needed, contact Dr for advice	Maximum every 2 hours
Start date	Signature	Pharm
1/3/13	A Doctor	

Figure 8.2 Examples of in-patient opioid prescriptions.

Opioid conversions

There are differences in the literature regarding opioid conversion ratios. An approximate guide to conversions between opioids is shown in Table 8.2. Patients metabolise medications in different ways, so conversions may need to be modified, and therefore analgesia must be regularly reviewed. If a patient has escalating pain, review the underlying cause and increase the dose as necessary.

Example: converting codeine to morphine
- Morphine is *ten times* as potent as codeine.
- If a patient is taking 2 x co-codamol 30/500 four times a day:
  - $60 \times 4 = 240$ mg codeine.
  - $240/10 = 24$ mg morphine *per day*.
  - Morphine is given twice a day 12 hours apart: 10–15 mg of morphine twice a day.
  - Breakthrough doses are a sixth of the total dose so if patient is taking 15 mg twice a day this is a total of 30 mg. $30/6 = 5$ mg immediate release morphine (Oramorph®).

Opioid switching
- If a patient suffers severe constipation and nausea with morphine, despite regular laxatives and anti-emetics, then an opioid switch can be considered. Other side effects which may lead to a change include hallucinations, excessive drowsiness and myoclonic jerks.
- An alternative oral opioid is oxycodone. OxyNorm® is the immediate release version and OxyContin® is the modified release (long-acting, 12-hour) preparation of oxycodone. OxyNorm® is available in liquid form (5 mg/5 ml or 10 mg/1 ml concentrations) or 20 mg immediate release capsules.
- Other reasons for switching include if a patient is unable to take medications orally and the opioid of choice is not available in a suitable format (e.g. codeine to morphine if unable to take codeine orally). If a patient is stable on a dose then consideration of a fentanyl patch may be appropriate.

Table 8.2 A guide to conversions between opioids.

Analgesic	To convert to oral morphine DIVIDE by
Codeine	10
Dihydrocodeine	10
Tramadol	5
Analgesic	**To convert to oral morphine TIMES by**
Oxycodone (oral)	1.5–2
SC Alfentanil	30
SC morphine	2

SC = Subcutaneous

Opioid patches

- Transdermal delivery of medications can be effective and ease tablet burden for patients with stable pain.
- Patients may feel that a patch delivers a less potent medication than an oral medication, but fentanyl is 100–150 times more potent than oral morphine.
- If patients are self-administering patches they must understand the potency and remove old patches when applying a new patch.
- See Tables 8.3, 8.4 and 8.5 for examples of patches available and the suggested doses for breakthrough pain.
- Transdermal patches should not be used on lymphoedematous areas due to poor adhesion and absorption.
- Heat increases drug absorption by increasing the microcirculation and skin permeability. Therefore, the dose delivery may not be reliable in patients who are pyrexial and an alternative method of administration should be used. Patients should also be advised not to apply heat pads to the area of skin with the patch on.

Table 8.3 Available fentanyl patches and breakthrough doses. Change patches every 72 hours (three days).

Patch strength micrograms per hour (mcg/hr)	Equivalent 24 hour dose of oral morphine*	Oral immediate release morphine dose (mg)
12	30–60	5–10
25	60–135	10–20
50	135–225	20–35
75	225–320	40–50
100	315–400	50–65
125	400–500	65–80
150	500–600	80–100
175	585–675	100–110
200	675–765	110–130
225	765–855	130–140

*The equivalent dose is presented as a range to represent the variation in conversion ratios in the literature 1:100–150 and the variance in selectivity at opioid receptors. Check units carefully – fentanyl is prescribed in micrograms (mcg), whereas morphine is prescribed in milligrams (mg)

Table 8.4 Available buprenorphine patches (Transtec®) and breakthrough doses. Change patches every 96 hours (four days).

Patch strength micrograms per hour (mcg/hr)	Oral immediate release morphine dose (mg)
32	5–10
52.5	15
70	20

Table 8.5 Available buprenorphine patches (BuTrans®) and breakthrough doses. Change patches every seven days.

Patch strength micrograms per hour (mcg/hr)	Codeine equivalence – mg per day	Breakthrough codeine	Breakthrough oral immediate release morphine dose (mg)
5	30–60 mg/day	15 mg	NA
10	60–120 mg/day	15–30 mg	2–3 mg
15	120–180 mg/day	30 mg	3–5 mg

Opioid toxicity

- If opioids are titrated carefully then toxicity is unlikely. Signs of toxicity include drowsiness, small pupils, myoclonic jerks, confusion or hallucinations and a decreased respiratory rate. There may be other reasons for these symptoms so a careful history and medication review is essential. Patients nearing the end of life may be confused, drowsy or agitated for other reasons.
- If a patient's respiratory rate is significantly depressed (< 8 breaths per minute), then opioid antagonists may be considered. However, it is important to remember that this will reverse all the effects of the medication and so if a patient had severe pain they are likely to regain these symptoms.
- Naloxone, naltrexone and methylnaltrexone are opioid antagonists:
  - Naloxone is most commonly used to reverse opioid toxicity and reverses respiratory depression.
  - The onset of action is 1–2 minutes if given IV and 2–5 minutes if given subcutaneously. Its half-life is one hour and the duration of action is 15–90 minutes so it may be necessary to start a naltrexone infusion.
  - For opioid overdose give 400 micrograms – 2 mg IV every 2–3 minutes and repeat as required based on patient symptoms and response, up to a maximum of 10 mg.
  - To reverse respiratory depression dilute a standard ampoule containing 400 micrograms of naloxone with 10 ml of sodium chloride 0.9%. Administer 0.5– 1 ml (20–40 micrograms) IV every 1–2 minutes until the patient's respiratory status is satisfactory.
  - Possible side effects from naloxone include nausea and vomiting and occasionally hypertension, pulmonary oedema, arrhythmias and cardiac arrest. Therefore it should only be given if a definite diagnosis of respiratory depression due to opioids is made.
- If toxicity is less overt and the patient's respiratory rate is preserved then monitor the patient. If they have taken a short-acting opioid then the effects may be short-lived. The metabolism of the medication will also depend on the patient's renal function if using morphine or oxycodone, so reviewing this is useful.

- A full medication review is then required. An opioid switch may reduce the unwanted side effects while preserving the analgesic effects.

Syringe pumps

- A syringe pump is also referred to as a continuous subcutaneous infusion (CSCI) or syringe driver. It is an effective method of delivering medications in palliative care. Indications for using a syringe pump include:
  - Patient too unwell to take medications via the oral route due to reduced conscious level
  - Severe nausea or vomiting
  - Problems with absorption, such as bowel obstruction
- Patients may worry that it is a sign that they are more unwell, but they can be used as an effective way of delivering medications which can lead to a vast improvement in symptoms, enabling medications to be delivered by the oral route again.
- They are small devices consisting of a pump with integrated syringe filled with medication that can be stored in a bag to make it portable and easy for patients to mobilise with. There is a small butterfly needle which is sited under the skin. The site should be regularly checked and changed as local reactions can occur.
- Common medications which are administered this way include analgesics such as morphine, anti-emetics such as metoclopramide, hyoscine to dry secretions and midazolam for agitation.
- Subcutaneous medication delivered this way takes 3–4 hours to achieve a steady state so patients may need immediate doses of medications when the pump is first initiated.
- Problems that may occur include compatibility of the drugs in the syringe, problems with the pump and local reactions at the site of the needle.
- Problems at the site may be due to glass particles from the ampoule, infection, sterile abscess, allergic response to nickel needle, chemical reaction in the subcutaneous tissue, tonicity of the solution and pH. Ways to improve this include dilution of the solution to as large a volume as practical, rotation of the site every 72 hours, use of a non-metal cannula, consider changing the drug combination, adding a small dose of dexamethasone (1 mg/24hrs) or applying hydrocortisone cream 1% to the affected area.

Starting a syringe pump

- To start a syringe pump review the 'as required' and regular medications used over the last 24 hours and convert this to the same drug and dosage form. The total is used to calculate the dose for the syringe pump. If a patient is still experiencing ongoing symptoms then the cumulative dose may need to be increased. For example if a patient is taking 20 mg BD of MST and has had 10 mg of Oramorph® orally in the last 24 hours this is: $20 + 20 + 10 = 50$ mg total oral morphine. To convert to subcutaneous morphine divide by 2: $50/2 = 25$ mg of morphine sulphate for injection over 24 hours.

- Drugs are usually diluted with water for injection and prescribed over 24 hours. Generally there are few compatibility problems with common two and three drug combinations containing:
  - Diamorphine
  - Cyclizine
  - Haloperidol
  - Metoclopramide
  - Levomepromazine
  - Hyoscine hydrobromide or butylbromide
  - Midazolam
- However, there can be problems with medications in which the pH varies and can cause the other medications to precipitate:
  - These include cyclizine (with diamorphine if diamorphine exceeds 200 mg/24 hours), ketorolac (a subcutaneous NSAID) and dexamethasone.
  - If there are no alternatives to the medication then two syringe pumps can be prescribed and administered at separate sites on the body.
  - Always consider if one drug can control more than one symptom, for example levomepromazine for agitation and nausea, or can be given as a separate subcutaneous stat dose, for example dexamethasone.

An example of a syringe driver prescription is shown below. Each trust will have its own prescription chart specifically for syringe drivers. It is good practice to write drug doses in figures and words to avoid drug errors.

Morphine sulphate 30 mg (thirty)
Midazolam 10 mg (ten)
Hyoscine hydrobromide 1.2 mg (one point two milligrams)

Diluent: water for injection
Give over 24 hours

End-of-life care

As people near the end of life there are common changes, such as sleeping for longer periods, reduced appetite and possible agitation or confusion. It is important to explain these changes to patients and relatives.

Advance care planning and NHS Continuing Healthcare funding

- Advance care planning focuses on establishing the patient's wishes regarding end-of-life care. Patients and their families should be supported in making decisions such as their preferred place/priorities of care. Discussions about 'do not attempt resuscitation' (DNAR) should also occur if appropriate.
- Many patients may wish to die at home or in a hospice, rather than in hospital. Timely discussions about patients' care preferences can enable the necessary support to be put in place, for example additional carers/equipment and anticipatory prescribing of medication.

- Good communication between the community and hospital teams, including making appropriate plans for emergency situations, is critical to preventing unnecessary hospital admissions.
- NHS Continuing Healthcare:
  - This is a package of care that is arranged and funded by the NHS (i.e. it is free of charge to the patient). Patients with cancer may be eligible for Continuing Healthcare, depending on their assessed health needs.
  - Patients who are rapidly deteriorating and may be entering the terminal phase are usually eligible for NHS Fast Track Continuing Healthcare funding. This facilitates the immediate provision of a package of support, for example to enable patients to die at home.

The Gold Standards Framework

The Gold Standards Framework represents a standard of excellence for end-of-life care across primary care, care homes and other areas. It is concerned with helping people to live well until the end of life and includes care in the final years of life for people with any end-stage illness in any setting. It includes:

- Communication
- Co-ordination
- Control of symptoms
- Continuity, including out of hours
- Continued learning
- Carer support
- Care in the dying phase

End-of-life care plans

- The Liverpool Care Pathway (LCP) is a guidance tool that aimed to standardise and deliver care at the end of life and was widely used in hospitals, the community and palliative care settings. This was phased out in July 2014 and replaced by individual personal care plans which vary locally but should incorporate principles included in the LCP.
- End-of-life care plans should provide guidance on support for relatives and care after death, as well as clinical advice. Patients should have undergone a multidisciplinary assessment and an assessment of whether they are dying. All reversible causes must have been considered and the patient should be regularly reviewed to see if other management should be considered.
- The initial assessment includes screening for common symptoms such as pain, agitation, nausea and dyspnoea.
- Patients' symptoms should be reviewed regularly by nursing staff and if they are not well controlled this should be recorded and the action taken should be documented.
- Consideration should be given to discontinuing patient observations and investigations (including blood tests) and emphasising symptom control.
- Non-essential medications should be stopped.
- Typical medications used for the management of symptoms at the end of life are shown in Table 8.6.

Table 8.6 Medications commonly used at the end of life.

Symptom	Drug	Dose	Alternatives
Terminal restlessness and agitation	Midazolam	2.5–5 mg SC PRN	
Pain (if opiate naive)	Diamorphine	2.5–5 mg SC PRN	Morphine sulphate for injection
Pain (if on opioid already)	Dose conversion to a syringe driver or a sixth of the total dose PRN		
Respiratory tract secretions	Hyoscine hydrobromide	400 micrograms PRN (max 1.2–2.4 mg in 24 hours)	Glycopyrronium 0.4 mg SC PRN (max 1.2 mg in 24 hours)
			Hyoscine butylbromide 20 mg PRN (max 120 mg in 24 hours for secretions – can give up to 300 mg for bowel colic)
Nausea and vomiting	Haloperidol	2.5–5 mg SC PRN	Cyclizine 50 mg SC PRN (max 150 mg in 24 hours)
			Levomepromazine SC 6.25 mg PRN
Dyspnoea	Diamorphine	2.5–5 mg SC PRN	If anxious midazolam 2.5–5 mg SC PRN

- Advice should be given to relatives regarding the dying process, including the natural loss of appetite. There can be many anxieties associated with patients not eating and drinking. As appetite decreases, patients feel less hungry and there is no evidence to support artificial hydration either helping symptoms or affecting prognosis.
- Secretions can sound distressing and anticipatory anti-secretory medicine (e.g. hyoscine hydrobromide or glycopyrronium depending on local formulary choice) should be prescribed. This is due to normal secretions not being swallowed and so pooling in the throat, leading to a louder breathing sound.
- Clear communication with patients and relatives is essential. It is important to explain that the patient has been assessed as dying, and that the aims are to deliver a good standard of care and to avoid discomfort or unnecessary tests at the end of life.

References

Dickman A, Schneider J, Varga J. *The Syringe Driver: Continuous Subcutaneous Infusions in Palliative Care*, second edition. Oxford University Press: Oxford. 2005.

The Gold Standards Framework. Available from: http://www.goldstandardsframework.org.uk (accessed 1 January 2014).

International Association for the Study of Pain. Available from: http://www.iasp-pain.org//
AM/Template.cfm?Section=Home (accessed 1 January 2014).

Joint Formulary Committee. *British National Formulary*. BMJ Group and Pharmaceutical Press:
London. Available from: http://www.medicinescomplete.com (accessed 1 January 2014).

National Institute for Health and Care Excellence. Opioids in palliative care: safe and effective
prescribing of strong opioids for pain in palliative care of adults (CG140). Available from:
http://publications.nice.org.uk/opioids-in-palliative-care-safe-and-effective-prescribing-of-
strong-opioids-for-pain-in-palliative-cg140 (accessed 1 January 2014).

Twycross R, Wilcock A. *Palliative Care Formulary*, fourth edition. Palliativedrugs.com Ltd:
Nottingham. 2011.

World Health Organisation. *WHO's Pain Ladder for Adults 2013*. Available from: http://www.
who.int/cancer/palliative/painladder/en/ (accessed 1 January 2014).

CHAPTER 9

Oncology procedures and their complications

Juanita Lopez

The Royal Marsden NHS Foundation Trust, UK

CHAPTER MENU

Ascitic drains (paracentesis)

Overview of paracentesis

- *Indications*: significant symptoms due to malignant ascites not responding to medical treatment.
- *Assess*: abdominal swelling, discomfort, decreased appetite, sense of fullness, shortness of breath, weight gain, ankle swelling; focus especially on duration and rapidity of symptom onset.
- *Investigations*: FBC, U&Es, albumin, BP, clotting.
- *Contraindications*: disseminated intravascular coagulation (DIC), massive ileus with bowel obstruction.
- Unfortunately there are no established evidence-based guidelines for the management of malignant ascites due to a lack of randomised controlled trials identifying optimal therapy, but the following guidelines are based on our local experience and review articles.

Clinical Problems in Oncology: A Practical Guide to Management, First Edition.
Edited by Sing Yu Moorcraft, Daniel L.Y. Lee and David Cunningham.
© 2014 John Wiley & Sons, Ltd. Published 2014 by John Wiley & Sons, Ltd.

Paracentesis procedure

- Ensure coagulation profile is satisfactory.
- Ultrasound marking of drain site is recommended.
- The procedure should be undertaken by experienced doctor/sonographer using strict aseptic technique.
- There is no consensus on the rate of drainage. Some local guidelines recommend that this should not exceed 1 L/hour and that the drain should be clamped following drainage of every 2 litres, with an hour's rest prior to recommencing drainage.
- IV fluids are not routinely required, but patient's symptoms, BP and urine output should be regularly assessed.
- IV albumin has no proven role as a means of maintaining intravascular volume during paracentesis of malignant ascites, but can be considered for patients with portal hypertension, or massive hepatic metastases that may be more at risk of hypovolaemia (100 ml human albumin solution (HAS) 20% stat every four hours or after every 2 L of ascites drained).

Complications and side effects

- Common side-effects (>5%) include:
  - Mild discomfort associated with the drain, for which simple analgesia can be prescribed.
  - Nausea.
  - Fatigue lasting 1–3 days.
  - Leakage of fluid from the drain site.
- Other potential complications:
  - Hypotension and renal impairment. The risk can be minimised by careful management of the rate of drainage, and judicious fluid management.
  - Bleeding.
  - Infection:
    - With strict aseptic technique, the risk of infection is rare (< 1%) unless the bowel is perforated, but should be considered if patient develops abdominal pain, fever, or signs of sepsis following a procedure.
    - Management: send ascitic fluid for microbiology and white cell count, and start broad spectrum antibiotics to cover both Gram positive and Gram negative bacteria.
  - Perforation of abdominal organs. The risk is minimised by the use of ultrasound marking of the ideal site for drainage.

Permanent indwelling catheter (PleurX® drain)

- *Indications*: patients who are experiencing distressing symptoms from the rapid re-accumulation of ascitic fluid despite fortnightly paracentesis. NICE recommends this for patients for whom there is a low likelihood of further successful systemic treatment, who have had at least three large-volume paracenteses.

- *Procedure*:
  - Inserted in interventional radiology suite under local anaesthetic.
  - Connection of a vacuum bottle to the drain allows the drainage of 1 L in 15 minutes.
  - Short in-patient stay for patient or carer to learn to manage drains aseptically. Thereafter patients can drain up to 2 L/day at home (often requires district nurse involvement).
- *Complications include*: infection, leakage, loculations, occlusion or drain displacement (all of these are rare, occurring in <2% of patients).

Other relevant sections of this book
Chapter 3, section on ascites

References

Chung M, Kozuch P. Treatment of malignant ascites. *Current Treatment Options in Oncology*. 2008. 9(2–3): 215–33.

Fleming ND, Alvarez-Secord A, Von Gruenigen V, Miller MJ, Abernethy AP. Indwelling catheters for the management of refractory malignant ascites: a systematic literature overview and retrospective chart review. *Journal pf Pain and Symptom Management*. 2009. 38(3): 341–9.

Keen A, Fitzgerald D, Bryant A, Dickinson HO. Management of drainage for malignant ascites in gynaecological cancer. *Cochrane Database of Systematic Reviews*. 2010. (1): CD007794.

National Institute for Health and Care Excellence. PleurX peritoneal catheter drainage system for vacuum assisted drainage of treatment-resistant recurrent malignant ascites (MTG9)2012. Available from: http://guidance.nice.org.uk/MTG9 (accessed 1 January 2014).

Biliary drains and stents

Overview of biliary stenting
- *Indications*: malignant biliary tract obstruction. Decompression of an obstructed biliary system can significantly improve a patient's quality of life, and therefore palliative intervention (either endoscopic or percutaneous) should always be considered.
- *Assess*: clinical signs of liver dysfunction, pain, fever or clinical signs of sepsis.
- *Investigations*: LFTs, WCC and CRP, U&Es and clotting.

Types of biliary stenting
1 **Endoscopic:**
  (a) *Indications*: mainstay treatment, less invasive than the percutaneous approach.
  (b) *Procedure*:
    (i) ERCP performed by a gastroenterologist in endoscopy suite under sedation.
    (ii) Self-expanding metal stents are usually inserted when unresectable malignant disease is present as these have lower rates of stent re-occlusion.

(iii) A stat dose of prophylactic antibiotics is given pre-procedure to patients with an obstructed biliary system due to malignancy.

(iv) The choice of antibiotic should be discussed with the local microbiologists and gastroenterologists, but should cover biliary flora, including enteric Gram negative organisms and enterococci (e.g. Tazocin® 1.5 g stat).

(v) Where biliary drainage is complete, continuation of antibiotics is not recommended.

(c) *Response:* normalisation of bilirubin can take up to one week.

2 Percutaneous

(a) *Indications:* patients not suitable for endoscopic intervention.

(b) *Procedure:*

(i) Percutaneous transhepatic cholangiography (PTC) and stent insertion performed by an interventional radiologist in intervention suite. May require the additional presence of an anaesthetist to monitor sedation or light anaesthesia.

(ii) Bile duct drainage may be external, or may be directed internally (in which case an external drain is usually left for at least 48 hours, then clamped to ensure patency).

Complications

- **Early complications of ERCP and biliary stenting:**
  - *Sepsis:* including cholangitis, cholecystitis, and pancreatitis:
    - Typically occurs 24–72 hours post procedure. More likely where there is incomplete drainage of the obstructed biliary system (90%).
    - Assess for fever, RUQ pain, worsening LFTs, clinical signs of shock. Blood cultures should be taken immediately and broad-spectrum antibiotics commenced as per current microbiology advice.
  - *Bleeding:* most commonly post-sphincterotomy (up to 5%) but usually mild and resolves spontaneously if clotting and coagulation profile corrected.
  - *Perforation:* very rare, but consider urgent imaging with erect CXR/AXR and CT if patient presents with severe acute abdominal pain and guarding.
- **Early complications of percutaneous biliary stenting:**
  - *Sepsis:* similar to post-ERCP
  - *Haemobilia:*
    - Rare, but classically presents with acute biliary colic, jaundice and upper GI bleeding due to communication of the PTC tract with a major vascular structure.
    - Image urgently with CT angiography and discuss definitive management with interventional radiologist.
- **Late complications of endoscopic or percutaneous biliary stenting:**
  - *Stent obstruction:*
    - Most commonly due to tumour regrowth, tissue hyperplasia, or biliary sludge.
    - Patients typically present with cholangitis and elevated liver enzymes.

○ *Stent migration*:
  ▪ More common in patients who had received a biliary sphincterectomy.
  ▪ ERCP will successfully remove >90% migrated stents and re-stent persistent lesions.
○ Metal stents have lower rates of recurrent obstruction; however, when infected or occluded they are less easily removed.

Other relevant sections of this book
Chapter 3, section on abnormal liver function tests

References

Chu D, Adler DG. Malignant biliary tract obstruction: evaluation and therapy. *Journal of the National Comprehensive Cancer Network.* 2010. 8(9): 1033–44.
van Delden OM, Lameris JS. Percutaneous drainage and stenting for palliation of malignant bile duct obstruction. *European Radiology.* 2008. 18(3): 448–56.

Central venous access devices

Overview of central lines
- *Indications*: inadequate peripheral access, chemotherapy regimes that include a sclerosing agent or long infusions, administration of total parenteral nutrition.
- *Assess*: peripheral veins by clinical exam; ensure no contraindications to line placement, for example previous axillary surgery, presence of a pacemaker.
- *Investigations:* FBC and clotting.
- The characteristics of the main different types of central venous access devices are summarised in Table 9.1 and an implantable port is shown in Figure 9.1.

Checking the position of a central venous line
- Ideally, the tip of a central venous line should lie in the long axis of the superior vena cava, always above the pericardial reflection.
- Catheter placement within the right atrium may cause arrhythmias.
- Tips that are too proximal can cause mechanical or chemical irritation of the vessel wall, leading to pain on injection of drugs, thrombosis and subsequent infection.
- The major radiological landmarks are shown in Figure 9.2. Once the carina is identified, catheter tips that lie vertically in the marked zone (2 cm above and 2 cm below the carina) are likely to be in a safe position.

Table 9.1 Types of central venous access devices.

	Percutaneous (e.g. PICC, see Figure 9.2)	**Tunnelled** (e.g. Hickman or Groshong)	**Implanted** (e.g. port, see Figure 9.1)
Insertion	Bedside placement	Inserted by radiologist or anaesthetists usually under sedation	Inserted by surgeons under general anaesthetic
Risk of infection	High	Medium	Low
Activity restrictions for patients	Yes	Yes	No
	Able to shower, but not immerse arm	Able to shower and bath, but not submerge chest	Able to bath and shower without restrictions
	Not able to swim	Not able to swim	Able to swim
Need for flushing and dressing change	Once a week	Once a week	Once a month
Need for needles	No	No	Yes – into port
Removal	Easy, will not leave scar	Local anaesthetic procedure, may leave a scar	Requires surgical removal, and will leave a scar

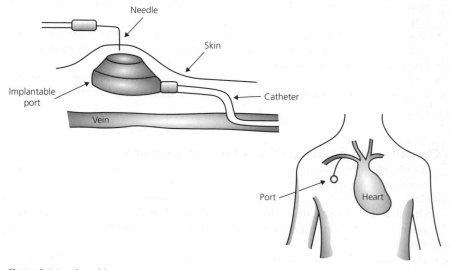

Figure 9.1 Implantable port.

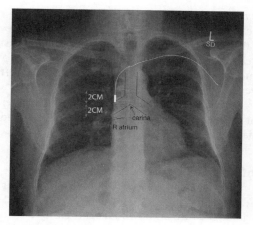

Figure 9.2 Ensuring the ideal position for the catheter tip for central venous access devices. The CXR shows a left-sided PICC line with its tip (white square) lying in the long axis of the superior vena cava (SVC) just above the carina. The boundaries of the safe zone are shown by the red dotted lines, lying 2 cm above and 2 cm below the carina respectively. To see a colour version of this figure, see Plate 9.2.

Complications of a central venous line and their management

1 Infective complications:
  (a) Extremely common, reported rates up to 30–60%.
  (b) *Colonised catheter*: growth of a microorganism from the catheter tip, but without any erythema or discharge. Treat with wound care and oral antibiotics.
  (c) *Exit-site infection*: erythema within 2 cm of exit site without purulent drainage or clinical signs of sepsis. Treat with wound care and oral antibiotics without removal of catheter, but monitor carefully.
  (d) *Tunnel infection*: tenderness, erythema and induration >2 cm from exit site and along subcutaneous tunnel without signs of sepsis. Treat with systemic antibiotics, and consider line removal.
  (e) *Pocket infection*: erythema and necrosis of skin over the reservoir of an implanted device, or purulent exudate in the subcutaneous pocket without signs of sepsis. Treat with systemic antibiotics, but likely to need line removal and drainage of infected site.
  (f) *Systemic line sepsis*: clinical signs of sepsis with positive blood cultures from the line. Treat with systemic antibiotics; consider line removal depending on response to treatment and guidance from local microbiologists.
2 Catheter-related thrombosis:
  (a) *Symptoms and signs*: pain, tenderness to palpation, swelling, warmth in upper limb where catheter is located; development of unilateral collateral vessels in respective limb, neck or side of the body.
  (b) *Investigations*: urgent USS, CT venogram or MRA.

(c) *Management*:
   (i) If the catheter is no longer required: LMWH for seven days prior to removal and then full anticoagulation for six months.
   (ii) If the catheter is required: full dose therapeutic LMWH for at least 6–12 months, followed by prophylactic dose LMWH until catheter is removed.

(d) *Long-term complications of catheter-related thrombosis include*: increased risk of subsequent catheter infections, PE, post-thrombotic syndrome and persistent vascular compromise.

Obstruction of venous devices

* Extremely common and can be related to thrombotic or non-thrombotic causes.
* Figure 9.3 provides guidance on how to diagnose the cause of obstruction and determine if the obstruction interferes with withdrawal and/or with infusion of fluids.
* *Thrombotic causes include*: fibrin sheaths or intra-luminal clot. Management: thrombolytics (e.g. Alteplase 2 ml at a concentration of 1 mg/1 ml placed within the catheter lumen and left for 120 minutes). Fibrin sheaths can sometimes be dislodged and removed by interventional radiologists.
* *Non-thrombotic causes include*: malpositioning, catheter kinking, luminal occlusion due to drug precipitation and fracture of the catheter. These may require the repositioning or removal of the catheter.

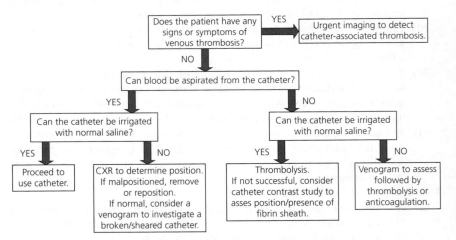

Figure 9.3 Flowchart for the investigation of occluded venous devices.

References

Baskin JL, Pui CH, Reiss U, Wilimas JA, Metzger ML, Ribeiro RC, *et al.* Management of occlusion and thrombosis associated with long-term indwelling central venous catheters. *Lancet.* 2009. 374(9684): 159–69.

Marcy PY. Central venous access: techniques and indications in oncology. *European Radiology.* 2008. 18(10): 2333–44.

Ponec D, Irwin D, Haire WD, Hill PA, Li X, McCluskey ER, *et al.* Recombinant tissue plasminogen activator (alteplase) for restoration of flow in occluded central venous access devices: a double-blind placebo-controlled trial – the Cardiovascular Thrombolytic to Open Occluded Lines (COOL) efficacy trial. *Journal of Vascular and Interventional Radiology.* 2001. 12(8): 951–5.

Schuster M, Nave H, Piepenbrock S, Pabst R, Panning B. The carina as a landmark in central venous catheter placement. *British Journal of Anaesthesia.* 2000. 85(2): 192–4.

Chemoembolisation

Background
- Chemoembolisation is based on the differential blood supply of both primary and secondary liver tumours from normal liver parenchyma.
- Tumours derive all their blood supply from the hepatic artery, while normal liver receives at least 50% of its blood supply from the portal vein.
- Selective cannulation of the hepatic artery enables the targeted delivery of chemotherapy and embolic material to liver tumours.

Overview of chemoembolisation
- *Indications (following discussion at a specialist liver MDT):*
  - Primary treatment for unresectable HCC.
  - Treatment for symptomatic liver metastases from neuroendrocrine carcinomas.
  - Being developed for the treatment of liver metastases from other primary cancers.
- *Contraindications:* thrombus in the main portal vein and portal vein obstruction, encephalopathy, biliary obstruction, Child-Pugh C cirrhosis.
- *Assess:* fitness to undergo procedure, Child-Pugh score.
- *Investigations:* FBC, LFTs, U&Es, albumin, clotting.

Procedure
- Performed in the angiography suite, with the patient under conscious sedation.
- Prophylactic antibiotics (e.g. Tazocin® 1.5 g stat), anti-emetics and analgesia are administered pre-procedure.
- Access is usually gained via the femoral artery, with the catheter threaded into the appropriate hepatic artery feeding the tumour, following which chemotherapy and embolic particles are injected.

Complications

- Post-embolic syndrome:
  - Occurs in 80–90% of patients.
  - *Symptoms*: RUQ pain, nausea, a moderate degree of ileus, fatigue, fever and transient elevation of LFTs (particularly transaminases). Symptoms are usually self-limiting, but can last up to ten days.
- Hepatic decompensation and liver failure: rarely occurs and is related to the pre-procedure hepatic function.
- Sepsis, for example acute cholecystitis, hepatic abscess:
  - Occurs in 2% of patients.
  - *Symptoms*: RUQ pain, worsening LFTs, clinical signs of shock.
  - *Management*: obtain multiple blood cultures when febrile and commence broad spectrum antibiotics (e.g. Tazocin® 1.5 g QDS).
- Injury to biliary tract, including the formation of subcapsular bilomas, focal stricturing of the hepatic or common bile duct occurs in < 2% of patients.
- Gastro-duodenal ulceration: occurs in < 5% of patients and is less common now that coil embolisation of the gastroduodenal vessels is performed to protect the stomach and duodenum from potential reflux of the chemoembolic agent.
- Although most of the chemotherapy is retained in the liver, there is a small amount of systemic exposure, so patients are at risk of nausea, vomiting and bone marrow suppression.

References

Memon K, Lewandowski RJ, Riaz A, Salem R. Chemoembolization and radioembolization for metastatic disease to the liver: available data and future studies. *Current Treatment Options in Oncology*. 2012. 13(3): 403–15.

Chest drains and pleurodesis

Overview of chest drainage

- *Indications*: significant symptoms due to malignant pleural effusion. Some malignant effusions due to lymphoma, ovarian or breast cancer may respond quickly to systemic treatment and will not need intervention unless patient develops significant symptoms.
- *Contraindications*: uncorrected bleeding diathesis, very small (< 1 cm) effusion.
- *Assess*: shortness of breath, pleuritic chest pain, cough, fever.
- *Investigations*: FBC, U&Es, albumin, BP, clotting, CXR.
- *Success rate*: unfortunately the recurrence rate for malignant effusions following drainage is > 95% at 30 days and definitive management should be discussed with the chest multidisciplinary team.

Chest drain procedure

- Ensure coagulation profile is satisfactory.
- The procedure should be undertaken by experienced practitioner using a strict aseptic technique.

- Ideally, the drain should be inserted under direct thoracic ultrasound guidance during working hours. The marking of a site for drainage for subsequent remote aspiration or chest drain insertion is not recommended.
- The Seldinger technique is most commonly used. Free aspiration of fluid must be ensured prior to drain placement:
  - The chest drain is then attached to an underwater seal bottle, and secured in place.
  - Portable chest drain systems utilising a drainage bag with a one-way valve are becoming more common. However, they have limited capacity (< 500 ml) and are only suitable for patients with small effusions who want to be more mobile.
- A CXR should be performed post procedure to document drain position and to exclude a pneumothorax.
- Ensure patients are prescribed regular analgesia, and encouraged to mobilise.

Monitoring
- Patients should be monitored closely following chest drain insertion.
- Assess symptoms, oxygen saturations, BP and chest drainage system:
  - Fluid within the tube should swing with normal respiration. Absence of swinging indicates the drain is occluded or is no longer in the pleural space.
  - Drains inserted for fluid drainage should never bubble. Bubbling in the underwater seal fluid chamber indicates an ongoing air-leak.
- *Rate of drainage*:
  - Drainage of a large pleural effusion should be controlled to prevent re-expansion pulmonary oedema.
  - A maximum of 1.5 L should be drained in the first hour following insertion of chest drain. The drain can then be clamped to control drainage rate.
  - Drains that are bubbling should *never* be clamped as the continuing air leak may lead to a tension pneumothorax.
- When a drain bottle is full, it should be temporarily clamped and changed using aseptic technique.

Chest drain removal
- Chest drains can be removed once there is:
  - No (or minimal, stable) pneumothorax
  - No air leak
  - Less than 200 ml fluid drained in last 24 hours
- A post-removal CXR should be performed to exclude residual pneumothorax. If the lung has not re-expanded ('trapped lung'), definitive management with the respiratory/thoracic team should be discussed.

Complications
- Common:
  - Pain associated with the chest drain.
  - Chest tube malposition. Image urgently and consult with respiratory physicians and thoracic surgeons prior to removal.

- Uncommon/rare:
  - Bleeding.
  - Infection:
    - Occurs in 1–3% of patients.
    - The longer the chest drain is left *in situ*, the greater the risk of developing empyema.
    - Prophylactic antibiotics are not indicated, but the patient's symptoms and respiratory observations must be closely monitored.
    - The drain exit site must be dressed regularly and swabbed at the earliest sign of infection.
  - Organ injury.
  - Re-expansion pulmonary oedema:
    - Can be potentially life-threatening.
    - Occurs after rapid drainage of large volumes of effusion.
    - *Symptoms*: cough, dyspnoea and hypoxia.
    - *Management*: supportive, with supplemental oxygen and ventilation if required.

Pleurodesis

This is the mainstay for the long-term management of malignant pleural effusion, but increasingly being replaced by indwelling PleurX® catheters.
- Most commonly, talc is instilled via a chest tube by respiratory physicians, or at thoracoscopy by thoracic surgeons.
- Contraindicated in patients with 'trapped' lungs.
- Significant complications, including fever and pain (very common) but also life-threatening ARDS (1%).

Permanent indwelling catheter (PleurX® drain)

- Increasingly common as less invasive than pleurodesis, with similar efficacy.
- PleurX® pleural catheters have a one-way valve that allows fluid drainage but does not allow air to enter the pleural space.
- Patients are able to shower when appropriate waterproof dressings are used.
- *Procedure*:
  - Inserted in interventional radiology suite under local anaesthetic.
  - Connection of a vacuum bottle allows the drainage of 500 ml of fluid.
  - Short in-patient stay for patient or carer to learn to manage drains aseptically, may require district nurse involvement.
  - Usual drainage rate is 500 ml every other day.
- *Complications include*: infection, leakage, blockage, loculations, occlusion or displacement (all of these are rare, occurring in <5% of patients).

Other relevant sections of this book

Chapter 3, section on breathlessness

References

Havelock T, Teoh R, Laws D, Gleeson F, B. T. S. Pleural Disease Guideline Group. Pleural procedures and thoracic ultrasound: British Thoracic Society pleural disease guideline 2010. *Thorax.* 2010. 65 (Suppl. 2): ii61–76.

Kaifi JT, Toth JW, Gusani NJ, Kimchi ET, Staveley-O'Carroll KF, Belani CP, *et al.* Multidisciplinary management of malignant pleural effusion. *Journal of Surgical Oncology.* 2012. 105(7): 731–8.

Roberts ME, Neville E, Berrisford RG, Antunes G, Ali NJ, B. T. S. Pleural Disease Guideline Group. Management of a malignant pleural effusion: British Thoracic Society pleural disease guideline 2010. *Thorax.* 2010. 65 (Suppl. 2): ii32–40.

Enteral feeding tubes

Overview of enteral feeding tubes
- *Indications*: providing enteral access for cancer patients who are unable to maintain oral intake.
- Percutaneous endoscopic gastrostomy (PEG) tubes are inserted by gastro-enterologists at endoscopy.
- Radiologically inserted gastrostomy (RIG) tubes are inserted by interventional radiologists.
- Both procedures are carried out under sedation.
- Patients who are known MRSA carriers should have completed nasal decontamination prior to the procedure.
- *Contraindications*: non-functioning GI tract, gross ascites.

Complications due to procedure
- Benign pneumoperitoneum (very common, occurring in >50% of patients) usually self-limiting and treated conservatively.
- Peri-stomal pain is very common post procedure.
- Abscess and wound infection:
  - Rarely occurs if peri-procedural antibiotics are given.
  - *Symptoms*: persistent or worsening peri-stomal pain.
  - *Management*: image urgently, antibiotics.
- Bowel injury or gastrocolocutaneous fistula (very rare). Assess urgently if patient develops signs of peritonitis and obtain an early surgical opinion.
- Intraperitoneal or retroperitoneal bleeding is very rare:
  - *Symptoms*: worsening abdominal pain, a clinically rigid abdomen, hypotension and a drop in Hb.
  - *Management*: image urgently and obtain a surgical opinion.

Late complications
- Tube blockage (common):
  - Due to thick enteral feeds and medication delivered through a narrow tube.

- Prevent blockages by flushing tube with 30–60 ml water using a large syringe after each use.
  - Liquid formulations of medications are preferred and solid formulations should be completely dissolved in water prior to administration.
  - Flushing with carbonated drinks or pineapple juice can sometimes restore patency of partially obstructed tubes.
- Tube dislodgement (rare):
  - When this occurs prior to a mature tract forming (usually one month, but sometimes longer in malnourished patients) assess urgently for signs of peritonitis and sepsis.
  - Dislodgement after the formation of a mature tract is less worrying. A Foley catheter (of the same size as the tube) should be inserted as soon as possible (otherwise the stoma will close) and a replacement procedure planned.

Other relevant sections of this book
Chapter 3, section on anorexia and nutrition

Nephrostomies and ureteric stents

Background
- There are no established evidence-based guidelines for the management of malignant ureteric obstruction.
- As patients can often be asymptomatic, the decision for intervention to decompress the upper tracts should always be taken in a multidisciplinary environment.

Overview of ureteric decompression
- *Indications*: avoiding the complications of renal insufficiency; allowing systemic treatment, particularly if nephrotoxic chemotherapy is being considered.
- *Contraindications*: severe bleeding disorders, hyperkalaemia (should be urgently corrected prior to contemplating a procedure).
- *Assess*: fitness to undergo procedure.
- *Investigations*: FBC, LFTs, U&Es and clotting.
- Ureteric decompression can either be performed anterogradely, with the insertion of a nephrostomy tube followed by an anterograde stent, or retrogradely. The choice of route for decompression should be discussed with both the urologists and the interventional radiologists.

Percutaneous nephrostomy and anterograde ureteric stenting
- The procedure is carried out in an interventional radiology suite under sedation.
- Prophylactic antibiotics are given prior to procedure (e.g. Ceftriaxone 1 g) and continued for 5–7 days pending results of urine culture.

- The collecting system is punctured under ultrasound guidance and a nephrostomy tube placed in the upper ureter and connected to an external drainage bag.
- The patient will usually return to interventional radiology a few days later to have an anterograde ureteric stent inserted, following which the nephrostomy tube will be clamped to ensure stent patency prior to removal.
- *Complications*:
  - Discomfort and bruising at insertion site (common).
  - A small amount of haematuria that is usually self-limiting within 24–48 hours (very common). Prolonged haematuria should alert the physician to the possibility of persistent bleeding from a vascular injury.
  - Brisk diuresis which requires careful fluid management.
  - Sepsis (common):
    - *Symptoms and signs*: fever, clinical signs of shock.
    - *Management*: ensure urine cultures and multiple blood cultures are sent for microbiology and commence broad spectrum antibiotics.
  - Nephrostomy tube kinking, obstruction or dislodgement: rare but may require repeat intervention.
  - Urinary leak (rare).
  - Pleural complications, for example pneumothorax, hydrothorax and haemothorax can occur very rarely.
  - Injury to inter-abdominal viscera can occur, also very rarely.

Retrograde ureteric stenting
- The procedure is performed by urologists in theatre under anaesthetic.
- Complications are similar to those for antegrade ureteric stenting.

Complications of ureteric stents
- Irritative symptoms (urgency, frequency, supra-pubic pain, haematuria). Tamsulosin may improve pain and voiding symptoms.
- Urinary tract infection (common). Repeated urinary tract infections may be due to encrusting of the stent *in situ* and an early stent change should be considered.
- Stent migration.
- Stent obstruction, for example due to encrusting, chronic infection or tumour progression.

Other relevant sections of this book
Chapter 3, section on renal failure and hydronephrosis

References

Allen DJ, Longhorn SE, Philp T, Smith RD, Choong S. Percutaneous urinary drainage and ureteric stenting in malignant disease. *Clinical Oncology* (R Coll Radiol). 2010. 22(9): 733–9.

Oesophageal stents and dilatation

Overview of oesophageal stents
- *Indications*:
  - ○ Symptom palliation for dysphagia due to unresectable advanced oesophageal cancer.
  - ○ Maintenance of oral intake for patients with locally advanced, but potentially resectable oesophageal cancer undergoing neoadjuvant chemotherapy.
- *Contraindications*: total oesophageal obstruction (but consider if the patient is suitable for a radiologically inserted gastronomy (RIG) tube).
- *Assess*: symptoms, nutritional state, weight loss, fitness to undergo procedure.
- *Investigations*: FBC, clotting, U&Es and LFTs.

Procedure
- Performed in endoscopy suite under sedation, usually takes < 1 hour.
- Post-procedure CXR performed to check position.
- Patient should always be upright prior to attempting any oral intake.
- Liquids can be consumed following a successful stenting procedure, then soft diet 24 hours post procedure. Fizzy drinks post meals are useful to wash down food remnants. High fibre foods should be avoided.
- Patients with stents across the GOJ should be commenced on pro-motility agents (e.g. metoclopramide 20 mg TDS) and high dose PPI (e.g. omeprazole 40 mg BD) to reduce reflux and risk of aspiration. They should not lie flat, and should sleep at a 30 degree angle.

Early complications
- *Chest pain*: can be prolonged in 10% patients, particularly if stent located in cervical oesophagus.
- *Bleeding*: a small amount of bleeding is very common for 24–48 hours due to direct trauma and stent expansion into friable tumour.
- *Gastro-oesophageal reflux*: particularly with stents placed across the GOJ.
- *Aspiration*: can occur during stent insertion, particularly when lower stents placed across the oesophageal sphincter.
- *Perforation*: occurs more frequently in patients whose tumours have been treated with chemotherapy or radiotherapy.
- Management:
  - ○ Urgent contrast study to confirm diagnosis.
  - ○ Patients should be made NBM immediately and commenced on parenteral nutrition, broad spectrum antibiotics (e.g. Tazocin® 1.5 g TDS) and an intravenous PPI.
  - ○ Definitive further management should be discussed with endoscopist and surgeons.

Delayed complications
- Half of patients will require a further intervention due to complications.

- *Stent obstruction*: most commonly due to tumour regrowth, reactive hyperplasia or food impaction. Tumour overgrowth at end of stent may be treated with ablative therapies, or deployment of second stent.
- *Stent migration*: more common when stents are placed across the GOJ. Common in patients receiving neoadjuvant chemotherapy where tumours have shrunk with treatment (30%), but will only need endoscopic retrieval if symptomatic; stent is otherwise removed at surgery.
- Bleeding due to stent erosion into vessels/tumour.
- Perforation due to pressure necrosis (rare).
- Fistula formation (rare).

Oesophageal dilatation
In the oncology setting, this is most often required by patients with early oesophageal cancer who have had an oesophagectomy complicated by the formation of an anastomotic stricture. Patients typically report dysphagia with each meal. Dilatation can result in sustained improvement, but multiple sessions may be required.

Other relevant sections of this book
Chapter 3, section on dysphagia

References

Kubba AK, Krasner N. An update in the palliative management of malignant dysphagia. *European Journal of Surgical Oncology*. 2000. 26(2): 116–29.

Radioembolisation (SIR-spheres®)

Background
- Similarly to chemoembolisation, radioembolisation utilises the differential blood supply of liver metastases and normal liver parenchyma to deliver focal radiation to tumours.
- Radioactive isotopes (90 Yttrium-tagged microspheres) are injected into the hepatic artery, where they preferentially lodge in the microvasculature surrounding metastatic deposits, thereby delivering high doses of radiation.
- Radioembolisation is more commonly referred to as SIR-Spheres®, after the trade name for the 90 Y-labelled biocompatible resin microspheres.

Overview of radioembolisation
- *Current indications*: the treatment of liver metastases from colorectal cancer following discussion at liver multidisciplinary meeting, but likely to expand to include metastases from other primary tumours.
- *Contraindications*: poor hepatic reserve, portal vein thrombosis, prior radiation to the liver, pre-treatment angiography that demonstrates abnormal blood flow to lungs or GI tract that places the patient at risk of radiation toxicity.

- *Assess*: fitness to undergo procedure.
- *Investigations*: FBC, clotting, U&Es and LFTs.

Procedure

- Performed in the angiography suite, with the patient under conscious sedation.
- Prophylactic antibiotics, anti-emetics and analgesia are administered pre-procedure.
- Access to the appropriate hepatic artery feeding the tumour is gained in a manner similar to chemoembolisation,
- A first stage planning procedure involves a hepatic angiogram to map vasculature. Any variant hepatic vessels that communicate with the GI tract will be coil embolised to prevent the radioactive microspheres damaging extra-hepatic tissues. A trial run for the definitive procedure is then carried out using a small amount of radioactive microspheres, with careful imaging to look for any shunting from the liver to the lungs.
- About 10–14 days following the planning procedure, the definitive SIR-Spheres® procedure is then carried out using the 90 Y-labelled microspheres.

Radiation safety

- 90 Yttrium is a beta emitter with limited tissue penetration; therefore no particularly burdensome safety precautions are necessary for healthcare workers, patients or their families.
- The angiography suite must be suitably shielded and radiation precautions strictly adhered to.
- Patients should be nursed in a side-room.
- Patients should be warned to avoid contact with bodily fluids for 24 hours (men need to sit to urinate, careful hygiene, double flushing).
- Pregnant staff and family members should be excluded from the procedural/post-procedural care of patients undergoing radioembolisation.

Complications

- Flu-like post-embolisation syndrome:
  - *Symptoms:* low-grade fever, malaise, chills, myalgia, pain and nausea.
  - Onset, on average, 1–2 days after ablation.
  - Common, normally self-limiting but can last up to 5–7 days.
- Hepatic dysfunction and liver failure.
- Septic complications, including biliary sepsis, hepatic abscesses and peritonitis.
- Injury to bile ducts and stricture formation (rare).
- Gastric and duodenal injury, manifesting as severe pain post procedure (rare). The incidence of this is reduced with careful pre-treatment angiography to identify and coil embolise variant vessels that supply the GI tract.
- Radiation pneumonitis (very rare, <1%). Patients with excessive shunting of blood from the liver to the lungs detected at the work-up phase are usually recommended not to undergo the procedure.

References

Memon K, Lewandowski RJ, Riaz A, Salem R. Chemoembolization and radioembolization for metastatic disease to the liver: available data and future studies. *Current Treatment Options in Oncology.* 2012. 13(3): 403–15.

Radiofrequency ablation (RFA)

Overview of radiofrequency ablation (RFA)
- Radiofrequency ablation (RFA) is a minimally invasive image-guided technique that produces cell death by coagulative necrosis using heat.
- *Indications*:
  - The treatment of liver metastases (three or fewer lesions that are 3 cm or less in diameter that are not located near major vascular structures).
  - The treatment of lung metastases.
  - The primary treatment for small renal cell carcinomas.
  - The treatment for primary bone malignancy.
- *Contraindications*: bleeding disorders, tumour too large (>3 cm), inability to safely access the tumour, pre-existing severe lung disease (for lung RFA).
- *Assess*: fitness to undergo procedure.
- *Investigations*: FBC, clotting, U&E and LFTs.

Procedure
- Performed in the angiography suite, with the patient under conscious sedation.
- Prophylactic antibiotics, anti-emetics and analgesia are administered pre-procedure.
- An ablation needle is placed directly into the target tissue, following which electrodes are deployed from the end of the needle into the tissue.
- Radiofrequency energy flows through the electrodes and heats them, damaging and killing target tissue.

Complications following RFA to liver metastases
- Focal discomfort at the probe entry site(s) is very common and resolves with simple analgesia.
- Flu-like post-ablation syndrome:
  - *Symptoms*: low-grade fever, malaise, chills, myalgia, delayed pain, nausea and vomiting.
  - *Onset*: on average, 1–2 days after ablation.
  - Common, normally self-limiting but can last up to 5–7 days.
- Septic complications including biliary sepsis, hepatic abscesses and peritonitis.
- Injury to bile ducts or major vessels.
- Biliary stenosis/obstruction (rare).
- Needle track seeding.

Complications following RFA to lung metastases
- Fever, pleurisy, and small reactive pleural effusions (common).
- Pneumothorax (in 30–40%) but only a small proportion of these will require insertion of a chest drain.
- Pneumonia, pulmonary abscess, and haemoptysis (rare).
- Formation of a bronchopleural fistula (very rare).

References

Gillams AR. The use of radiofrequency in cancer. *British Journal of Cancer*. 2005. 92(10): 1825–9.

CHAPTER 10

Cancer drug development and funding

Sing Yu Moorcraft

The Royal Marsden NHS Foundation Trust, UK

Clinical trials

Research is an important part of oncology and a significant number of patients are enrolled into clinical trials. Trial methodology is evolving in order to try to shorten the time (and cost) involved in establishing if a drug is effective. However, in general, research can be categorised into the following phases:

- **Preclinical**: testing that is performed before the treatment is tried in humans.
- **Phase I**: aims to establish the dose and schedule of the experimental agent and to assess toxicity, i.e. *'what dose should we use?'*
  - Usually single arm studies (i.e. all patients receive the same experimental agent).
  - Usually involves small numbers of patients with a good performance status for whom there is no standard treatment option.
  - Involves progressively increasing the dose of a drug in small cohorts of patients until the dose cannot be escalated any higher due to toxicity.
  - Not designed to assess the efficacy of the drug and so only a small number of patients are expected to show any response (although this is improving with the development of targeted therapies).
- **Phase II**: aims to assess the activity, safety and feasibility of the new treatment, i.e. *'does the treatment work and are the side effects tolerable?'*
  - May be a single arm study or involve randomisation of patients to the new treatment, the standard treatment or to a number of new treatments. The

Clinical Problems in Oncology: A Practical Guide to Management, First Edition.
Edited by Sing Yu Moorcraft, Daniel L.Y. Lee and David Cunningham.
© 2014 John Wiley & Sons, Ltd. Published 2014 by John Wiley & Sons, Ltd.

randomisation is not for statistical comparison of treatments, but rather to ensure that the patient population in each cohort is similar.
- Often open-label (and therefore not blinded).
- **Phase III**: aims to establish the efficacy and toxicity of a new treatment compared to an existing treatment (which might be observation/best supportive care if there is no current standard treatment), i.e. *'Is the new treatment any better than our existing treatments?'*
  - Usually randomised in order to minimise bias.
  - Usually involves large numbers of patients to ensure sufficient statistical power to detect differences in outcomes between treatments. This is very expensive and often involves multiple centres and international cooperation.
  - Many newer drugs are molecularly targeted and involve screening patients for specific biomarkers that may be predictive of response. For targeted drugs, the number of patients in the trial may be lower.
- **Phase IV**: aims to learn more about toxicity and long-term risk-benefits. Post-marketing studies in oncology patients rather than within the context of a clinical trial.

All trials should be conducted according to good clinical practice (GCP). This is an international standard that aims to protect patient safety and confidentiality. Oncology research nurses and doctors need to undergo regular GCP training. All staff involved in a clinical trial should receive training regarding the trial and sign a delegation log, detailing their trial responsibilities. A doctor should not prescribe trial treatment for a patient unless they are on the delegation log.

Trial terminology

Randomisation: patients are randomly allocated into different groups/arms. This can be done in a variety of different ways and aims to minimise the effects of potential confounding variables (e.g. age). Patients do not get a choice of which treatment they receive and unless the trial is a crossover trial there is no guarantee that they will receive the experimental treatment.

Crossover: patients are switched to another treatment part way through the study.

Blinding: helps to minimise bias. In double blind studies, neither the researchers nor the patients know what treatment the patient is receiving. In single blind studies, either the researchers or the patients (usually the researchers) know what treatment the patient is receiving.

Open-label: both researchers and patients know what treatment is being administered.

Placebo-controlled: one group of patients receives the active drug whereas another group receives an inactive substance (placebo).

Protocol: the plan for the trial. This details the trial objectives, design and methodology and includes information such as trial eligibility and exclusion criteria and the schedule of treatments, tests, procedures and follow-up.

Endpoint: an overall outcome that the study is designed to evaluate. Common endpoints include progression-free or overall survival.

Safety reporting

It is important to remember to inform the hospital research team of any untoward events that occur in patients who are on a clinical trial as they may need to be reported to the regulatory authorities (usually by the trial sponsor) within a specific time period. The sponsor may not be the hospital in which the trial is being conducted (e.g. a pharmaceutical company may be the trial sponsor). Therefore, adverse events/reactions need to be reported in a timely manner to the sponsor so that they can report the event to the regulatory authorities within the specified time limits.

There are a number of different types of adverse event/reactions:

- *Adverse event (AE)*: any untoward medical occurrence encountered by a patient during the course of the trial. This can include the exacerbation of a pre-existing condition and is not necessarily related to the trial treatment.
- *Serious adverse event (SAE)*: any AE that:
  ○ Results in death
  ○ Is life-threatening
  ○ Requires in-patient hospitalisation or prolongation of existing hospitalisation
  ○ Results in persistent or significant disability/incapacity
  ○ Is a congenital abnormality/birth defect
  ○ Is of medical importance

SAEs should be reported immediately to the trial sponsor unless they are specified in the trial protocol or in the Summary of Product Characteristics or the Investigator's brochure as not requiring immediate reporting.

- *Adverse reaction (AR)*: an AE where there is a reasonable possibility that the event may be related to the trial treatment (i.e. a relationship between the adverse event and the treatment cannot be ruled out).
- *Serious Adverse Reaction (SAR)*: any SAE where there is a reasonable possibility that it has been caused by the study treatment. Some of these might be reasonably expected when taking into account the known side effects of the treatment or the likely cause of the patient's disease.

SARs must be reported to the Medicines and Healthcare products Regulatory Agency (MHRA) and the relevant ethics committee as part of the annual safety report.

- *Suspected Unexpected Serious Adverse Reaction (SUSAR)*: a SAR which was not expected from what was known about the trial treatment at that time.

SUSARs should be reported to the ethics committee and regulatory authorities according to specified timelines. In the UK, fatal and life-threatening SUSARs must be reported by the trial sponsor within seven days of awareness and within 15 days for other categories of SUSARs.

References

Medicines and Healthcare products Regulatory Agency. Clinical trials for medicines: Safety reporting – SUSARs and DSURs 2013. Available from: http://www.mhra.gov.uk/ Howweregulate/Medicines/Licensingofmedicines/Clinicaltrials/Safetyreporting-SUSARs andASRs/index.htm (accessed 1 January 2014).

National Institute for Health Research. Clinical Trials Toolkit 2013. Available from: http://www. ct-toolkit.ac.uk/home (accessed 1 January 2014).

Funding of cancer drugs

Cancer drugs are becoming increasingly expensive. For example, vemurafenib (a drug for melanoma) has a net cost of £1,750 per week. In the USA, more than 90% of drugs approved by the Food and Drug Administration (FDA) in recent years cost more than US$20,000 for a 12-week course. It is therefore becoming increasingly important to consider the cost of cancer drugs and the different ways in which patients can access them. It is also important to bear in mind the time lag between the publication of trial results and obtaining marketing authorisation, as well as the lag time between marketing authorisation and approval for NHS use.

National Institute for Health and Care Excellence (NICE)
- Develops evidence-based guidelines for diagnosis, treatment and prevention of diseases.
- Appraises new drugs and technologies and makes recommendations that take into account both clinical effectiveness and cost effectiveness. NICE decides which treatments are available on the NHS in England and Wales (not Scotland).
- If a treatment is approved by NICE then the NHS has to find the money to fund it and make it available to patients. However, even if a high-cost drug is NICE approved some NHS trusts require a form to be completed on an individual patient basis to ensure that the patient meets specific criteria.
- Other organisations which have similar roles to NICE:
  - Wales: All Wales Medicines Strategy Group
  - Scotland: NHS Quality Improvement for Scotland, Scottish Intercollegiate Guidelines Network (SIGN), Scottish Medicines Consortium

Cancer Drugs Fund (CDF)
- The CDF is a pot of money that the government specifically sets aside to facilitate access to cancer drugs that have not been approved by NICE (e.g. because they have not yet been assessed or because they are not cost effective).
- The CDF was introduced in England (not Wales or Scotland) in 2011, but its long-term future is uncertain.
- Each cancer network developed its own list of CDF approved drugs, leading to regional variations in access to drugs.
- Funding requests usually involve an oncology doctor completing a 'tick-box' style form and funding decisions are normally made within a few days.

Individual funding requests (IFR)
- These are requests to Clinical Commissioning Groups (which replaced Primary Care Trusts) to fund a treatment that is not within the range of commissioned services and treatments.

- IFRs are usually used for patients with rare cancers or patients with a more common cancer who are 'exceptional' in some way.
- In order to show that a patient is exceptional, details need to be provided explaining both of the following:
  - Why they are significantly different from the general population of patients with their cancer.
  - Why they are likely to gain significantly more benefit from the treatment than might normally be expected for patients with their cancer. This should be supported by evidence from published research.
- Requests are made on an individual patient basis (usually by an oncology doctor) by completing a relatively lengthy form. It may take weeks to hear the outcome of the funding decision.

Private healthcare

- This usually involves paying the whole cost of a patient's medical care and drugs (including drugs not approved by NICE).
- Can be extremely expensive (costing thousands of pounds) and the healthcare provider may request a substantial deposit to ensure that funds are available to cover the estimated treatment costs.
- Health insurance policies usually do not include complementary therapies or prostheses (e.g. wigs, external breast prostheses), may not include certain cancer treatments and may not fund more than one course of treatment.

Co-payment

- This is when a patient receiving NHS treatment pays privately to have a treatment that is not funded by the NHS (either by paying the cost themselves or through an existing health insurance policy).
- The cost includes the drug itself, as well as any associated costs (e.g. the cost to administer the drug and any additional blood tests or scans that are required).
- The NHS care and the private care must be given separately. Therefore, patients may receive their standard NHS treatment in one day unit/ward and then go to another unit (which may or may not be part of the same hospital) for the private part of their treatment.

Clinical trials and expanded access programmes

- Drugs may be available through clinical trials (e.g. some quality of life studies involve all the patients in the study receiving the new drug). Other trials may involve randomising patients to treatments which are not otherwise available on the NHS.
- In some cases there may be an 'expanded access' programme, which is when a pharmaceutical company allows access to promising drugs outside of a clinical trial (e.g. in the lag time before granting of a marketing authorisation or to allow patients in a clinical trial to continue on treatment once the trial has finished).

References

Cancer Research UK. Cancer Drugs Fund 2012. Available from: http://www.cancerresearchuk. org/cancer-help/about-cancer/cancer-questions/cancer-drugs-fund (accessed 1 January 2014).

Jackson DB, Sood AK. Personalized cancer medicine – advances and socio-economic challenges. *Nature Reviews Clinical Oncology.* 2011. 8(12): 735–41.

Joint Formulary Committee. *British National Formulary* (online). BMJ Group and Pharmaceutical Press: London. Available from: http://www.medicinescomplete.com (accessed 1 January 2014).

National Institute for Health and Care Excellence. About NICE 2012. Available from: http:// www.nice.org.uk/aboutnice/about_nice.jsp (accessed 1 January 2014).

The NHS Confederation. *Priority Setting: Managing Individual Funding Requests.* NHS Confederation Publications: London. 2008.

Personalised medicine

Advances in the understanding of molecular changes seen in cancer have led to the development of therapeutic agents that target cell signalling pathways, for example by targeting specific receptors or kinases (enzymes). This means that oncology treatments are becoming more personalised, with patient stratification according to the molecular characteristics of their tumours. Molecular testing is therefore becoming increasingly important in oncology.

Different tumour lesions in the same patient can have different molecular characteristics. Furthermore, the molecular characteristics can change over time (e.g. progesterone receptor expression is lost in approximately 40% of breast tumours when they metastasise) and so repeat molecular testing may be warranted.

Biomarkers may be prognostic or predictive:
- *Prognostic biomarkers* provide information about the patient's overall outcome, regardless of treatment, for example risk of recurrence.
- *Predictive biomarkers* provide information on the effect of a therapeutic intervention, for example predict which patients will respond to a given treatment.

New targets for treatment and biomarkers are continually being developed. A comprehensive review of new targets and biomarkers is beyond the scope of this book, but promising molecular markers include FGFR, IGF and MET.

Molecular tests that may currently influence patient management outside of clinical trials
ALK gene rearrangement (EML4-ALK)
NSCLC
Around 3–5% of patients have oncogenic rearrangements of the ALK gene and may benefit from crizotinib.

BRAF mutations

- BRAF is a serine/threonine kinase that activates MAP/ERK kinase signalling. It is currently most relevant in patients with metastatic melanoma, but is increasingly being tested for in other tumour types.
- Approximately 60% of melanomas have mutations in BRAF (usually V600E mutations) and may be suitable for treatment with BRAF inhibitors such as vemurafenib.

BRCA1/BRCA2

- The BRCA1 and BRCA2 genes encode components of the DNA-repair pathway and mutations in these genes lead to increased cancer susceptibility.
- PARP is an enzyme involved in DNA repair. Breast cancer cells with BRCA mutations are highly sensitive to PARP inhibitors, which are currently in clinical trials.

EGFR

- EGFR is a member of the HER/ERB family of receptor kinases and activates a signalling pathway involving KRAS, RAF and PI3K.
- EGFR is overexpressed and mutated in a variety of cancers, including colorectal cancer and NSCLC.
- EGFR tyrosine kinase inhibitors (TKIs) (gefitinib and erlotinib) and anti-EGFR monoclonal antibodies (cetuximab and panitumumab) are in clinical use.
- NSCLC:
  - Patients should be tested for the presence of EGFR activating mutations, which occur in approximately 10% of patients. These patients tend to be female, Asian, non-smokers with adenocarcinoma.
  - Patients with activating EGFR mutations have better outcomes if treated with gefitinib or erlotinib, whereas patients without these mutations do better with chemotherapy.
- Colorectal cancer:
  - EGFR mutations are not routinely tested for as they are rare and do not predict for response to anti-EGFR therapy.
  - However, the presence of RAS mutations is predictive of response to anti-EGFR therapy (see below).
- Some patients with glioblastoma also have EGFR overexpression, but response to erlotinib or gefitinib seems to be independent of EGFR expression and is associated with co-expression of PTEN.

Oestrogren receptor (ER) and progesterone receptor (PR)

- ER and/or PR expression is a prognostic factor in breast cancer. Patients with ER and/or PR positive tumours have a better survival than patients with hormone receptor negative tumours.
- High cellular expression of ER and PR predicts benefit to endocrine therapies.

HER2/neu

- HER2 is a growth factor receptor that is overexpressed in approximately 20–25% of breast and gastric cancers. All patients with breast cancer and patients with metastatic gastric/GOJ cancer should be tested for HER2.
- HER2 positive breast tumours are more aggressive than HER2 negative tumours and without targeted therapy patients have a worse prognosis.
- HER2 is measured by immunohistochemistry (IHC):
  - 0–1+ means no expression (i.e. HER2 negative).
  - 3+ means high expression (i.e. HER2 positive).
  - 2+ means borderline expression. FISH should be performed to determine positivity/negativity.
- Trastuzumab (Herceptin®) is a monoclonal antibody that targets the HER2 protein. Trastuzumab is used in HER2 positive (IHC3+ or IHC2+ FISH positive) breast cancer and HER2 positive (IHC3+ only) metastatic gastric/GOJ cancers.
- Not all HER2 positive patients will respond to trastuzumab and both primary and secondary resistance can develop.
- Lapatinib is a dual TKI of HER2 and EGFR and is used in HER2 positive patients with breast cancer.

Ki-67

- Ki-67 is a marker of proliferative activity and may be performed in a number of cancer types, for example to aid decision-making in breast cancer management.
- There is a lack of standardisation of Ki-67 pathological assessment but one panel of experts used the following index:
  - ≤15% = low proliferation
  - 16–30% = intermediate proliferation
  - >30% = high proliferation

KIT

- Imatinib is a TKI that inhibits KIT and is used in patients with GIST (85–95% of patients with GIST have KIT mutations).
- Some acral and mucosal melanomas also have KIT mutations and so imatinib may be a treatment option in these patients.

KRAS and NRAS

- KRAS and NRAS are proteins involved in the EGFR signalling pathway. RAS mutations lead to continuous signalling independently of EGFR activation.
- KRAS mutations occur in 34–45% of patients with colorectal cancer and 15–30% of patients with lung adenocarcinoma.
- Patients with KRAS or NRAS mutations do *not* respond to anti-EGFR therapy (e.g. cetuximab, panitumumab). Therefore, patients who are considered for these drugs should have RAS mutation testing performed and only patients who are RAS wild-type (i.e. patients who do not have an activating mutation in KRAS or NRAS) receive these treatments.

- In lung cancer, KRAS mutations are usually seen in heavy smokers and are predictive of poor prognosis and treatment failure on EGFR TKIs.
- Just because a patient is KRAS wild-type does not mean they will definitely respond to anti-EGFR therapies, as up to 50–65% of patients with wild-type tumours are also resistant.

Microsatellite instability

- Cancers with a defective DNA mismatch repair (MMR) mechanism accumulate mutations at a faster rate, leading to variability in the length of DNA microsatellites. This is called microsatellite instability (MSI).
- The majority of hereditary non-polyposis colorectal cancers and 10–15% of sporadic cases show MSI.
- Colorectal tumours with MSI have a better prognosis and lower risk of recurrence.
- Patients with MMR-deficient tumours do not benefit from adjuvant chemotherapy with 5-FU. Therefore some centres routinely test for MMR-deficiency in patients with stage II colorectal cancer and do not recommend adjuvant chemotherapy for patients who are MMR deficient.

Other molecular tests (not currently in routine clinical use)

- OncotypeDx

An assay that tests for overexpression of 21 genes to determine the risk of breast cancer recurrence in order to aid decision making regarding adjuvant therapies.

- PIK3CA

PIK3CA mutations are associated with resistance to anti-EGFR therapies in colorectal cancer and to trastuzumab in breast cancer.

- PTEN

Low levels of PTEN are associated with resistance to trastuzumab and cetuximab.

References

Alymani NA, Smith MD, Williams DJ, Petty RD. Predictive biomarkers for personalised anti-cancer drug use: discovery to clinical implementation. *European Journal of Cancer*. 2010. 46(5): 869–79.

Cappetta A, Lonardi S, Pastorelli D, Bergamo F, Lombardi G, Zagonel V. Advanced gastric cancer (GC) and cancer of the gastro-oesophageal junction (GEJ): focus on targeted therapies. *Critical Reviews in Oncology/Hematology*. 2012. 81(1): 38–48.

De Roock W, De Vriendt V, Normanno N, Ciardiello F, Tejpar S. KRAS, BRAF, PIK3CA, and PTEN mutations: implications for targeted therapies in metastatic colorectal cancer. *Lancet Oncology*. 2011.12(6): 594–603.

Deschoolmeester V, Baay M, Specenier P, Lardon F, Vermorken JB. A review of the most promising biomarkers in colorectal cancer: one step closer to targeted therapy. *Oncologist*. 2010. 15(7): 699–731.

Jonat W, Arnold N. Is the Ki-67 labelling index ready for clinical use? *Annals of Oncology*. 2011. 22(3): 500–2.

La Thangue NB, Kerr DJ. Predictive biomarkers: a paradigm shift towards personalized cancer medicine. *Nature Reviews Clinical Oncology*. 2011. 8(10): 587–96.

Oldenhuis CN, Oosting SF, Gietema JA, de Vries EG. Prognostic versus predictive value of biomarkers in oncology. *European Journal of Cancer*. 2008. 44(7): 946–53.

Shi C, Washington K. Molecular testing in colorectal cancer: diagnosis of Lynch syndrome and personalized cancer medicine. *American Journal of Clinical Pathology*. 2012. 137(6): 847–59.

Appendices

Sing Yu Moorcraft[1] and Daniel L.Y. Lee[2]

[1] The Royal Marsden NHS Foundation Trust, UK
[2] St James' Institute of Oncology, UK

Chemotherapy regimes

Chemotherapy regimes are often abbreviated. Each drug is identified by a letter. In some cases this is the first letter of the drug name (e.g. B for bleomycin). In other cases this may reflect a drug's trade name. Common trade names include: Xeloda® (capecitabine), Adriamycin® (doxorubicin), Taxol® (paclitaxel), Taxotere® (docetaxel) and Herceptin® (trastuzumab). Some letters represent different drugs in different regimes, for example the C in CMF stands for cyclophosphamide, whereas the C in ECX stands for cisplatin. Table 1 shows some of the more frequently used abbreviations. This list is not comprehensive, particularly as institutions may use their own local abbreviations.

References

All Wales Clinical Coding Service. OPCS-4.6 Chemotherapy Regimen List April 2011 (version1.2) 2012. Available from: http://www.wales.nhs.uk/sites3/docmetadata.cfm?orgid=920&id=171364 (accessed 1 January 2014).

The Christie NHS Foundation Trust. Chemotherapy Information Sheets 2012.. Available from: http://www.christie.nhs.uk/the-foundation-trust/patient-information/chemotherapy-information-sheets.aspx (accessed 1 January 2014).

Macmillan Cancer Support. Combination chemotherapy regimen 2013. Available from: http://www.macmillan.org.uk/Cancerinformation/Cancertreatment/Treatmenttypes/Chemotherapy/Combinationregimen/Combinationregimen.aspx (accessed 1 January 2014).

Drug toxicities

Anti-cancer drugs may be given as a single agent or in combination with other drugs. Although combinations are usually devised to minimise overlapping of toxicities, this is not always possible. In some cases it can be relatively easy to identify the cause of toxicity (e.g. peripheral neuropathy in patients on capecitabine and oxaliplatin (CAPOX) is most likely to be caused by oxaliplatin). In

---

Table1 Commonly used abbreviations for chemotherapy regimes.

Abbreviation	Chemotherapy regime
5-FU	5-fluorouracil
ABVD	doxorubicin, bleomycin, vinblastine, dacarbazine
AC	doxorubicin, cyclophosphamide
ADE	cytarabine, daunorubicin, etoposide
AIDA	idarubicin, tretinoin, mitoxantrone
BEACOPP	bleomycin, cyclophosphamide, doxorubicin, etoposide, prednisolone, procarbazine, vincristine
BEAM	carmustine, etoposide, cytarabine, melphalan
BevIrMdG	bevacizumab, irinotecan and modified de Gramont
BevOxMdG	bevacizumab, oxaliplatin and modified de Gramont
BCNU	carmustine
BD	bortezomib, dexamethasone
BEP	bleomycin, etoposide, cisplatin
BOP	bleomycin, cisplatin, vincristine
BR	bendamustine, rituximab
CAP	cisplatin, doxorubicin, cyclophosphamide
CAPOX	capecitabine, oxaliplatin
CarboEtop (E-carboplatin)	carboplatin, etoposide
Carbo MV	carboplatin, methotrexate, vinblastine
CAV	cyclophosphamide, doxorubicin, vincristine
CBOP/BEP	carboplatin, bleomycin, vincristine, cisplatin/bleomycin, etoposide, cisplatin
CCNU	lomustine
CETIRI	cetuximab, irinotecan
ChIVPP	chlorambucil, vinblastine, procarbazine, prednisolone
CHOP	cyclophosphamide, doxorubicin, vincristine, prednisolone
CMF	cyclophosphamide, methotrexate, 5-fluorouracil
CMV	cisplatin, methotrexate, vinblastine
CODOX-M	cyclophosphamide, vincristine, doxorubicin, cytarabine, methotrexate
CTD	cyclophosphamide, thalidomide, dexamethasone
CVAD	cyclophosphamide, dexamethasone, doxorubicin, vincristine
CVP	cyclophosphamide, vincristine, prednisolone
DA	daunorubicin, cytarabine
De Gramont	folinic acid, 5-fluorouracil
DHAP	dexamethasone, cytarabine, cisplatin
DTIC	dacarbazine
EC	epirubicin, cyclophosphamide
E-Carbo-F	epirubicin, carboplatin, 5-fluorouracil
E-Carbo-X	epirubicin, carboplatin, capecitabine
ECF	epirubicin, cisplatin, 5-fluorouracil
E-CMF (Epi-CMF)	epirubicin, cyclophosphamide, methotrexate, 5-fluorouracil
ECX	epirubicin, cisplatin, capecitabine
EOX	epirubicin, oxaliplatin, capecitabine
EP	etoposide, cisplatin

Continued

Table 1 Continued

EPOCH	etoposide, prednisolone, vincristine, cyclophosphamide, doxorubicin
ESHAP	etoposide, methylprednisolone, cytarabine, cisplatin
FC	fludarabine, cyclophosphamide
FCR	fludarabine, cyclophosphamide, rituximab
FCiSt	folinic acid, 5-fluorouracil, cisplatin, streptozocin
FEC	5-fluorouracil, epirubicin, cyclophosphamide
FEC-D (or FEC-T)	5-fluorouracil, epirubicin, cyclophosphamide followed by docetaxel
FLA	fludarabine, cytarabine
FLAG	fludarabine, cytarabine, GCSF
FLAG-Ida	fludarabine, cytarabine, GCSF, idarubicin
FMD	fludarabine, mitoxantrone, dexamethasone
FOLFIRI	folinic acid, 5-fluorouracil, irinotecan
FOLFIRINOX	folinic acid, 5-fluorouracil, irinotecan, oxaliplatin
FOLFOX	5-fluorouracil, oxaliplatin
GemCap	gemcitabine, capecitabine
GemCarbo	gemcitabine, carboplatin
GemCis	gemcitabine, cisplatin
GEMOX	gemcitabine, oxaliplatin
Hyper-CVAD	cyclophosphamide, vincristine, doxorubicin, dexamethasone
ICE	ifosfamide, carboplatin, etoposide
IdaRAM	idarubicin, cytarabine, methotrexate
IVAC	ifosfamide, etoposide, cytarabine, methotrexate
IVE	epirubicin, etoposide, ifosfamide, mesna
LD	lenalidomide, dexamethasone
MACE	amsacrine, etoposide, cytarabine
Mayo	folinic acid, 5-fluorouracil
MIC	mitomycin C, ifosfamide, cisplatin
MIDAC	mitoxantrone, cytarabine
Mini-BEAM	carmustine, cytarabine, etoposide, melphalan
MitoCap	mitomycin C, capecitabine
MF	mitomycin C, 5-fluorouracil
MM	methotrexate, mitoxantrone
MMM	mitomycin, methotrexate, mitoxantrone
Modified de Gramont (MdG)	folinic acid, 5-fluorouracil
MOPP	mustine, vincristine, doxorubicin, cisplatin
MP	melphalan, prednisolone
MPT	melphalan, prednisolone, thalidomide
MVAC	methotrexate, vinblastine, doxorubicin, cisplatin
MVP	mitomycin C, methotrexate, vinblastine, cisplatin
OX	oxaliplatin, capecitabine
PAM or MAP	cisplatin, doxorubicin and high-dose methotrexate
PC	paclitaxel, carboplatin
PCV	procarbazine, lomustine, vincristine

Continued

Table 1   Continued

Abbreviation	Chemotherapy regime
PemCarbo	pemetrexed, carboplatin
PemCis	pemetrexed, cisplatin
PMB	cisplatin, methotrexate, bleomycin
PMitCEBO	prednisolone, mitoxantrone, cyclophosphamide, etoposide, bleomycin, vincristine
POMB/ACE	cisplatin, vincristine, methotrexate, bleomycin/actinomycin D, cyclophosphamide, etoposide
R-CHOP	rituximab, cyclophosphamide, doxorubicin, vincristine, prednisolone
R-CVP	rituximab, cyclophosphamide, vincristine, prednisolone
R-DHAP	rituximab, dexamethasone, cytarabine, cisplatin
R-ESHAP	rituximab, etoposide, methylprednisolone, cytarabine, cisplatin
R-Gem-P	rituximab, gemcitabine, cisplatin, methylprednisolone
R-ICE	rituximab, ifosfamide, carboplatin, etoposide
TAC	docetaxel, doxorubicin, cyclophosphamide
TC	docetaxel, cyclophosphamide
TCCape	trastuzumab, carboplatin and capecitabine
TCH	docetaxel, carboplatin, trastuzumab
TD	thalidomide, dexamethasone
TIP	paclitaxel, ifosfamide, cisplatin
TPF	docetaxel, cisplatin, 5-fluorouracil
VIDE	vincristine, ifosfamide, doxorubicin, etoposide
VIP	etoposide, ifosfamide, cisplatin
VAI	vincristine, actinomycin D, ifosfamide
VMP	bortezomib, melphalan, prednisolone
Xeliri	capecitabine, irinotecan
XELOX	capecitabine, oxaliplatin

other cases, the toxicities overlap and identifying the causative drug can be more difficult (e.g. FOLFIRI contains 5-FU and irinotecan, both of which can cause diarrhoea).

Table 2 provides a guide to some of the toxicities of individual anti-cancer therapies. It is important to remember that drug toxicity is affected by other factors such as the dose, method of administration (e.g. bolus, infusion, oral), renal/liver impairment and whether the drug is used in combination with other agents. Local guidelines/consent forms and patient information sheets provide more detailed information on the toxicities associated with specific drug regimes.

Table 2 Drug toxicities.

Drug	Alopecia	Cardiovascular toxicity	Diarrhoea	Hearing loss	Hypertension	Infusion reactions	Liver toxicity (inc. elevated LFTs)	Lung toxicity (inc. SOB, cough)	Myelosuppression	Nausea or vomiting	Neuropathy or CNS effects	Renal or bladder toxicity	Skin toxicity	Notes
Alemtuzumab	-	+	+	-	-	++	-	+	++	+	-	-	+	
Bendamustine	+/-	+/-	+	-	+/-	+	-	+/-	++	+	-	-	+/-	
Bevacizumab	-	+/-	+/-	-	++	+	-	+	-	-	-	+	-	Thromboembolism, GI perforation, bleeding
Bleomycin	++	-	-	-	-	-	-	++	-	+	-	-	++	Fever, rigors
Busulphan	+	+/-	++	-	-	+	+	+	++	++	++	+	+	Alopecia at high dose
Cabazitaxel	+	+/-	++	-	-	-	-	++	++	++	+	++	-	Hypotension
Capecitabine	+/-	+/-	+	-	+/-	oral	+/-	+/-	+	+/-	-	-	++	Chest pain
Carboplatin	-	-	+	+	-	+/-	+/-	+/-	++	++	+	+	-	Renal toxicity is not usually dose-limiting
Carmustine	-	-	+	-	-	+/-	+/-	+/-	++	++	-	+/-	+/-	Carmustine implant associated with diabetes
Cetuximab	-	-	+	-	-	++	+	+/-	-	+	-	-	++	Hypomagnaesaemia, conjunctivitis, hair changes
Chlorambucil	-	-	+	-	-	oral	+/-	+/-	++	+	+/-	-	+/-	Seizures
Cisplatin	-	+/-	+/-	++	-	+/-	-	-	+	++	++	++	-	Electrolyte disturbances
Crizotinib	-	+	++	-	-	oral	+	+	++	++	+	-	+	Vision disorders, QT prolongation, oedema
Cyclophosphamide	++	+	+	-	+/-	-	+/-	+/-	++	++	-	++	+/-	Risk of second malignancies
Cytarabine	+/-	+	+	-	-	-	+/-	+/-	++	++	+/-	+/-	+/-	Conjunctivitis, high doses - cerebellar/cerebral effects

Continued

Table 2 Continued

Drug	Alopecia	Cardiovascular toxicity	Diarrhoea	Hearing loss	Hypertension	Infusion reactions	Liver toxicity (inc. elevated LFTs)	Lung toxicity (inc. SOB, cough)	Myelosuppression	Nausea or vomiting	Neuropathy or CNS effects	Renal or bladder toxicity	Skin toxicity	Notes
Dacarbazine	+/-	-	+/-	-	-	+/-	+/-	-	++	+	-	-	+/-	
Dactinomycin	++	-	+	-	-	-	+	+/-	++	++	-	-	+	
Dasatinib	+	+	++	-	+	oral	-	+	++	++	+	+/-	+	Headache, bleeding, oedema, arthralgia
Daunorubicin	++	++	+	-	-	-	-	-	++	++	-	+	+	Red colouration of urine, nephrotic syndrome
Docetaxel	++	+	++	-	+/-	+	-	-	++	+	+	-	++	Oedema
Doxorubicin	++	++	+	-	-	-	-	-	++	++	-	+	+	Red colouration of urine, mucositis
Liposomal doxorubicin (Caelyx®)	++	+	+	-	-	+/-	+	-	+	+	+	+	+	Red colouration of urine, mucositis
Eribulin	++	+/-	+	-	-	-	+/-	+	++	+	++	+/-	+	Arthralgia, QT prolongation, constipation
Epirubicin	++	+/-	+/-	-	-	-	-	-	++	++	-	-	+/-	Red colouration of urine
Erlotinib	+/-	-	++	-	-	oral	+	+	-	+	-	-	++	Conjunctivitis, hair changes
Etoposide	++	+/-	+	-	-	+	+	-	++	++	+/-	-	+/-	Hypotension, rarely loss of vision
Everolimus	-	-	+	-	+	oral	-	+	+	+	+/-	-	+	Hypercholesterolaemia, seizures, bleeding
5-fluorouracil	+/-	+	++	-	-	-	+/-	-	++	+	+/-	-	+	Diarrhoea and mucositis may be life-threatening
Fludarabine	-	+/-	+	-	-	-	+/-	+	++	+	+	+/-	+	Visual disturbances, rarely loss of vision
Gemcitabine	+/-	-	+	-	-	-	++	++	++	+	-	+	+	Peripheral oedema, flu-like symptoms

Drug													Notes
Gefitinib	+/-	-	++	-	-	oral	+	+	-	+	-	+/-	Conjunctivitis, hair changes, bleeding
Idarubicin	++	+	+	-	-	-	+	+	++	++	-	+	Red colouration of urine
Ifosfamide	++	+/-	-	-	-	-	+/-	+/-	++	++	++	++	Encephalopathy, haematuria
Imatinib	-	-	+	-	-	oral	+	+/-	++	+	-	-	Peripheral oedema
Interferon	+/-	+	++	-	-	+	-	-	++	++	+	-	Autoimmune disorders (rare), flu-like symptoms, mood changes
Interleukin–2	+	++	++	-	+	++	+	++	++	++	++	++	Capillary leak syndrome, hypothyroidism, mood changes
Ipilimumab	+	-	++	-	-	-	+	+	+	++	+	-	Hypotension, Stevens-Johnson syndrome, hypothyroidism, hypopituitarism
Irinotecan	++	+/-	++	-	-	+	++	-	++	++	+	+	Cholinergic syndrome, acute and delayed diarrhoea
Lapatinib	+/-	+	+	-	-	oral	+	++	-	++	-	-	Reduction in LVEF
Lomustine	-	-	+	-	-	oral	+	-	++	+/-	+/-	-	Leucopenia
Melphalan	++	-	++	-	-	-	+/-	+/-	++	++	-	+/-	Isolated limb perfusion not considered in this table
Methotrexate	+/-	-	++	+/-	-	+/-	++	+/-	++	+	+	+	Dose-dependent side effect profile. Intrathecal toxicity not considered in this table.
Mitomycin C	+/-	+/-	+	-	-	-	+/-	+/-	++	++	-	+/-	Bladder toxicity with intravesical treatment. Haemolytic uraemic syndrome.
Mitotane	-	-	++	-	-	oral	++	-	++	++	-	+/-	Can cause adrenal insufficiency
Mitoxantrone	+/-	+/-	+	-	-	-	+	+	++	++	+	+	May cause blue-green discoloration of urine
Oxaliplatin	++	-	++	+	+	+	+	++	++	++	++	+	Peripheral neuropathy, haematuria
Paclitaxel	++	+	++	-	-	++	-	-	++	++	++	-	Hypersensitivity, hypotension, arthralgia

Continued

Table 2 Continued

Drug	Alopecia	Cardiovascular toxicity	Diarrhoea	Hearing loss	Hypertension	Infusion reactions	Liver toxicity (inc. elevated LFTs)	Lung toxicity (inc. SOB, cough)	Myelosuppression	Nausea or vomiting	Neuropathy or CNS effects	Renal or bladder toxicity	Skin toxicity	Notes
Panitumumab	++	+	++	–	–	+	–	++	+	++	+	–	++	Anaemia, hypersensitivity, tachycardia, hypomagnesaemia, conjunctivitis
Pazopanib	++	–	++	–	++	oral	+	+	+	++	+	+	++	Hypothyroidism, proteinuria
Pemetrexed	++	–	++	–	–	–	+	+/–	++	++	++	+	++	Avoid NSAIDs
Procarbazine	–	–	+	–	–	oral	+	–	+	++	+	–	+	Tyramine reaction with tyramine containing foods
Raltitrexed	+	–	++	–	–	–	++	–	++	++	+	–	++	
Rituximab	+	+	+	–	+	++	–	+	++	++	+	–	+	Infusion related reactions
Sorafenib	++	+	++	+ (tinnitus)	++	oral	+	–	+/++	++	+	+	++	Hypophosphataemia, haemorrhage
Sunitinib	+	+	++	–	++	oral	–	+	++	++	+	+	++	Haemorrhage and tumour bleeding, reduced LVEF and QT prolongation, hypothyroidism
Temsirolimus	–	–	++	–	+	+	+	++	++	++	+	+	++	Hypersensitivity, pneumonitis, intracranial haemorrhage, hyperglycaemia and electrolyte imbalance
Temozolamide	++	–	+	+	–	oral	+	+	+	++	+	+	++	Headache, visual change, constipation, allergy
Thiotepa	++	++	++	++	++		++	++	++	++	++	++	+	Encephalopathy, convulsions, haemorrhagic cystitis

Drug											Notes
Topotecan	++	–	++	+	–	+	+/–	++	++	–	+	Neutropenic colitis, interstitial lung disease
Trabectedin	+	–	+	+/–	++	+	++	++	+	–	–	Anorexia, insomnia, headache
Trastuzumab	+	++	++	+	++	+	++	+	+	+/++	+	Arthralgia, febrile neutropenia, cardiotoxicity (reduction in LVEF)
Treosulphan	++	+/–	–	+	–	–	+/–	++	++	–	+/–	Bronze skin pigmentation (++), treatment related secondary malignancies
Vinblastine	+	+/–	+	+	–	–	–	++	+	+/–	+	Leucopenia, most SE last <24hours
Vemurafenib	++	+	++	Oral	++	–	–	+	++	+	++	Hypersensitivity reactions, Stevens-Johnson syndrome, QT prolongation
Vincristine	–	+/–	+/–	+	–	+/–	+/–	+	+	+	+/–	FOR INTRAVENOUS USE ONLY. Leucopenia, SIADH (rare). Infusion reaction (bronchospasm/SOB) with mitomycin C co-administration.
Vinorelbine	++	+/–	–	–	–	++	+	++	++	++	+/–	Constipation and paralytic ileus (rare)

– rare, +/– uncommon (or rare but significant), + common, ++ very common (or common and potentially severe)

References

electronic Medicines Compendium, 'Summaries of Product Characteristics'. Available from: http://www.medicines.org.uk/EMC/default.aspx (accessed 1 January 2014).

Macmillan Cancer Support, 'Cancer Treatment' http://www.macmillan.org.uk/Cancer information/Cancertreatment/Treatments.aspx (accessed 1 January 2014).

Useful resources

There are many useful oncology websites (some of which are detailed below), many of which offer similar resources in slightly different ways.

- **Adjuvantonline**: www.adjuvantonline.com
  Free registration online tool to assist decision making regarding adjuvant treatment for breast cancer (includes endocrine therapy and chemotherapy but does not currently take HER2 status into account), colon cancer and non-small cell lung cancer. Also has a tool to calculate the estimated benefits of additional therapy after five years of tamoxifen for breast cancer. Calculates both mortality and relapse estimates.
- **American Association for Cancer Research (AACR)**: http://www.aacr.org/default.aspx
  Members (subscription required, which is low if in training) gain benefits such as reduced subscriptions to journals such as *Clinical Cancer Research* and the opportunity to attend week-long intensive summer educational workshops.
- **American Society for Radiation Oncology (ASTRO)**: https://www.astro.org/
  Online resources, including links to guidelines and patient information leaflets (American-orientated). Can also subscribe to the society (free if in training). Members have access to journals, newsletters and e-learning resources.
- **American Society of Clinical Oncology (ASCO)**: http://www.asco.org/
  Large oncology society with more than 30,000 members. The website contains links to clinical guidelines. Membership (which is free if in training) provides discounted rates to a number of resources such as the ASCO slide library and the *Journal of Clinical Oncology*.
- **Association of Cancer Physicians (ACP)**: http://www.cancerphysicians.org.uk/
  The speciality association for medical oncologists in the UK (small annual subscription). Online resources, including conference updates. Free annual training weekend for trainees and New Consultants' Group weekend.
- **British National Formulary (BNF)**: http://www.bnf.org
  Authoritative and practical information on medicines prescribed in the UK. Free registration for users in the UK and specific developing nations.
- **Cancer.net**: http://www.cancer.net/
  Patient information from ASCO, including information on cancer types, statistics, treatment and end-of-life care.

- **Cancer Research UK**: http://www.cancerresearchuk.org/home/
  Patient information (including cancer types and treatment), cancer statistics for the UK and information for cancer researchers regarding grants, etc.
- **Clinical Care Options**: www.clinicaloptions.com/oncology
  Free registration oncology website with lots of useful resources, including downloadable PowerPoint slide sets, guidelines, an online textbook, interactive cases and treatment and conference updates.
- **ClinicalTrials.gov**: http://clinicaltrials.gov/
  Registry and results database of clinical trials worldwide.
- **E-learning for Healthcare (e-LfH)**: http://www.e-lfh.org.uk/index.html
  E-learning programs which are free to anyone with an NHS email address, including modules on end-of-life care and radiotherapy.
- **Electronic Medicines Compendium (eMC)**: http://www.medicines.org.uk/EMC/default.aspx
  Free website with information about medicines licensed for use in the UK. Provides patient information leaflets and summaries of product characteristics (SPCs). SPCs contain a lot of useful information, including details on contraindications, side effects (including their frequency), drug interactions, pharmacokinetics, pharmacodynamics and details of clinical trial results.
- **European Organisation for Research and Treatment of Cancer (EORTC)**: http://www.eortc.org/
  Information on EORTC clinical trials.
- **European Society for Medical Oncology (ESMO)**: http://www.esmo.org/
  The leading European Oncology Society. Members (subscription fee required) have a number of benefits, including free subscription to *Annals of Oncology* and access to educational resources. These include targetscapes (maps of cell signalling pathways) and a database of biomarkers.
- **Individualised Melanoma Patient Outcome Prediction Tools**: http://www.melanomaprognosis.org/
  Free online tool for predicting the clinical outcome for patients with localised or regional cutaneous melanoma. Provides estimated one, two, five and ten-year survival rates.
- **International Society of Geriatric Oncology**: http://www.siog.org/
  Membership provides free access to the *Journal of Geriatric Oncology* and *Critical Reviews in Oncology/Hematology*.
- **Macmillan Cancer Support**: http://www.macmillan.org.uk/Home.aspx
  Provides lots of information for patients and healthcare professionals, including patient information leaflets on chemotherapy regimes, types of cancers and social issues such as financial support.
- **MDLinx**: http://www.mdlinx.com/
  Free email newsletters with oncology news and links to journal articles. Daily oncology quiz.

- **Medscape**: www.medscape.com/oncology
  Free email newsletters, which include drug and clinical trial news as well as conference coverage. Also has a large number of e-learning modules, reference articles and an online tool for checking drug interactions.
- **My Cancer Genome**: http://www.mycancergenome.org
  Free online cancer resource providing information on mutations and related therapeutic implications. Matches tumour mutations to therapies, including lists of clinical trials of drugs targeting specific mutations and has links to lots of useful journal articles.
- **National Cancer Institute**: http://www.cancer.gov/cancertopics/pdq
  Comprehensive free cancer database with summaries on a wide range of cancer topics, a registry of open and closed clinical trials and dictionaries of cancer terms, genetics terms, statistics and drugs.
- **National Institute for Health Research Cancer Research Network**: http://www.ncrn.org.uk/
  Information on UK local cancer research networks, clinical trials units, clinical studies groups and a database of clinical trials.
- **National Institute for Health and Care Excellence (NICE)**: http://www.nice.org.uk/
  Provides evidence-based guidelines on the most effective ways to prevent, diagnose and treat disease and ill health.
- **NHS Choices**: http://www.nhs.uk/Pages/HomePage.aspx
  Lots of patient information on numerous topics and a searchable database of clinical trials in the UK.
- **Office for National Statistics**: http://www.ons.gov.uk/
  Provides UK statistical information, including cancer registration, mortality and survival.
- **OncLive**: http://www.onclive.com/
  The official website of the Oncology Specialty Group. Online resources include conference coverage. Free registration for email-based oncology newsletters. Also has an oncology nursing news section.
- **OncoLink**: www.oncolink.org
  American-based online resources for medical professionals and patients, including details on chemotherapy drugs, patient information leaflets and e-learning modules.
- **Oncologyeducation.com**: http://www.oncologyeducation.com
  Online resources, including conference updates, links to key journal articles, guidelines and prediction tools.
- **Oncology Nursing Society**: http://www.ons.org/
  Free nursing-orientated clinical practice resources. There are also members-only benefits (subscription required) such as journal subscriptions.
- **Patient.co.uk**: www.patient.co.uk
  Information for patients and health professionals, including information leaflets and links to guidelines.

- **PracticeUpdate**: www.practiceupdate.com
  Free registration website, providing email newsletters with up-to-date oncology news, journal article summaries in your area of interest and conference coverage.
- **Predict**: http://www.predict.nhs.uk/
  Free online computer program designed to assist decision making regarding adjuvant treatment for breast cancer (incorporates HER2 status and method of detection into the program). Calculates five and ten-year survival estimates with and without adjuvant therapy (endocrine therapy, chemotherapy and trastuzumab).
- **The Royal College of Radiologists**: http://www.rcr.ac.uk/section.aspx? pageID=10
  All UK Clinical Oncology trainees are expected to enrol as trainee members of the college. Access to radiotherapy and radiology e-learning resources.
- **Surveillance Epidemiology and End Results (SEER)**: http://seer.cancer.gov/
  Provides information on cancer statistics in the USA, including fact sheets on different cancer types and the facility to create tables and graphs of SEER and US cancer statistics.
- **UpToDate**: http://www.uptodate.com/index
  Online evidence-based clinical decision support system authored by physicians and available to subscribers. Articles summarise the evidence on numerous medical specialties, including oncology.

Index

Page numbers in *italics* refer to illustrations, those in **bold** refer to tables

Clinical Problems in Oncology: A Practical Guide to Management, First Edition.
Edited by Sing Yu Moorcraft, Daniel L.Y. Lee and David Cunningham.
© 2014 John Wiley & Sons, Ltd. Published 2014 by John Wiley & Sons, Ltd.